FETAL ALCOHOL SPECTRUM DISORDERS

Fetal alcohol spectrum disorders (FASDs) have emerged as a major phenomenon within the education, health, criminal justice and social care systems of many countries, with current prevalence figures suggesting that one in a hundred children and young people have FASDs. In this publication academics, professionals and families from around the world share expertise and insights on FASDs. Their combined interdisciplinary perspective makes an invaluable contribution to how we understand and address the complex social, educational and health needs associated with this growing group of children and young people.

Articulating fundamental knowledge, cutting edge initiatives and emerging trends in FASDs, this book provides an evidence base that will enable services to identify and respond to the need for action on FASDs. It recognizes that families – natural, foster or adoptive – are at the heart of this process, and that their rich knowledge base, grounded in their lived experience, is crucial.

Any education, social care, criminal justice or health professional working with children and young people with FASDs and their families will find this book a seminal and authoritative resource.

Barry Carpenter OBE holds Honorary Professorships at the universities of Worcester (UK), Limerick (Ireland), Hamburg (Germany) and Flinders (Australia). His original research on children with FASD stemmed from his time as a Fellow at the University of Oxford, UK.

Carolyn Blackburn is a member of the early childhood research group and a Visiting Lecturer at Birmingham City University, UK, where she teaches on research practice, inclusion and diversity to early childhood students.

Jo Egerton is a Research Project Coordinator for SSAT (The Schools Network) Ltd and Lead Research Coach for their Research Charter Mark Award.

FETAL ALCOHOL SPECTRUM DISORDERS

Interdisciplinary perspectives

Edited by
Barry Carpenter, Carolyn Blackburn and
Jo Egerton

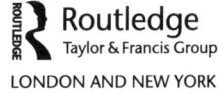

LONDON AND NEW YORK

First Published in 2014
by Routledge
2 Park Square, Milton Park, Abingdon, Oxon OX14 4RN

Simultaneously published in the USA and Canada
by Routledge
711 Third Avenue, New York, NY 10017

Routledge is an imprint of the Taylor & Francis Group, an informa business

© 2014 Barry Carpenter, Carolyn Blackburn and Jo Egerton

The right of the editor to be identified as the author of the editorial material, and of the authors for their individual chapters, has been asserted in accordance with sections 77 and 78 of the Copyright, Designs and Patents Act 1988.

All rights reserved. No part of this book may be reprinted or reproduced or utilised in any form or by any electronic, mechanical, or other means, now known or hereafter invented, including photocopying and recording, or in any information storage or retrieval system, without permission in writing from the publishers.

Trademark notice: Product or corporate names may be trademarks or registered trademarks, and are used only for identification and explanation without intent to infringe.

British Library Cataloguing in Publication Data
A catalogue record for this book is available from the British Library

Library of Congress Cataloging in Publication Data
A catalog record for this book has been requested

ISBN: 978-0-415-67015-9 (hbk)
ISBN: 978-0-415-67016-6 (pbk)
ISBN: 978-1-315-88966-5 (ebk)

Typeset in Bembo
by Saxon Graphics Ltd, Derby

Remember to look up at the stars and not down at your feet. Try to make sense of what you see and wonder about what makes the universe exist. Be curious. And however difficult life may seem there is always something you can do and succeed at. It matters that you don't just give up.

(Professor Stephen Hawking, seventieth birthday speech)

Until the great mass of the people shall be filled with the sense of responsibility for each other's welfare, social justice cannot be attained.

(Helen Keller, 'In behalf of the IWW [Industrial Workers of the World]', *The Liberator*, 1 (March 1918): 13)

CONTENTS

List of figures   *xi*
List of tables   *xiii*
Contributors   *xv*
Foreword – Dame Philippa Russell   *xxiii*
Acknowledgements and dedication   *xxvii*

PART I
Introduction   1

1   A brief introduction to fetal alcohol spectrum disorders   3
Barry Carpenter, Carolyn Blackburn and Jo Egerton

2   International overview: The challenges in addressing fetal alcohol spectrum disorders   14
Elizabeth J. Elliott

3   Fetal alcohol syndrome: The causal web from disadvantage to birth defect   27
Ron Gray

4   Women's alcohol consumption in the UK   39
Moira Plant

PART II
Families – living with FASDs — 51

5 Fetal behaviour and the effect of maternal alcohol consumption — 53
Peter G. Hepper

6 Parenting in the early years — 65
Simon Brown and Julia Brown

7 Life as we know it: A perfectly normal family — 71
Sarah Muir-Timmins and John Timmins

8 Fetal alcohol spectrum disorders and children in care: Good care makes a difference — 80
Kevin Williams

PART III
Education — 89

9 Fetal alcohol spectrum disorders: Knowledge and referral pathways in early childhood settings in Western Australia — 91
Kate Frances

10 Walking through a moonless night: Fetal alcohol spectrum disorders and early childhood intervention — 102
Carolyn Blackburn

11 Evolving pedagogy for children and young people with fetal alcohol spectrum disorders — 123
Barry Carpenter

12 A step in time: Fetal alcohol spectrum disorders and transition to adulthood — 141
Jo Egerton

PART IV
Interdisciplinary perspectives — 159

13 Fetal alcohol spectrum disorders: Diagnosis and complexities — 161
Raja A.S. Mukherjee

14 Building a community of care through diagnosis of fetal alcohol
    spectrum disorders in Aotearoa New Zealand   174
    Christine Rogan and Andi Crawford

15 The Baby Bundle Project: Midwives on the front line of fetal alcohol
    spectrum disorders prevention   183
    Susan Fleisher

16 Fetal alcohol spectrum disorders and criminal responsibility   199
    Julian Killingley

17 Social Care and fetal alcohol spectrum disorders in the UK   207
    Alison McCormick

18 The effects of prenatal alcohol exposure on brain and behaviour   219
    Tanya T. Nguyen and Edward P. Riley

19 Developmental psychiatric disorders in children, adolescents and
    young adults with fetal alcohol spectrum disorders: A transgenerational
    approach to diagnosis and management   241
    Kieran D. O'Malley

PART V
International perspectives   263

20 North American perspectives on fetal alcohol spectrum disorders   265
    Therese M. Grant and Sterling K. Clarren

21 Fetal alcohol spectrum disorders: European perspectives   277
    Diane Black

22 Fetal alcohol spectrum disorders: The current situation in South Africa   288
    Denis Viljoen

23 Fetal alcohol spectrum disorders: Australian perspectives   294
    Elizabeth J. Elliott

24 The way forward for fetal alcohol spectrum disorders: Diverting bleak
    outcomes   306
    Barry Carpenter, Carolyn Blackburn and Jo Egerton

Epilogue. Finding inspiration: 'I Will', a poem written by
Jennifer Woodward who is diagnosed with a fetal alcohol
spectrum disorder 313
Jennifer Woodward

Index *314*

FIGURES

10.1	An ecological model of fetal and early childhood development and intervention for children with FASDs	105
11.1	Comparison between the brain of a typically developing baby and that of a baby with FAS	124
11.2	Developmental profile of an 18-year-old with an FASD	125
11.3	Accessible research cycle	132
11.4	Graph showing Naseem's Engagement for Learning outcomes monitored using the Engagement Profile and Scale	135
13.1	Lip philtrum guidance	162
13.2	Normal distribution curve	163
13.3	(a) Railroad ears and (b) Hockey-stick palmar crease	165
13.4	Diagram showing developmental periods for different organ systems during pregnancy	167
13.5	Relationship between symptoms, phenomenology and aetiology	168
13.6	Diagrammatic comparison between a genetic risk and syndrome (fragile X) and prenatal alcohol to highlight relationship between risk, syndrome and outcome	169
15.1	Comparison between the brain of a typically developing baby and that of a baby with FAS	184
15.2	The impact of alcohol consumption on the fetus through pregnancy	185
15.3	Characteristic facial features in FAS	192
15.4	National Organisation on Fetal Alcohol Syndrome UK (NOFAS-UK) booklet for fathers	195
15.5	NOFAS-UK information booklet for midwives	196
17.1	Perceptions and experiences of the 38 parents of 57 children with FASDs of the Social Care support they received	215
18.1	Maps of the mean difference in cortical thickness in the brains of subjects with FASDs compared to control subjects. Increases in cortical thickness of up to 1.2 mm were observed in subjects with FASDs in most regions of the lateral brain surface, including frontal, temporal, occipital and parietal cortices	221

18.2 The isthmus of the corpus callosum in alcohol-exposed individuals
with dysmorphic features showed significantly lower FA values than these
of the control individuals   222
18.3 An illustration of a prototypical tower task commonly used to assess
problem-solving and planning skills   225
18.4 Representative designs on Delis–Kaplan Executive Function System
(D-KEFS)   226
18.5 Responses of two nine-year-old children on a clock-drawing task   228
18.6 Regions of dorsolateral frontal parietal activation patterns during a
spatial working memory task relative to vigilance   231

TABLES

5.1	The gestational age at which movements are first observed	55
5.2	The behavioural parameters and their combination in the four fetal behavioural states	55
9.1	Survey sample and response rates per sector	93
9.2	Self-reported knowledge of FASDs by type of setting	95
9.3	Self-assessment of amount of knowledge of FASDs	95
9.4	Knowledge of effects of maternal alcohol consumption during pregnancy on the developing fetus	96
9.5	Working with children who have FASDs	97
9.6	Type of suspicions which alerted participants to possible FASDs	97
9.7	Frequency of referrals by participants	98
9.8	Possible resources/resource issues suggested by participants	99
10.1	Emerging FASD approaches and implications for practice	114
11.1	Possible impairments experienced by children and young people with FASDs	126
11.2	Trials of educational and social programmes with positive outcomes	129
12.1	Examples of possible small steps towards adult skills	147
12.2	FASD-associated difficulties within the workplace: outcomes and solutions	150
13.1	Summary of the different diagnostic tools and the criterion broadly used in each	163
13.2	Sensitivity and specificity of a test to establish a characteristic being looked for	164
13.3	Summary of common physical features seen in people prenatally exposed to alcohol	165
13.4	List of conditions known to overlap physical characteristics with FASDs	166
15.1	Overlapping behavioural characteristics and related mental health diagnoses in children	193
19.1	Percentages of psychiatric disorders found in children, adolescents and adults with FASD in certain research populations	246
22.1	FASDs in school-entry children	291

CONTRIBUTORS

Diane Black is the adoptive mother of three children with FASDs, the chairperson of the European FASD Alliance and a member of the board of the Fetal Alcohol Syndrome Foundation of the Netherlands. One of her main interests is the role of nutrition in the management of FASDs. She holds a PhD from Purdue University (1986), and has previously held various positions as researcher at the University of San Diego, Hoefer Scientific (San Francisco), INSERM (Strasbourg) and Marion Merrell Dow Research Institute (Strasbourg). Since the adoption of three children with disabilities, she has devoted her time to them and other FASD-related activities.

Carolyn Blackburn is a member of the Early Childhood Research Group at Birmingham City University, UK, where she is also a visiting lecturer on the Early Childhood Education Studies degree course. Carolyn's doctoral research reflects her interest in child development, developmental differences and bio-ecological theory in relation to vulnerable children and families. Carolyn has been Lead Researcher for two projects investigating the educational implications of FASDs (NOFAS-UK) and early childhood practitioner knowledge of FASDs (Worcester Local Authority/Sunfield). Her work for the latter project won the Nursery World Editor's Choice Award. She is the lead author of the first UK text on the educational needs of children and young people with FASDs and a reviewer for the *International Journal of Alcohol and Drugs Research*.

Simon Brown and Julia Brown are the adoptive parents of a daughter with an FASD. They are also foster carers for their local authority, working with children who have challenging behavioural and emotional difficulties. They run the FASD Trust, a charity based in the UK, which they founded to support those with FASDs, their families and carers. They also provide information to professionals of all disciplines seeking to work alongside those with FASDs.

Barry Carpenter holds the iNet International Chair in Special and Inclusive Education, and Honorary Professorships at the Universities of Worcester (UK), Limerick (Ireland), Hamburg (Germany), and Flinders (Australia). In 2009, he was appointed by the UK Secretary of State for Education as National Director of the Complex Learning Difficulties and Disabilities Research Project, and is currently co-authoring a book on the education of children with complex needs. He oversaw the development of national online training materials for teachers of children with severe, profound and complex learning disabilities. His post-doctoral research at the University of Oxford explored the educational needs of children with FASDs, and he directed NOFAS-UK's FAS-eD Research Project, which developed UK curriculum frameworks for children with FASDs, and co-authored the first British and European text on the education of children and young people with FASDs. In a career spanning more than 30 years, he has held many leadership positions in special education. He lectures internationally on SEN, including FASDs, and acts as Lead Consultant to the South Australian Department of Education and Children's Services. He has published extensively in SEN. He is a fellow of the Royal Societies of Arts and of Medicine, and was awarded an OBE for services to children with special needs.

Sterling K. Clarren is the Scientific Director of the Canada FASD Research Network and a Clinical Professor of Pediatrics within the Division of Developmental Pediatrics and the Child Development and Rehabilitation Program at the University of British Columbia Faculty of Medicine and a Clinical Professor of Pediatrics at the University of Washington. He developed one of the first paediatric clinics focused on the difficult diagnosis of FAS and related conditions in 1978. As the founding director of the Washington State FAS Diagnostic and Prevention Network he led the team that developed the 4-Digit Diagnostic Code for FAS and has refined the clinical approach over many years. In 2001 he was given the Henry Rosett Award by the Fetal Alcohol Study Group of the Research Society on Alcoholism in recognition of 'outstanding clinical insight, leadership and research'. In 2006, he received the Award for Career Excellence from the National Organization for FAS in Washington, DC.

Andi Crawford qualified as a Clinical Psychologist at Victoria University, Wellington, in 2003. Since then she has completed specialist training in the diagnosis and treatment of FASDs both in New Zealand and Canada. Andi currently works in the Child Development Service at Hawke's Bay District Health Board, New Zealand and speaks regularly to raise awareness of FASDs in the health, education, justice and social development sectors. She is embarking on a doctorate with the University of Auckland researching into executive functioning, adaptive behaviour and social cognition of children with FASDs. Previously she has worked in Child and Adolescent Mental Health and Maternal Mental Health services. Andi is a member of the New Zealand College of Clinical Psychologists and of the Paediatric Society of New Zealand.

Jo Egerton is a Research Project Coordinator for SSAT (The Schools Network) Ltd and the lead Research Coach for the SSAT's Research Charter Mark Award. She previously worked on SSAT's Complex Learning Difficulties and Disabilities Research Project funded by the Department for Education. Jo has contributed to two educational research projects on FASDs, and led research into the use of interactive whiteboards with students with severe learning difficulties and ASD. She has a PGCE, and an MSc in Learning Disability Studies. Her most recent co-written/co-edited books are *Educating Children and Young People with Fetal Alcohol Spectrum Disorders* and *Creating Meaningful Inquiry in Inclusive Classrooms,* both published by Routledge.

Elizabeth J. Elliott AM is Professor in Paediatrics and Child Health at the University of Sydney, Consultant Paediatrician at the Children's Hospital at Westmead, Sydney, and a National Health and Medical Research Council of Australia (NHMRC) Practitioner Fellow. She is Founder/Director of the Australian Paediatric Surveillance Unit, established in 1993 for the study of rare childhood diseases, and heads the Centre for Evidence Based Paediatrics, Gastroenterology and Nutrition in Sydney. She also leads an education programme in Maternal and Child Health in Vietnam. Elizabeth has been involved in clinical service delivery, research and policy development regarding FASDs. She is a Chief Investigator for a government-funded project to develop national screening and diagnostic tools for FASDs; for the Lililwan Project, addressing prevalence of FASDs in remote Aboriginal communities in Western Australia; and for two birth cohort studies evaluating child outcomes of alcohol and other substance use in pregnancy. She was a member of The Royal Australasian College of Physicians' Alcohol Policy Working Party; the Intergovernmental Committee on Drugs Working Party on FASD; and the NHMRC committee to review the Australian Alcohol guidelines published in 2009. In 2008 she was made a Member of the Order of Australia for services to paediatrics and child health.

Susan Fleisher is Executive Director and Founder of NOFAS-UK (National Organisation for Fetal Alcohol Syndrome) and the International FASD Medical Advisory Panel. She is a Board Member of the European FASD Alliance and publisher of the international e-publication, *Fetal Alcohol Forum*. In addition she is a member of the UK Department of Health Advisory Group on Fetal Effects of Alcohol, and of the Alcohol Health Alliance (Royal College of Physicians) and the adoptive mother of a 24-year-old daughter with FAS.

Kate Frances, Research Fellow, has been working in the *Prevention, Early Intervention and Inequality* programme at the National Drug Research Institute, Curtin University, Perth, Western Australia since 2008. She has experience of working on a range of academic and applied research projects, including evaluations of programmes for Indigenous and non-Indigenous women and children experiencing drug and alcohol problems. Since 2009 she has been evaluating Save the Children Australia's *Communities for Children* early intervention initiatives for children and families in East Kimberley, and more recently working on projects on FASDs and their impact in health, and early learning and care settings in Western Australia and nationally.

Therese M. Grant is an epidemiologist who has worked in the field of substance abuse research and intervention at the University of Washington School of Medicine for over 25 years. She is the Ann Streissguth Endowed Professor in Fetal Alcohol Spectrum Disorders in the Department of Psychiatry and Behavioral Sciences and directs the Fetal Alcohol and Drug Unit in the Alcohol and Drug Abuse Institute. She serves as an adjunct associate professor of epidemiology, and is a research affiliate with the Center on Human Development and Disability. Since its inception in 1991, she has directed the Parent–Child Assistance Program (PCAP), an award-winning, evidence-based intervention model working with mothers who abuse alcohol and drugs during pregnancy. PCAP sites are now located throughout Washington State, and at over three dozen locations in the US and Canada. She has published and spoken widely on fetal alcohol spectrum disorders, effects of prenatal alcohol and drug exposure, and intervention with high-risk mothers and their children.

Ron Gray is Senior Clinical Research Fellow at the University of Oxford's National Perinatal Epidemiology Unit. He graduated in medicine from Glasgow University in 1982. After postgraduate training in psychiatry, he worked as a Consultant Psychiatrist for eight years. In 1999 he started training in public health medicine, completing a Master of Public Health in 2000. Between 2002 and 2003, he was a Commonwealth Fund Harkness Fellow in International Health Care Policy based at Harvard School of Public Health. He joined the National Perinatal Epidemiology Unit at Oxford University as a Senior Clinical Research Fellow in October 2003. He is also an Honorary Consultant in Public Health. He has published extensively on prenatal alcohol exposure, and his work in this area has been supported by research grants from the Department of Health in England and the Wellcome Trust.

Peter G. Hepper is a Chartered Psychologist and Fellow of the British Psychological Society. He was made a Professor of Psychology at Queen's University Belfast in 1993. He is Director of the Fetal Behaviour Research Centre at the Royal Jubilee Maternity Service, Belfast. His research interests centre around the impact of prenatal experiences on the fetus and development and behaviour after birth. Of particular interest is the examination of the effects of maternal alcohol consumption on the fetus and its behaviour to enable an understanding of the impact of alcohol exposure on the fetus's brain. He was awarded The Thomas R. Verny Award for Outstanding Contributions to Prenatal and Perinatal Psychology and Health by the American Association of Pre- and Perinatal Psychology and Health in 2007 for his work on the adverse effects of alcohol and smoking on the human fetus.

Julian Killingley is Professor of American Public Law at Birmingham City University's School of Law. He was formerly a solicitor and partner in West Yorkshire law firms for 12 years, where he mainly handled criminal and family law matters. Since joining the university in 1990 he has specialized in American constitutional and criminal law and is a member of the American National Association of Criminal Defense Lawyers (NACDL). He has worked closely with Amnesty International and the Law Society and Bar of England and Wales Human Rights Committees in organizing amicus curiae briefs in cases pending before the US Supreme Court. He has taken a particular interest in litigation involving juveniles and defendants suffering from learning difficulties. In 2005 he received a commendation from NACDL President Barry Scheck for organizing the NACDL's amicus brief in Deck v. Missouri. In 2011 he helped organize Amnesty International's amicus brief to the US Supreme Court in Miller v. Alabama protesting Alabama's imposition of life without possibility of parole sentences on 14-year-old juvenile defendants for homicide offences.

Alison McCormick is a qualified, currently registered, Postgraduate Social Work Consultant. She has given up her professional social work and financial income to care for her three adopted children, all diagnosed with FASD. She has extensive social work experience and was previously a Children's Guardian, advising and advocating for the legal rights of children in Care Proceedings. She has a special interest in FASDs and voluntarily coordinates the eastern branch of the charity FASawareUK. She chaired the Birmingham Independent Review Mechanism (IRM) Panel, on behalf of the Department for Children, Schools and Families, for eight years, and has the one-off accolade of chairing both the first ever adoption and fostering IRM panels in the country. She has recently been awarded the Directorship and Decision Maker Role for a fostering agency. Alison is an NHS NICE guideline Stakeholder Advisor in the UK. Drawing on her extensive theoretical and experiential knowledge, she advises, lectures, trains and writes on FASD, its prevention, education and support, as well as on social care, fostering and adoption. She has worked in statutory, independent, voluntary, legal and medical settings. She has a history of challenging injustice to improve people's lives, especially those of her children and others with FASD. She was nominated for and won the prestigious *Best Magazine* Bravest Woman of the Year Award 2010 for her voluntary work involving awareness raising, advocating and supporting families across the UK to access services suitable for their needs. Alison has fostered 35 children, is an adoptive mother of five (aged between 8 and 25 years), a birth mother of two, and a grandmother of five.

Raja A.S. Mukherjee is a Neurodevelopmental Consultant Psychiatrist for Surrey and Border's Partnership NHS Foundation Trust and lead clinician for the only NHS national FASD specialist behaviour clinic. Having trained in the various techniques used in the specialist clinic, he leads a team of psychology, speech and language therapy, and occupational therapy professionals to deliver comprehensive assessment and management guidance for individuals with FASD and behaviour difficulties. Since starting in September 2009, over 100 cases have been seen. Dr Mukherjee has researched and published research articles and edited a multi-professional clinical pathways document for FASD in the UK. Some of these are contributing to his PhD on Fetal Alcohol Syndrome, which is currently being completed. He has also acted as an invited advisor on FASDs to the British Medical Association Board of Science, the Department of Health and the World Health Organization. He continues to be an active member on the international scientific panel on FASDs for NOFAS-UK, for Vancouver's biennial international conference on FASDs, and for European meetings related to FASDs. Alongside colleagues he helped set up the first professional network in the UK on FASDs to improve training and knowledge.

Tanya T. Nguyen is undertaking doctoral studies at the San Diego State University/ University of California, San Diego Joint Doctoral Program in Clinical Psychology under the mentorship of Jennifer Thomas and Edward Riley. Her research interests involve understanding the neuropsychology of developmental disorders and utilizing this information to develop potential interventions in these clinical populations. Her research now combines experiences in both the basic and clinical sciences to better understand the effect of alcohol on the brain and neurocognition with the hopes of developing feasible interventions to improve the cognitive and motor abilities of individuals who have been prenatally exposed to alcohol. In particular, she is interested in exploring various models of nutritional interventions for use in children with FASDs. She has been the recipient of a T32 training grant from the National Institute on Alcohol Abuse and Alcoholism and recently received an individual fellowship (F31) from the same organization.

Kieran D. O'Malley is Consultant Child and Adolescent Psychiatrist at Our Lady's Children's Hospital, Crumlin/Charlemont Clinic, Dublin, Ireland. He has worked with psychiatric disorder and developmental (intellectual) disability patients for over 20 years in Canada, the USA, the UK and Ireland. He has published, lectured and researched extensively on FASDs, including nine years with Professor Ann Streissguth's research group at the University of Washington Seattle. Recently he received the International Starfish Award for his work in this area. He is a board member of the Society for the Study of Behavioural Phenotypes (SSBP). His medical training was undertaken at University College Dublin. He received postgraduate public health training at Guy's and Bromley Health Districts in London, and general practice training and practice in Edmonton, Canada. His child and adolescent psychiatry training was undertaken at McGill University Montreal, the University of Alberta Edmonton, Cornell Medical School New York and Alberta Children's Hospital Calgary. Kieran returned to Ireland in 2006 to take up an Adolescent Psychiatric Consultant post in Belfast, and has been working in Dublin for the last three years, where he divides his time between consultation liaison psychiatry and an all-Ireland consultation clinic for developmental psychiatric disorders, especially FASDs. He is a Fellow of the Royal Society of Medicine, London.

Moira Plant is Emeriti Professor of Alcohol Studies at the University of the West of England Bristol. Her main work focus relates to alcohol and gender. In collaboration with her husband Martin, she has conducted studies of HIV/AIDS risks in relation to the sex industry, nurses and stress, drinking in pregnancy, alcohol-related fetal harm, alcohol and drug problems among anaesthetists, and the mental health needs of prison inmates. She is Director of the UK and Isle of Man sections of a 40-country collaborative study, *Gender, Alcohol and Culture: an International Study* (GENACIS). Her publications include many articles in peer-reviewed journals and she has authored or co-authored the books *Women, Drinking and Pregnancy* (1985), *Risktakers: Alcohol, drugs, sex and youth* (1992), *Women and Alcohol: Contemporary and historical perspectives* (1997), *Binge Britain* (2006) and *Drug Nation* (2011). She acts as an advisor to the UK and other governments on issues such as women and alcohol, drinking in pregnancy, and alcohol-related fetal harm. Moira is the UK consultant to the US National Institute of Alcohol Abuse and Alcoholism's Collaborative Initiative on FASD. In addition to being a researcher, Moira is a psychotherapist, counsellor and supervisor. She is an accredited member of the British Association of Counselling and Psychotherapy (BACP).

Edward P. Riley is a Distinguished Professor of Psychology and Director of the Center for Behavioral Teratology at San Diego State University. He has authored over 250 scientific papers and reviews and served as Chair of the US National Task Force on FAS/FAE from 2000–2004. He currently serves on the Expert Panel for the SAMHSA FASD Center for Excellence and previously served as Chair of this committee. He is a past President of the Research Society on Alcohol (RSA), the Fetal Alcohol Study Group of the Research Society on Alcoholism, and the Behavioral Teratology Society. He is the current President of the International Society for Biomedical Research on Alcoholism. He has been a member of the National Institute on Alcohol Abuse and Alcoholism Council and a member of the Behavioral and Social Advisory Council of the ABMRF/The Foundation for Alcohol Research. He has received numerous awards for his scholarship and contributions to the alcohol field, including the RSA Distinguished Researcher Award, the National Organization on Fetal Alcohol Syndrome Research Recognition Award, and, most recently, the Frank Seixas Award from the RSA. His work on FASDs has been continually funded by the National Institute on Alcohol Abuse and Alcoholism since 1978.

Christine Rogan is a Health Promotion Advisor for Alcohol Healthwatch Trust, an evidence-based public health agency funded by the New Zealand Ministry of Health to reduce alcohol-related harm. Her primary role is the National Coordinator of the Fetal Alcohol Network NZ (FANNZ). Her work involves projects that raise awareness, build workforce skill and responsiveness and facilitate multi-sector connectedness, including affected families. Having worked to increase capacity for FASD prevention and intervention at all levels for more than 15 years, she draws on a considerable body of knowledge and experience when working with others to achieve positive and sustainable outcomes for FASDs. Christine has a bachelor degree in sociology.

Dame Philippa Russell has chaired the Standing Commission on Carers since 2007. Her term as Chair has recently been extended to 2014. She was previously Disability Policy Adviser to the National Children's Bureau, a Commissioner with the Disability Rights Commission and Director of the Council for Disabled Children. She is also the parent of a son with a learning disability. Her DBE was awarded for services to disabled children, young people and family carers and she also holds an OBE and CBE for her work with children/people with special educational needs and disabilities (SEND) and their families. Other awards related to SEND include the Rose Fitzgerald Kennedy Centenary International Award, the 4Children Lifetime Achievement Award, the RADAR (Royal Association of Disability and Rehabilitation) Lifetime Achievement Award. She is an Honorary Fellow of the Royal College of Paediatrics and Child Health and of the Royal College of Psychiatrists and a Fellow of the Royal Society of Arts. She has Honorary Doctorates from the Universities of Lincoln, York and King Alfred's College of Higher Education, Winchester and is an Honorary Fellow of the University of Central Lancashire. She is a trustee of the National Family Carers Network, the National Development Team for Inclusion and is Chair of the MOVE Partnership. She is also a member of Think Local Act Personal Partnership's (TLAP) Programme Board and of their National Co-production Advisory Group, representing carers' interests. She was also a member of the UK's National Health Service Future Forum and is a member of the Department of Health Ministerial Advisory Group on the Mental Health Strategy.

Sarah Muir-Timmins and John Timmins have been married for 15 years. Both were born and educated in South London before moving out to the countryside nearly 20 years ago. Sarah is one of three children and after completing a degree and postgraduate qualifications she worked as a child care social worker. Following the adoption of their two children Sarah became a full-time mum and carer, but has now returned to work part-time for a children's charity. She enjoys running, reading and lazy family days – although there are not many of those! John is one of five children and has 14 nephews and nieces. He enjoys large family celebrations. John has worked in electrics, lighting and sound for theatres and event management. He enjoys golf, reading and coaching their son's cricket team. He would always like more time to play golf, but still manages a weekend away with his brothers once a year. John enjoys cooking, and Sarah enjoys eating.

Denis Viljoen was born and educated in Rhodesia. His medical degree was awarded at the Godfrey Huggins School of Medicine in 1970, following which he joined the Rhodesian Air Force and became Senior Medical Officer. In 1979 he left the Air Force in order to specialize in paediatrics at the University of Cape Town (UCT). He trained at the Red Cross War Memorial Children's Hospital. He was awarded fellowship in paediatrics in 1985 and commenced training in the subspecialty of medical genetics. His doctoral thesis, entitled Pseudoxanthoma Elasticum in South Africa, led to the award of an MD in 1992. Denis was elected an Associate Professor at UCT Department of Medical Genetics soon thereafter, and appointed Head of Human Genetics at the Department of Human Genetics, South African Institute of Medical Research (now National Health Laboratory Service), University of the Witwatersrand in 1998. He established the Foundation for Alcohol Related Research (FARR) in 1995 of which he is the Chairperson and Chief Executive Officer. Denis has written 12 chapters for medical textbooks and more than 150 manuscripts for peer-reviewed journals, mainly on subjects related to FASDs. He has received several awards for research and prevention of FASDs, the most recent of which is the Henry Rosett Award in 2012 for international contributions to the field of FASD.

Kevin Williams was appointed Chief Executive Officer (CEO) of The Adolescent and Children's Trust (TACT), a national charity for children in care, in 2001. Previously he was employed in the public sector, where he had a career in social services, mainly working with children in care in relation to child protection. Since his appointment as CEO, TACT has grown from a small charitable fostering agency to a national children's charity working with and for children in care. Kevin initially qualified as a teacher before moving into social work. Over his 30-year career, he has always had a strong drive to improve the life chances of society's most disadvantaged people. He spent five years on the Board of British Association for Adoption and Fostering, and founded the 'Fostering through Social Enterprise' (FtSE) Group. He sits on the Advisory Board of Research in Practice and was the first Chair of the Nationwide Association of Fostering Providers. He has been a member of a number of UK government and Department for Education working groups. He is on the Advisory Editorial Board of Children and Young People Now and is a Fellow of the Royal Society of Arts. He regularly talks at international and national conferences and frequently comments in the media and elsewhere on issues affecting Looked After Children.

Jennifer Woodward. My name is Jennifer Woodward. I am 31 years old, and I have an FASD. Edith and Harold Woodward, also foster parents at that time, adopted me at the age of six. I had exhausted every foster home in Northern Alberta. Edith knew something was wrong with me, but couldn't identify it. So years later, many frustrating years later, testing was done and it came back as FASD. That was at the Hospital for Sick Kids in Toronto, Ontario, Canada, when I was 13. It now had a name. A name or label I grew to hate. To me I wasn't normal, and all I ever wanted to be was normal. Failure after failure, painful mistake after mistake, I grew up. I learned how to drive at 26. I showed all the doctors who said, 'She won't learn anything after reaching a grade 5 level.' But I did. My saying I use is 'Watch me, I will.' It was hard on everyone. I would lash out at whatever was in my way. I couldn't understand simple things; learning was very difficult. In a way everyone was learning how to cope with FASD. School equalled bullying. I remember when I came home crying, begging my mom to take me out of school in grade one. My favourite hobby is writing – there is where I can put down on paper what I can't say through my mouth. After the years we learned and cried and loved so firmly, maybe I am a little normal.

FOREWORD
Dame Philippa Russell

The past decade has seen major advances in the early identification of and interventions for young disabled children. However, while mortality rates have greatly improved, there is growing concern about the possible *prevention* of the increased prevalence of children with very complex physical and cognitive impairments and also growing awareness of the linkages between maternal lifestyle and good outcomes for pregnancy. Sadly the past decade has also seen growing anxiety about the attitudes to alcohol in young women, with many health education programmes apparently going unnoticed, and with schools and other services for children and families increasingly concerned about the implications of alcohol for the 'new generation' of children with complex needs. Fetal alcohol spectrum disorders (FASDs) are now probably the fastest rising cause of childhood disability and special educational needs. They also present a unique twenty-first century challenge of addressing a complex cluster of disabilities and special educational needs which, to paraphrase Professor Barry Carpenter (2010), require a new pedagogy and some very different approaches to the identification, assessment and teaching skills in order to achieve best results for the children.

I warmly welcome this book, which offers us both international perspectives and shared solutions to what are only now recognized as new challenges. To cite Professor Carpenter again, until 2007 we were looking at a 'blank sheet of paper' with regard to the education of children and young people with FASDs. Now we are developing a robust evidence base both about prevention (challenging because of the drinking culture that has not only become widely tolerated but also socially accepted in many communities) and importantly about intervention. Children with FASDs face multiple physical and intellectual challenges. Those challenges, often representing an 'umbrella' of different disorders, also face their teachers and very importantly the families who can struggle with children who, as one mother put it recently, 'seem to be wired differently'.

Meeting the needs (socially and educationally) of children who are 'wired differently' – children with FASDs, for example – is not resource neutral. At a time of economic tension across the global economies, we have to justify the efficient use of resources (which means in turn agreeing outcomes, working across agencies and raising the profile of the 'atypical' children who need new forms of investment).

As the Nuffield Bioethics Committee commented in 2006, when reviewing policy and practice in the treatment of very young children in neonatal services:

> At present we note the inconsistency of investing heavily in high cost medical interventions to ensure the survival of the children with the most complex needs and then discharging that growing population of children with major difficulties without proper investment in an infrastructure to support them and most importantly their families in addressing their often very complex and long-term additional needs.
> *(Nuffield Council on Bioethics Working Party on Decision-Making in Neonatal Medicine 2006, in Russell 2011: 109)*

This book offers us important messages as to what that infrastructure might be and also what new skills teachers, child care workers and others need to acquire in order to appropriately assess, plan and provide the right support.

All children with disabilities and special educational needs present challenges. At a recent conference for parents of children with special educational needs, one mother talked about her child:

> I sometimes think of him like a changeling, a very nice, very beautiful changeling but someone who is also like a jigsaw, so many different pieces and nobody seems to have the time to put the picture together and see the whole child!
> *(Parent of a child with an FASD, Every Disabled Child Matters event, pers. comm. 2012)*

Precisely because children with FASDs have such complex needs, we must share knowledge, research findings and look for some common solutions in order to ensure that the children (and families) do not feel like dismantled jigsaws. Also, as another mother sadly put it:

> We'd like to have a life instead of the almost daily phone calls from the school about what he has done – or not done – during the school day.
> *(Parent of a child with an FASD, Every Disabled Child Matters event, pers. comm. 2012)*

A significant message from this book is that we need strategies to address what might be described as layered needs, that is to say an often complex profile of mental and physical health problems, social, behavioural and communication issues and frequently cognitive impairments. Meeting those needs cannot be the responsibility of education alone. Children with FASDs will frequently require transdisciplinary support – a constellation of interconnected professionals unified in their service delivery approach – to develop not only personalized pathways for physical and educational development but also to inform and support teachers, care workers, other professionals and families to share in the learning process.

This group of children may of course be doubly disadvantaged by family circumstances. They may experience multiple breakdowns in care and successful family placements in long-term foster or adoptive families will require considerable support to ensure success. As one foster family said of an eight-year-old child with an FASD:

> He is such a lovely child, so articulate, so eager to please and try anything new – but then you realise he has no idea of safety, he tries things and then forgets. The words flow but he forgets what he has said in an hour or so. He has a school now which does understand him. They work together but his teacher said that he is not like any child she has ever taught before. It's like learning to read again, she said.
>
> *(pers. comm.)*

That child is flourishing, with much sharing of ideas, expertise and mutual understanding from multiple agencies. The school and the foster parent are confident but, as the mother added:

> It was like a new route map. We needed a lot of professionals to mark the roads and deal with the disasters on the way. But now we have the pathway. These are new children and we need new solutions to some very new problems.
>
> *(pers. comm.)*

Not only do we need new solutions, we also need an international sharing of issues, ideas and solutions. This international perspective offers that opportunity, recognizing not only the challenges of working with this group of children but also how we may actually prevent a second generation emerging. We must continue to endeavour to change the cultural acceptability (in some cases almost a social requirement) of excessive alcohol consumption in young women across the world. We must also address the stigma that often accompanies FASDs. I was saddened recently to hear an adoptive mother of a young woman with an FASD say that she had been saddened by some of the attitudes she encountered, either implicitly blaming her (assuming she was the natural mother) or expressing amazement that she would adopt a child from 'that background'. Her daughter, 'Susie' (not her real name), was married last month. She has done well, a charming young woman albeit with some problems which she herself acknowledges and copes with well. But, as her mother says:

> It was such a battle; I had to be her advocate on so many occasions. We must work together around Foetal Alcohol Spectrum Disorders. The school, the GP, the speech and language therapist and others all worked together but we were so often struggling in the dark. We must demystify Foetal Alcohol Syndrome in the way that we have demystified (and de-stigmatised) so many other conditions and illnesses in the past decade. We also have the big challenge of society itself being willing to change to prevent it in the future. Susie has a good life, but the story could have been so different
>
> *(pers. comm.)*

I feel very privileged to have been invited to write a foreword for this book. As Professor Elliott says in her chapter on the Australian experience, we need a *'whole population perspective'* on a very important challenge of our time.

There is an urgent need for educational opportunities for teachers, lawyers, health and social care professionals, correction services and other professionals to increase understanding of FASDs and the needs of affected individuals.

This is a particularly important book. It both addresses the sensitive subject of prevention (inevitably meaning exploring and changing the lifestyles of a wide range of citizens around the world) *and* explores the challenges around a complex set of cognitive and physical impairments in children (and the adults they will become) who will challenge our existing knowledge and expertise. It is also a reminder that together we can find new, effective and innovative solutions to a major challenge.

As Dr Ron Gray notes (Chapter 3, this publication) FASDs are an equality issue:

> one could certainly argue that, through FAS, social injustice is causing considerable childhood disability and is destroying the lives of children and their families on a major scale.

In effect, FASDs are all our business and this book enables us to take a broader perspective and to acknowledge Dr Gray's arguments about social justice in developing a new repertoire of teaching skills (and preventive strategies) to ensure that this group of children can achieve good lives within supportive families and communities. 'Susie', cited above, has such a good life, but it should have been neither such a challenge nor such a steep learning curve for those trying to support her.

Dame Philippa Russell
Chair, Standing Commission on Carers, UK

References

Carpenter, B. (2010) *Children with Complex Learning Disabilities: A 21st century challenge*, London: SSAT.

Russell, P. (2011) 'Building brighter futures for all our children: education, disability, social policy and the family', in S. Haines and D. Ruebain (eds) *Education, Disability and Social Policy*, Bristol: The Policy Press.

ACKNOWLEDGEMENTS AND DEDICATION

It is our experience that all professionals can remember with vivid clarity the first time they heard about the range of effects resulting from prenatal exposure to alcohol that comprise fetal alcohol spectrum disorders (FASDs). Inevitably as a collective of caring professionals, they wonder how we have reached the twenty-first century with so little knowledge available, not only to women about healthy pregnancies and specifically the irreversible effects of FASDs, but also to the range of professionals whose duty it is to inform and support them.

It was our privilege to co-author the first British and European text relating to the educational needs of children and young people with FASDs (also published by Routledge). It is now an honour to co-edit the enormous wealth of knowledge that inheres in this publication.

As an editorial team, we are grateful to the professionals who raised our awareness of FASDs and the children, young people and families who inspired us to share our collective knowledge, alongside other contributors.

In particular we would like to thank the parent support groups who operate as charitable organizations, both in the UK and internationally, and who work tirelessly to raise awareness and provide a valuable chain of support for vulnerable families.

We are also grateful to Alison Foyle and Rhiannon Findlay and their colleagues at Routledge for their enduring patience and support.

This book is dedicated to the numerous children, young people and families we have met and worked with who live with the effects of prenatal exposure to alcohol.

We hope that, in some small way, the words on these pages support you on your journey for and with those affected by prenatal exposure to alcohol.

Barry Carpenter, Carolyn Blackburn and Jo Egerton

PART I
Introduction

1

A BRIEF INTRODUCTION TO FETAL ALCOHOL SPECTRUM DISORDERS

Barry Carpenter, Carolyn Blackburn and Jo Egerton

Many disabilities have an unknown etiology or cause, but fetal alcohol spectrum disorders (FASDs) are known to be associated with prenatal alcohol exposure, which can cause lifelong, permanent, physical and intellectual disabilities in an unborn child. It is 100 per cent preventable. While FASDs are predominantly associated with maternal alcohol consumption during pregnancy, there are also indications that fathers who are heavy drinkers produce infants with lower birth weight and increased likelihood of heart defects (Cleaver *et al.* 2011).

The association between alcohol use in pregnant mothers and poor outcomes for children and young people has been recognized for centuries, from Plato (429–347 BC; see University of Chicago 2009) to Bacon (1627) and Sullivan (1899). However, it is only in recent years that researchers and professionals have begun to understand the full impact of a mother's alcohol use on her developing baby in the womb.

It is well established that alcohol affects the fetus differently depending on the stage of pregnancy and how much the mother drinks (Warren *et al.* 2011). However, there is risk not only in heavy or binge drinking, but also in moderate to low levels of maternal alcohol use (Gray *et al.* 2009; Lewis *et al.* 2012; May *et al.* 2011; Mukherjee *et al.* 2005; O'Connor *et al.* 2006). Other factors, such genetic make-up and maternal age, also influence the outcome for the baby (Jonsson *et al.* 2009; Mattson and Riley 2011; Morleo *et al.* 2011). It is therefore impossible to predict how an unborn child will be affected even by a single drink. Only one message gives a 100 per cent guarantee of no alcohol damage for the fetus: 'Women who are pregnant or trying conceive should avoid alcohol'. Based upon current research, men should also avoid alcohol while trying to conceive (Cleaver *et al.* 2011).

Public misconceptions and low levels of FASD awareness mean that many birth mothers of children and young people with FASDs who drank alcohol in pregnancy were unaware of the potential harm to their child. MacKinnion (in Mukherjee *et al.* 2006) found that although 97 per cent of a group of US teenagers realized that alcohol affected an unborn baby, 48 per cent thought this meant that the baby was addicted to alcohol, and over 50 per cent thought any damage could be cured. BBC One's *Inside Out* (2009) found similar beliefs among UK teenagers. One way to address this is by training midwives to give accurate information and effective support to mothers who are likely to drink during their pregnancy (Fleisher, Chapter 15, this publication).

Prenatal alcohol exposure and its historic impact

A characteristic pattern of abnormalities in children born to mothers who used alcohol in pregnancy was first documented by Lemoine (Lemoine *et al.* 1968) and then by Jones and Smith (1973), who coined the term 'fetal alcohol syndrome'. Jones and Smith were the first to describe in detail a consistent characteristic pattern of impairments associated with prenatal alcohol exposure and to propose diagnostic criteria (Hoyme *et al.* 2005; see also Elliott, Chapter 2, this publication).

'Fetal alcohol spectrum disorders' (FASDs) is an umbrella term, first used by Streissguth and O'Malley (2000), which encompasses the range of possible outcomes of prenatal alcohol exposure, including fetal alcohol syndrome (FAS), partial fetal alcohol syndrome (pFAS), alcohol-related neurodevelopmental disorder (ARND) and alcohol-related birth defects (ARBD) (Bertrand *et al.* 2005; BMA 2007; Mattson and Riley 2011; see also Mukherjee, Chapter 13, this publication). These effects may include physical, mental, behavioural and/or learning disabilities with lifelong implications (Bertrand *et al.* 2005).

Only FAS can be formally diagnosed using the criteria within the *International Classification of Diseases (ICD-10-CM)* (WHO 2011), and is the only FASD that can be diagnosed without confirmation of maternal alcohol use during pregnancy. The easiest time to identify FAS is in early childhood when a child is aged between six months and three years and facial and growth differences are most pronounced; for other fetal alcohol exposure conditions, the early school years, when the child is six or seven years old, may be better (Chandrasena *et al.* 2009; May 2009).

The presence of three key characteristics can lead to a diagnosis of FAS (Gray and Mukherjee 2007; WHO 2011):

- Facial differences – flattening of the mid-line groove between nose and mouth (philtrum), a thin upper lip (vermillion border), and narrowing of the opening between upper and lower eyelids (small palpebral fissures)
- Delayed growth – below average height, weight, or both (< 10th percentile)
- Central nervous system (CNS) abnormalities – structural, neurological, functional or a combination These may include microcephaly, learning disabilities, developmental delay, hyperactivity disorders, seizures and brain structure abnormalities.

Other common non-diagnostic differences include organ and skeletal malformations, sensory impairments, muscle tone and coordination difficulties and otherwise unexplained behavioural and cognitive issues. Although the core diagnostic features may seem unequivocal, non-specialists should not assume a child has FAS based upon these features; they are also found in conditions unrelated to maternal alcohol use (e.g. Williams syndrome, Noonan's syndrome) (Chudley *et al.* 2005; Hoyme *et al.* 2005).

The facial differences associated with FAS form during a specific development window in the first trimester (first three months) of pregnancy (Mattson and Riley 2011; Streissguth and O'Malley 2000). The heart and other organs, including the bones are also at risk at this time. In the early weeks of pregnancy, and during the second trimester, the fetus has an increased risk of spontaneous abortion. In the third trimester, the effects of alcohol on the fetus include impaired height, weight and brain development (Chudley *et al.* 2005). However, the fetal CNS (including eyes and ears) remains very vulnerable to the effects of alcohol throughout pregnancy (Mattson and Riley 2011; US Department of Health and Human Services *et al.* 2008).

Although the associated physical differences make FAS easier to diagnose than other FASDs, if there is evidence of the mother's alcohol intake during pregnancy and detailed historical, biological, neurobehavioural, social and physiological evidence, it is possible to identify children and young people on the wider fetal alcohol spectrum (Gray and Mukherjee 2007; Mukherjee *et al.* 2005; see also Mukherjee, Chapter 13, this publication).

Differences across the lifespan

The cognitive and behavioural profiles of infants, children and young people with FASDs change over time. One study indicates impaired information processing before birth may have longer term consequences for the ability to learn after birth (see Hepper, Chapter 5, this publication). Riley (2011) notes that newborn babies with FASDs are frequently hyper-reactive to stimulation and have arousal and dysregulation issues. He also mentions 'high activity levels, disturbed sleep patterns, trouble feeding, and, in extreme cases, a neonatal withdrawal syndrome'. Older babies may have motor problems, developmental delay, language and cognition issues (Riley 2011; see also Nguyen and Riley, Chapter 18, this publication). Learning, behavioural/emotional and social difficulties typically become more evident as the children and young people progress through school. The learning needs of primary and secondary students with FASDs are subtly different from one another. For teenagers, issues around emotions, friendships and sexual behaviour, independence and achievement compound their primary impairments (Connor and Huggins 2005; see also Egerton, Chapter 12, this publication).

Prevalence of FASDs

In the UK, there are currently no reliable prevalence figures for FAS or FASDs as they are not routinely collected or recorded by the British Paediatric Surveillance Unit (BMA 2007). The most quoted prevalence figure is that given by the Institute of Medicine in the USA – about 0.5 to 3 children and young people with FAS per 1,000 of population, and, for those with FASDs, 10 in 1,000. The prevalence of FAS/FASDs is energetically debated, and Gray *et al.* (2009) point out the need for caution and further research before these figures can be confirmed. However, based on current research among representative populations in Italy, May and his colleagues believe accepted rates for the US and Europe are low. He states:

> We believe that the prevalence of FAS is closer to 2 to 7 per 1,000; and rather than FASD existing at 1 per cent, we believe that the rates of FASD ... are between 2 per cent and 5 per cent in the general population of developed countries.
>
> *(May 2009: 21)*

Many researchers and clinicians also report that children with FASDs are often misdiagnosed with conditions such as attention deficit hyperactivity disorder, reactive attachment disorder and oppositional defiant disorder, among others (Coles 2011; Dubovsky 2009; FASCETS 2010; Mukherjee et al. 2006; O'Malley 2007).

Prevalences of FASDs among populations with traditionally high alcohol use are much greater. Golden (2005) reports one in 170 live births among aboriginal populations in New Zealand, Australia and the United States (see also Elliott, Chapter 23, this publication, for a discussion of most recent Australian findings), while in certain very high-risk South African communities, the prevalence has been estimated at 68.0–89.2 per 1,000 (see also Viljoen, Chapter 22, this publication). Elevated prevalence is also seen in moderate alcohol-using communities – 3.7–7.4 per 1,000 children and young people, and 20.3–40.5 per 1,000 for FASDs in some Italian populations (May et al. 2006). Gray (see Chapter 3, this publication) describes how alcohol in three populations has given rise to increased risk of FASDs and a cycle of deprivation and disadvantage.

Responding to FASDs

Early childhood intervention (ECI) is now well documented as providing both developmental and economic benefits for vulnerable children (see also: Blackburn, Chapter 10, this publication; Frances, Chapter 9, this publication). Moreover, children's rights to ECI are embodied within the Convention on the Rights of the Child and the Convention of the Rights of Persons with Disabilities for State Parties, and it is quite simply 'the right thing to do' (Brown and Guralnick 2012: 283).

Early diagnosis and intervention for children and young people with FASDs are crucial so that an effective network of professional and social support can be put in place from an early age to support both the children and their families (Benz et al. 2009; Mattson and Riley 2011; May 2009). However, the current situation is far from ideal. Families describe the unrelenting battle for services and the hardships, alongside the joys, of parenting children with FASDs (see also: Brown and Brown, Chapter 6, this publication; Muir-Timmins and Timmins, Chapter 7, this publication; McCormick, Chapter 17, this publication). These interventions will require an ongoing interdisciplinary approach to assessment, diagnosis and support, as FASDs are not only complex and multi-factoral, but change and evolve as children mature into adults (see also O'Malley, Chapter 19, this publication). Without diagnosis and support, unrealistic expectations from themselves and others may lead to children and young people developing serious defensive behavioural, cognitive and psychological secondary disabilities leading to mental health problems, disrupted school experience, trouble with the law, inappropriate sexual behaviour, addiction, problems with independent living and attempted suicide (Baer et al. 2003; Kelly 2009; O'Connor et al. 2002; Riley 2003; Streissguth and O'Malley 2000; Streissguth et al. 1996).

Some people oppose diagnosing children and young people with FASDs because they believe it stigmatizes them and their families, but as Substance Abuse and Mental Health Services Administration (SAMHSA 2010) points out:

> inaccurate diagnosis can be harmful. Persons with an undiagnosed FASD may be mislabeled as noncompliant, uncooperative, or unmotivated. In addition, treatments are selected on the basis of the diagnosis. If the diagnosis is not correct, the treatment

will not be correct. For example, medications for ADHD may not help a person whose attention deficits stem from prenatal alcohol exposure.

Morgan Fawcett, a young man with an FASD, also emphasizes the importance of diagnosis:

> I had no clue [that] I was struggling because parts of my brain didn't develop … so I simply felt stupid. But the more I read [about FAS], the more I … understood why I did or didn't think in certain ways, why I did or didn't understand certain subjects, and that was huge. It was like 1,000 lbs was lifted off my shoulders.
>
> I can't tell you how many times people have said to me, 'Well, I don't want to label my child' … Well, denial doesn't help. But acceptance and knowing that you have a disability … not only brings relief, but it also gives you a base of where you can need help. Knowing and understanding where your deficits lie helps you build upon your strengths
>
> *(NOFAS 2012)*

So what do we need?

Today, there are major societal issues surrounding excessive consumption of alcohol (see Plant, Chapter 4, this publication), and the increase in the identification of FASDs in children is widely reported (BMA 2007). Regularly, the popular press reports growing concerns regarding the fast-growing 'binge-drinking culture'. In developed countries, this phenomenon is causing political and social concern (see Black, Chapter 21, this publication, for a discussion of the European response to FASDs). In alcohol awareness education in schools, we educate young people to 'know your limits', and to take 'personal responsibility' for identifying their own safe levels of alcohol consumption. Public Health campaigns reflect a similar message, with television and media campaigns giving a focus to issues such as drink-driving at peak times such as Christmas. What none of these campaigns or educational programmes truly address is the toxic impact of alcohol-fuelled socializing and unplanned pregnancy on the life of an unborn child.

Although some drinks companies voluntarily badge alcohol with a 'no alcohol in pregnancy' logo (mandatory in the USA), and, in the UK, Diageo has funded FASD training for midwives (see Fleisher, Chapter 15, this publication), the message needs to be stronger and more consistent. Our politicians need to stand up, advocate and act on behalf of the thousands of children born each year with 100 per cent avoidable, lifelong disabilities due to prenatal alcohol exposure (see Elliott, Chapter 2, this volume). They should stand in spite of recrimination from the alcohol industry and the vitriol of public opinion from those who maintain a dangerous 'love affair' with alcohol. As O'Malley (Chapter 19, this publication) states, it is up to us – Society – to take the proverbial ball and run with it.

As a society, we need to address the ever-growing tranche of children whose lives have been affected, in varying degrees, by alcohol while *in utero*. These children are 'at risk'; potentially vulnerable from the moment of birth – socially, emotionally and intellectually. For young children with FASDs the need for bonding and emotional stability, to nurture their already fragile and compromised brain development, is very great. However, as Williams (Chapter 8, this publication) documents, children and young people with FASDs are the largest group being placed in fostering and adoption services. If the physical health, mental state or social circumstances of a birth mother results in her alcohol-affected child being placed in foster care, how will these fragmented very early childhood experiences affect the child emotionally? We know that attachment issues are significant for children whose early childhood was not always stable (Bomber 2007). High-quality early childhood experiences are crucial to the positive, holistic well-being and development of the young child with an FASD (see also Blackburn, Chapter 10, this publication), but, once again, perverse social circumstances threaten, or deprive them of, that vital opportunity.

Beyond early childhood, our education/school systems may not be well prepared to accommodate the unique learning needs, style and pattern of a child with an FASD. While Canada and parts of the USA have long-established, well-structured social and educational support for children and young people with FASDs, in many countries teachers are ill equipped to deliver meaningful, relevant learning experiences for children with FASDs. Curriculum design can often compound that inaccessibility (see also Carpenter, Chapter 11, this publication).

There are, however, some signs of an emerging response from governments to assimilate the learning needs profile of children and young people with FASDs into the school system. An example of this is the guidance recently issued by the Department of Children's Services (DECS), in South Australia, to its school principals on how to manage the learning environment for children and young people with FASDs.[1]

By the time children with FASDs enter the secondary phase of education they often find themselves disenfranchised from the school experience, finding it overly demanding and unresponsive to their individual needs. For some, school becomes intolerable and they 'drop out'. Lost in an inflexible system, and struggling with the rollercoaster emotions of adolescence and peer pressure, some young people with FASDs turn to criminal activities. Often they do not realize the consequences of their actions. Just as in school they failed to grasp the fundamentals of the classroom routines, they do not always appreciate the 'rules of the game' as young adults, and commit a whole series of social misdemeanours, which bring them into contact with the law.

Miers (2008 pers. comm.) has reported that young people with FASDs form the largest percentage group of young people entering the criminal justice system. She describes them as 'revolving door prisoners'. Like our education system, the justice system – ill prepared, ill equipped – is only beginning to be aware of FASDs and its impact (see also: Killingley, Chapter 16, this publication; Rogan and Crawford, Chapter 14, this publication). This example further illuminates how, for such a major social issue, society has failed to respond and address the needs of this ever-growing group of children, young people and adults with FASDs. As Grant and Clarren advocate (Chapter 20, this publication), with 90 per cent of adults with FASDs experiencing mental health problems, we need to look at the whole life trajectory of children with FASDs (see also O'Malley, Chapter 19, this publication).

Examining the life trajectory of children and young people with FASDs as they face adult life threatens bleak outcomes. If the purpose of school-based education is preparation for adulthood, then clearly it has failed! (See also Egerton, Chapter 12, this publication.) With the notable exception of Canada and parts of North America, school systems have not redesigned to include children and young people with FASDs. Yet the universal cry of education is for inclusive systems that embrace every child, regardless of disability, or social circumstances (UNESCO 1994). In the case of learners with FASDs they are being denied this opportunity or entitlement. They are, as yet, under the radar of the education systems of many countries.

Why interdisciplinary perspectives?

The three editors of this text are all educationalists. That children and young people with FASDs face such bleak outcomes after their time in a system in which we are involved weighs heavy on our own collective conscience. Having written our previous book *Educating Children and Young People with Fetal Alcohol Spectrum Disorders* (Blackburn et al. 2012), we felt that, while we had articulated a much-needed pedagogy based on a framework for learning for these students, there was still a need for something more. This was the need for a holistic, interdisciplinary response to supporting the needs of children, young people and adults with FASDs.

As Elliott and Bower (2008: 236) state:

> The causal pathway to FASD is complex and prevention of the effects on the fetus of alcohol intake during pregnancy will require collaboration across health, community and education sectors.

We offer you this book with that hope, with that aspiration, in the belief that you, the reader, can be a cog in that wheel of change. Each discipline represented in this book has its own literature on FASDs. What we lack is a truly interdisciplinary text which says loudly, clearly and strongly that together we can improve the life chances of those born with FASDs.

The chapters in this publication represent an interdisciplinary wealth of FASD knowledge, research, practice and experience from families, professionals and academics in education, health and social care. In terms of professional practice, it is evident that the identification, assessment, diagnosis and ongoing support of FASDs through the lifespan require an interdisciplinary approach (Blackburn *et al.* 2012, Winstone 2012). Bronstein (2003: 304) notes the benefits of such practice for vulnerable individuals:

> in an elementary school when a school social worker decides to accommodate parents' requests for help with their children's homework, and the social worker elicits teachers' input for how to structure the homework in order to maximize participation and results. In a rehabilitation hospital optimal collaboration may occur when an interdisciplinary team of social worker, doctor, nurse and speech and language therapist meet regularly for case conference that each looks forward to as a place to find solutions for clients that they have been struggling with alone. In an in-patient unit of a community mental health centre, collaboration occurs when a family member calls the unit with a request that any of the professionals feel comfortable responding to in a way that makes the family members feel respected and a part of the team.

The impacts of interdisciplinary collaboration and multiple perspectives are many, often resulting in (Carpenter 2010; Fergusson and Carpenter 2010):

1. creative solutions to intellectual, social and practical problems;
2. important contributions by 'disciplinary immigrants';
3. illumination of previously undetected anomalies and oversights;
4. exploring topics of research which fall into the interstices of traditional disciplines;
5. greater research responsiveness and flexibility; and

6. bridging interdisciplinary communication gaps to mobilize and share resources in the cause of greater social rationality and justice.

This book celebrates the global FASD community of families, researchers and practitioners which serves those with FASDs, and in which families and professionals are equal partners. In this 'community of practice' (Lave and Wenger 1991), we work towards developing joint aims, a common language, collaboration and information sharing not only across disciplines but across socio-cultural and global landscapes. Our common understanding of core cultural values will support the transfer and sharing of knowledge and practice through Vygotskyian notions of socially constructed activity.

Just as the editors and contributors for this publication come to the community of FASDs from different disciplines, cultures, countries and levels of knowledge, we hope that readers will be from equally diverse backgrounds. More importantly we hope that each and every reader will join our community of practice and share our passion and endeavour to improve the knowledge about FASDs in both professional practice and society. In doing so, we can improve the potential for full participation and inclusion in social, educational and employment opportunities for those affected by prenatal alcohol exposure.

Note

1 Capital Programs & Asset Services Fact Sheet: SU001 Facilities for Children and Young People Foetal Alcohol Spectrum Disorder, available at: http://decd.sa.gov.au/assetservices/pages/topiclisting/FASD/.

References

Bacon, F. (1627) *Sylva Sylvarum: or a naturall historie in ten centuries*, London: William Lee.
Baer, J.S., Sampson, P.D., Barr, H.M., Connor, P.D. and Streissguth, A.P. (2003) 'A 21 year longitudinal analysis of the effects of prenatal exposure on young adult drinking', *Archives of General Psychiatry*, 60, April, 377–85.
BBC One (Cambridgeshire, East) (2009) 'Julie Reinger meets the families living with the consequences of Foetal Alcohol Syndrome', *Inside Out*, 23 November,7:30 PM.
Benz, J., Rasmussen, C. and Andrew, K. (2009) 'Diagnosing fetal alcohol spectrum disorder: history, challenges and future directions', *Paediatric Child Health*, 14(4): 231–7.
Bertrand, J., Floyd, R.L. and Weber, M.K. (2005) 'Guidelines for identifying and referring persons with fetal alcohol syndrome', *Morbidity and Mortality Weekly Report*, 54 (RR-11), 1–10 [online at: www.cdc.gov/mmwr/pdf/rr/rr5411.pdf; accessed: 25 September 2011].
Blackburn, C., Carpenter, B. and Egerton, J. (2012) *Educating Children and Young People with Fetal Alcohol Spectrum Disorders*, Abingdon: Routledge.
Bomber, L. (2007) *Inside I'm Hurting: Practical strategies for supporting children with attachment difficulties in schools*, Richmond: Worth Publishing.
BMA (British Medical Association) (2007) *Fetal Alcohol Spectrum Disorders: A guide for healthcare professionals*, London: British Medical Association.
Bronstein, L.R. (2003) 'A model for interdisciplinary collaboration', *Social Work*, 48(3): 297–306.
Brown, S.E. and Guralnick, M.J. (2012) 'International human rights to early intervention for infants and young children with disabilities: tools for global advocacy', *Infants and Young Children*, 25(4): 270–85.
Carpenter, B. (2010) 'Disadvantaged, deprived and disabled', *Special Children*, 193: 42–5.
Chandrasena, A.N., Mukherjee, R.A.S. and Turk, J. (2009) 'Fetal alcohol spectrum disorders: an overview of interventions for affected individuals', *Child and Adolescent Mental Health*, 14(4): 162–7.
Chudley, A.E., Conry, J., Cook, J.L., Loock, C., Rosales, T. and LeBlanc, N. (2005) 'Fetal alcohol spectrum disorders: Canadian guidelines for diagnosis', *Canadian Medical Association Journal*, 172(5

suppl), S1–S21 [online at: www.cmaj.ca/content/172/5_suppl/S1.full.pdf; accessed: 17 September 2011].

Cleaver, H., Unell, I. and Aldgate, J. (2011) *Children's Needs – Parenting Capacity. Child Abuse: Parental mental illness, learning disability, substance misuse and domestic violence* (2nd edition), London: The Stationery Office.

Coles, C.D. (2011) 'Discriminating the effects of prenatal alcohol exposure from other behavioral and learning disorders', *Alcohol Research and Health*, 34(1): 42–50 [online at: http://pubs.niaaa.nih.gov/publications/arh341/42-50.htm; accessed: 26 September 2011].

Connor, P.D. and Huggins, J. (2005) 'Prenatal development: fetal alcohol spectrum disorders', in: K.M. Thies and J.F. Travers (eds) *Handbook of Human Development for Healthcare Professionals*, Sudbury, MA: Jones and Bartlett Publishers [online at: http://books.google.co.uk/books?id=CkbMiPxwvBQC; accessed: 20 April 2009].

Dubovsky, D. (2009) 'Co-morbidities with mental health for an individual with FASD'. In: E. Jonsson, L. Dennett and G. Littlejohn (eds) *Fetal Alcohol Spectrum Disorder (FASD): Across the Lifespan (Proceedings from an IHE Consensus Development Conference 2009)*. Alberta, Canada: Institute of Health Economics [online at: www.ihe.ca/documents/FASDproceedings.pdf; accessed: 17 September 2011].

Elliott, E.J. and Bower, C. (2008) 'Alcohol and pregnancy: the pivotal role of the obstetrician', *Australian and New Zealand Journal of Obstetrics and Gynaecology*, 48(3): 236–9.

FASCETS (Fetal Alcohol Syndrome Consultation, Education and Training Services, Inc.) (2010) 'FASCETS conceptual foundation: a neurobehavioral construct for interventions for children and adults with fetal alcohol spectrum disorders (FASD)'; 'Understanding FASD (Fetal Alcohol Spectrum Disorders)' [online at: www.fascets.org/conceptualfoundation.html and www.fascets.org/info.html; accessed: 11 September 2011].

Fergusson, A. and Carpenter, B. (2010) *Professional Learning and Building a Wider Workforce*, London: SSAT.

Golden, J.L. (2005) *Message in a Bottle: The making of fetal alcohol syndrome*, Cambridge, MA: Harvard University Press.

Gray, R. and Mukherjee, R.A.S. (2007) 'A psychiatrist's guide to fetal alcohol spectrum disorders in mothers who drank heavily during pregnancy', *Advances in Mental Health and Learning Disabilities*, 1(3): 19–26.

Gray, R., Mukherjee, R.A.S. and Rutter, M. (2009) 'Alcohol consumption during pregnancy and its effects on neurodevelopment: what is known and what remains uncertain', *Addiction* 104(8): 1270–3.

Hoyme, H.E., May, P.A., Kalberg, W.O., Kodituwakku, P., Gossage, J.P., Trujillo, P.M., Buckley, D.G., Miller, J.H., Aragon, A.S., Khaole, N., Viljoen, D.L., Jones, K.L. and Robinson. L.K. (2005) 'Clarification of the 1996 Institute of Medicine criteria: a practical clinical approach to diagnosis of fetal alcohol spectrum disorders', *Pediatrics*, 115(1): 39–47.

Jones, K.L. and Smith, D.W. (1973) 'Recognition of the fetal alcohol syndrome in early infancy', *Lancet*, 2(7836): 999–1001.

Jonsson, E., Dennett, L. and Littlejohn, G. (eds) (2009) *Fetal Alcohol Spectrum Disorder (FASD): Across the lifespan (Proceedings from an IHE Consensus Development Conference 2009)*. Alberta, Canada: Institute of Health Economics [online at: www.ihe.ca/documents/FASDproceedings.pdf; accessed: 17 September 2011].

Kelly, K. (2009) 'Is foetal alcohol spectrum disorder linked to anti-social behaviour?' *Woman's Hour*, Radio 4, 20 April, 10–11 AM [online at: www.bbc.co.uk/radio4/womanshour/03/2009_16_mon.shtml; accessed: 20 April 2009].

Lave, J. and Wenger, E. (1991) *Situated Learning: Legitimate peripheral participation*, Cambridge: Cambridge University Press.

Lemoine, P., Harouusseau, H. and Borteyru, J.P. (1968) 'Les enfants de parents alcooliques: anomalies observées, à propos de 127 cas', *Ouest Médical*, 21: 476–82.

Lewis, S.J., Zuccolo, L., Davey Smith, G., Macleod, J., Rodriguez, S., Draper, E.S., Barrow, M., Alati, R., Sayal, K., Ring, S., Golding, J. and Gray, R. (2012) 'Fetal alcohol exposure and IQ at Age 8: evidence from a population-based birth-cohort study', *PLoS ONE*, 7(11): e49407.

Mattson, S.N. and Riley, E.P. (2011) 'The quest for a neurodevelopmental profile of heavy prenatal alcohol exposure', *Alcohol Research and Health*, 34(1): 51–5.

May, P. (2009) 'Prevalence and incidence internationally', in: E. Jonsson, L. Dennett and G. Littlejohn (eds) *Fetal Alcohol Spectrum Disorder (FASD): Across the lifespan (Proceedings from an IHE Consensus Development Conference 2009)*. Alberta, Canada: Institute of Health Economics [online at: www.ihe.ca/documents/FASDproceedings.pdf; accessed: 17 September 2011].

May, P.A., Fiorentino, D., Gossage, P.J., Kalberg, W.O., Hoyme, E.H., Robinson, L.K., Coriale, G., Jones, K.L., del Campo, M., Tarani, L., Romeo, M., Kodituwakku, P.W., Deiana, L., Buckley, D. and Ceccanti, M. (2006) 'Epidemiology of FASD in a province in Italy: prevalence and characteristics of children in a random sample of schools', *Alcoholism: Clinical and Experimental Research*, 30(9): 1562–75.

May, P.A., Fiorentino, D., Coriale, G., Kalberg, W.O., Hoyme, E.H., Aragón, A.S., Buckley, D., Stellavato, C., Gossage, J.P., Robinson, L.K., Lyons Jones, K., Manning, M. and Ceccanti, M. (2011) 'Prevalence of children with severe fetal alcohol spectrum disorders in communities near Rome, Italy: new estimated rates are higher than previous estimates', *International Journal of Environmental Research and Public Health*, 8(6): 2331–51 [online at: www.ncbi.nlm.nih.gov/pmc/articles/PMC3138028/pdf/ijerph-08-02331.pdf; accessed: 25 September 2011].

Morleo, M., Woolfall, K., Dedman, D., Mukherjee, R., Bellis, M.A. and Cook, P. (2011) 'Under-reporting of foetal alcohol spectrum disorders: an analysis of hospital episode statistics', *BMC Pediatrics*, 11(14) [online at: www.biomedcentral.com/1471-2431/11/14; accessed: 11 September 2011].

Mukherjee, R.A.S., Hollins, S. and Abou-Saleh, M.T. (2005) 'Low level alcohol consumption and the fetus', *British Medical Journal*, 330: 375–6.

Mukherjee, R.A.S., Hollins, S. and Turk, J. (2006) 'Fetal alcohol spectrum disorder: an overview', *Journal of the Royal Society of Medicine*, 99(6): 298–302 [online at: www.intellectualdisability.info/mental_phys_health/fetal_alcohol_mukherjee.htm; accessed: 19 April 2009]

NOFAS (National Organization on Fetal Alcohol Syndrome) (2012) 'Morgan Fawcett on living with FASD' (video), Washington, DC: NOFAS [online at: www.youtube.com/watch?v=K0VrkLQfkFg; accessed: 3 June2013].

O'Connor, M.J., Shah, B., Whaley, S., Cronin, P., Gunderson, B. and Graham, J. (2002) 'Psychiatric illness in a clinical sample of children with prenatal alcohol exposure', *American Journal of Drug and Alcohol Abuse*, 28(4): 743–54.

O'Connor, M.J., Frankel, F., Paley, P., Schonfeld, A.M., Carpenter, E., Laugeson, E.A. and Marquardt, R. (2006) 'A controlled social skills training for children with fetal alcohol spectrum disorders', *Journal of Consulting and Clinical Psychology*, 74(4): 639–48.

O'Malley, K. (2007) *ADHD and Fetal Alcohol Spectrum Disorders*, Hauppauge, NY: Nova Science Publishers.

Riley E. (2003) 'FAE/FAS: prevention, intervention and support services: commentary on Burd and Juelson, Coles and O'Malley and Stressguth', in: R.E. Tremblay, R.G. Barr and R.D.V. Peters (eds) *Online Encyclopaedia on Early Childhood Development* [online: www.child-encyclopedia.com/documents/RileyANGxp.pdf; accessed 14 June 2010].

Riley, E. (2011) 'Foetal alcohol syndrome', *Web Chats* (6 July). Hosted by the National Organization on Fetal Alcohol Syndrome (NOFAS) [online at: www.talkingalcohol.com/index.asp?pageid=134; accessed 9 September 2011].

SAMHSA (Substance Abuse and Mental Health Services Administration) (2010) 'Fetal Alcohol Spectrum Disorders (FASD): the basics' (PowerPoint version), [online at: http://fasdcenter.samhsa.gov/educationTraining/fasdBasics.aspx; accessed: 3 June 2013].

Streissguth, A.P. and O'Malley, K. (2000) 'Neuropsychiatric implications and long-term consequences of fetal alcohol spectrum disorders', *Seminars in Clinical Neuropsychiatry*, 5(3): 177–90.

Streissguth, A., Barr, H., Kogan, J. and Bookstein, F. (1996) *Understanding the Occurrence of Secondary Disabilities in Clients with Fetal Alcohol Syndrome (FAS) and Fetal Alcohol Effects (FAE. Final Report: Centers for Disease Control and Prevention Grant No. 04/CCR008515)*, Seattle, WA: University of Washington Fetal Alcohol and Drug Unit.

Sullivan, W. (1899) 'A note on the influence of maternal inebriety on the offspring', *Journal of Mental Science*, 45: 489–503.

UNESCO (United Nations Educational, Scientific and Cultural Organization) (1994) *The Salamanca Statement and Framework for Action on Special Needs Education*, Paris: UNESCO.

University of Chicago (2009) 'Greek texts and translations: Plato's Laws' [online at: http://perseus.uchicago.edu/perseus-cgi/citequery3.pl?dbname=GreekFeb2011&getid=1&query=Pl.%20Leg.%20776a; accessed: 15 September 2011].

US Department of Health and Human Services, Centers for Disease Control and Prevention, National Center on Birth Defects and Developmental Disabilities, FASD Regional Training Centers, and the National Organization of Fetal Alcohol Syndrome (2008) *Fetal Alcohol Spectrum Disorders Competency-Based Curriculum Development Guide for Medical and Allied Health Education and Practice* [online at: www.cdc.gov/ncbddd/fasd/curriculum/FASDguide_web.pdf; accessed 22 September 2011].

Warren, K.R., Hewitt, B.G. and Thomas, J.D. (2011) 'Fetal alcohol spectrum disorders: research challenges and opportunities', *Alcohol Research and Health*, 34(1): 4–14.

Winstone, A. (2012) 'FASD: are we getting the message across?', presentation at the 'Missing a Trick: Stepping up to the Challenge of FASD' Conference, Coventry, September.

WHO (World Health Organization) (2011) *International Classification of Diseases: 10th revision, clinical modification (ICD-10-CM)*. Geneva: WHO [online at: www.icd10data.com/ICD10CM/Codes/Q00-Q99/Q80-Q89/Q86-/Q86.0; accessed: 20 September 2011].

2

INTERNATIONAL OVERVIEW

The challenges in addressing fetal alcohol spectrum disorders

Elizabeth J. Elliott

Alcohol does not discriminate: its use during pregnancy can damage any child, anywhere

The birth of a child with one of the fetal alcohol spectrum disorders (FASDs) should be seen as a failure of society. FASDs are a group of preventable disorders that persist throughout life, with devastating impacts on health and development. They limit life choices and cause immeasurable suffering to individuals living with FASDs, their families and communities. In economic terms, FASDs are very costly; however no dollar, pound, euro, rand, yen, or any other currency value, can be placed on their human toll.

In an era when rates of risky drinking in women continue to rise, when a binge drinking mentality has taken hold of our teenagers, and when almost half of all pregnancies are unplanned, health professionals and teachers can expect to see more children with FASDs. International data from every stratum of society suggest that rates of FASDs are increasing and that in some countries FASDs are now the most common cause of intellectual impairment.

Babies born with FASDs, with brains irreversibly damaged by alcohol exposure *in utero*, are denied some of the most basic of human rights – the rights to health and normal development. Although we must identify and help these children reach their potential, prevention is the only acceptable future solution to FASDs. This is not easily achieved: it requires not only that we prevent alcohol use in pregnancy, but that we address wider issues, such as society's dependence on, and tolerant attitudes to, alcohol and that we break the cycle of social and economic disadvantage that underpins its use. In this chapter I will provide a brief historical context, outline the nature and frequency of FASDs and highlight common challenges we face as an international society in addressing and, most importantly, preventing FASDs. Rather than provide a comprehensive review of the international literature, I will use examples to illustrate key issues and challenges ahead.

FASDs in a historical context

The effects of alcohol use in pregnancy were recognized long before Fetal Alcohol Syndrome (FAS) was described in the *Lancet* by Jones and Smith in 1973 (Jones and Smith 1973). Ancient Greek and Roman writings associated alcohol use in pregnancy with congenital abnormalities and newlyweds were forbidden to drink on their wedding night; Aristotle (384–322 BC) suggested that children of 'drunken women' were often 'morose and languid'; and in the Bible's book of Judges pregnant women were advised to 'drink no wine or strong drink'.

As outlined in an online training course on FASDs (US Department of Health and Human Services *et al.* 2012), the link was made in the early eighteenth century between the 'gin epidemic' in the UK (associated with decreased alcohol taxes and ready availability of low cost gin) and the birth of children looking 'starved, shrivelled and imperfect' and who failed to develop normally. Modern governments should take a lesson from the British parliament of the time, which recognized price as a driver of alcohol consumption. In 1751 it imposed restrictions on gin sales to decrease high rates of morbidity and birth defects in children of 'alcoholic' women (US Department of Health and Human Services *et al.* 2012). Adverse effects of alcohol on pregnancy outcomes – miscarriage, stillbirth, birth defects, and prematurity were also recorded. In 1968 in France, Lemoine published a case series of children born to alcoholic mothers. They had a distinctive appearance that he called 'alcoholic embryopathy' (Lemoine *et al.* 1968). Jones and Smith in 1973 first gave a name to the 'pattern of malformations' that constituted 'Fetal Alcohol Syndrome' (Jones and Smith 1973; Jones *et al.* 1973). FAS became widely recognized internationally and by 1981 the US Surgeon General released an Advisory, warning about the harms of alcohol use in pregnancy. In 1988 the Alcoholic Beverage Labelling Act mandated warning labels about the potential for harm to the fetus for all alcohol beverages in the US.

In 2000, use of the term FASDs recognized that 'prenatal alcohol exposure can cause a whole spectrum of central nervous system sequelae that persist throughout the life span and manifest in a spectrum of effects from clinically indistinguishable to severely impairing' (Streissguth and O'Malley 2000: 177). Although 40 years have passed since FAS was named, recognition, and capacity for accurate diagnosis of FASDs remains a barrier to identifying and assisting children. This can be attributed in part to lack of knowledge and training of health professionals but also to lack of uniformity in the diagnostic criteria used internationally.

Alcohol and the rise of feminism

Accompanying the rise of feminism and equality of gender rights, the last few decades have seen increasing use of alcohol by women in most of the developed world, including 'risky' or 'binge' drinking. This modelled 'male' behaviour is paralleled by high rates of alcohol use in pregnancy. For example, between 30–60 per cent of women in Australia (Colvin *et al.* 2007; Peadon *et al.* 2010), 28 per cent in New Zealand (Ho and Jacquemard 2009) and 8 per cent in the US (Marchetta *et al.* 2012) report using alcohol during pregnancy, similar to other high-income settings. These figures may be misleading however, because the amount of alcohol consumed by *individual* women varies considerably, as does the prevalence of alcohol use *within* countries. In the US, for example, there is considerable variation by state in the proportion of women of childbearing age who report recent alcohol use, from 68 per cent in Wisconsin to 28 per cent in Tennessee, and this variation is likely reflected in pregnancy (CDC 2010). In the

US, alcohol use in pregnancy is highest in women aged 35–44 years (14.3–17.7 per cent), college graduates (10.0–14.4 per cent), employed (9.6–13.7 per cent) and unmarried (13.4 per cent) women (Denny *et al.* 2009; Marchetta *et al.* 2012). Binge drinking (five or more drinks at one time) is reported by 1.4–1.9 per cent, most commonly those aged 18–24 years.

In Australia, the overall rate of alcohol use in pregnancy is similar in Indigenous and non-Indigenous women; however, their pattern of drinking differs significantly. In a recent study in the remote Fitzroy Valley in Western Australia, 50 per cent of Aboriginal women reported alcohol use during pregnancy; however, over 90 per cent drank at risky levels (Elliott *et al.* 2012; Fitzpatrick *et al.* 2012). Similarly, in Cape Province in South Africa, where alcohol was historically exchanged as the 'wage', its use in pregnancy is higher than elsewhere in the country (May *et al.* 2007). Not surprisingly, FASDs rates are also higher in such 'high-risk' communities than elsewhere.

Alcohol toxicity and the unborn child

When consumed by a pregnant woman, alcohol readily crosses the placenta into the fetal circulation, exposing the unborn child to blood alcohol levels similar to those in their mother. Alcohol is a teratogen, a toxic substance that can disrupt development of the embryo and fetus, resulting in damage to the brain and other organs and impairing their function (Elliott and Peadon 2011). A challenge for clinicians is predicting the level of risk in an individual pregnancy. In general, the risk of damage to the unborn child increases with the quantity of alcohol consumed, but the pattern of exposure (this depends on the frequency, timing *and* amount of alcohol consumed) also has a bearing on the risk to the fetus. Other factors, such as maternal age, health, genetics and liver function are also important in determining the peak maternal blood alcohol concentration, and hence the level to which the fetus is exposed. For these reasons, no safe level of alcohol consumption can be established. Whenever alcohol is used during pregnancy there is *potential* for fetal damage, including FASDs, and to prevent FASDs the precautionary principle 'no alcohol, no harm' has been adopted internationally as the safest approach (NHMRC 2009).

Alcohol and its metabolites particularly target the rapidly multiplying cells of the developing brain and may disrupt brain structure and function. At the sub-clinical level, alcohol kills brain cells, interrupts migration of neural pathways, and interferes with production of neurotransmitters – the chemicals that transmit messages from one nerve cell to another. Because the brain continues to develop throughout pregnancy, exposure to alcohol at any time during gestation may be hazardous and the child may be born with a small brain (microcephaly) or structural abnormalities of the brain (Elliott and Peadon 2011). As a consequence, impairment in development may occur across multiple functional domains. This can result, for example, in problems with memory, cognition, executive function, attention and hyperactivity, motor function and communication. Functional impairment may also occur in the absence of evident structural damage to the central nervous system. Ability is variable in children with FASDs: while one child may have profound intellectual impairment, another may have a normal IQ but significant learning difficulties and behavioural problems (Elliott and Peadon 2011).

Increasingly, use of sophisticated neuroimaging is allowing us to identify the parts of the brain damaged by alcohol and their relationship with neurocognitive and behavioural problems in individuals with FASDs. For example, a recent paper from Riley's group demonstrated an association between decreased volume of the caudate nucleus and impaired cognitive performance and verbal learning in youth with heavy alcohol exposure *in utero* (Fryer *et al.* 2012). Structural brain abnormalities are also associated with dysmorphic facial features: in one study youth with heavy alcohol exposure *in utero* had inferior frontal cortical thickening, which correlated with reduced palpebral fissure length and neurocognitive impairment (Yang *et al.* 2012).

In addition to damaging the central nervous system, alcohol exposure may impair prenatal or postnatal growth, hearing and vision and cause a range of birth anomalies. Alcohol is associated with increased rates of miscarriage, prematurity, stillbirth, low birth weight and cerebral palsy. Abnormal development of the face and other organs reflects alcohol exposure during first trimester, the temporal relationship between exposure and the phase of embryological development being critical in determining the pattern of birth defects (Elliott and Peadon 2011).

A significant challenge for families and communities is managing children with FASDs as they become adults and experience the secondary disabilities that result from limited education, limited intellectual capacity and limited social skills. Few adults with FASDs are able to live and work independently and many remain dependent on families for life. Rates of mental illness, psychosis, sexual and social problems, suicide and use of drugs and alcohol are significantly higher than in the general population. Contact with the law and imprisonment is common, particularly for Indigenous youth living in settings where incarceration is the only option for detention. A lack of understanding of right and wrong and failure of the legal system to account for intellectual impairment often results in a cycle of offending, re-offending and recurrent arrest for people with FASDs and results in detention in settings that pose considerable physical and emotional risk to the vulnerable.

The challenges in addressing FASDs

We face a number of challenges in addressing FASDs, most of which are applicable internationally and include:

- overcoming scepticism about FASDs;
- documenting alcohol use in pregnancy;
- establishing FASDs prevalence;
- making an early diagnosis;
- providing evidence-based health care and education;
- educating and upskilling professional groups;
- supporting parents and care-givers;
- developing and disseminating consistent, evidence-based, alcohol policy for pregnancy;
- prevention of FASDs;
- a coordinated national approach to FASDs.

Overcoming scepticism about FASDs

Remarkably, scepticism is still expressed by members of the community (including some health professionals and members of the alcohol industry) that alcohol use in pregnancy is damaging to the fetus. Clinicians who place undue emphases on trying to establish a 'safe' level for alcohol consumption and give advice that 'a few drinks won't hurt', and those who believe it is paternalistic to advise pregnant woman about alcohol use, undermine public health messages that abstinence is safest.

Documenting alcohol use in pregnancy

To prevent FASDs it is important not only to establish the prevalence of alcohol use in pregnancy in each of our countries, but to identify high-risk groups and their location and characteristics. This enables targeted prevention programmes and treatment services. It is also crucial to understand the socio-economic factors that underpin drinking behaviour during pregnancy. Frequently these factors align with the 'causal pathway' to disadvantage, which is difficult to address, requiring action from several government portfolios including, but not limited to, health, education, employment and housing (Elliott and Bower 2004). For example, Australian Aboriginal women living in remote settings identify stress as trigger for alcohol use and say stress results from: loss of traditional land, language and culture; domestic violence; lack of access to education, health services and housing; and the legacy of colonization and 'the stolen generation' (D'Antoine, pers. comm.).

Understanding the risk factors associated with alcohol consumption in individual women allows clinicians to identify women at risk of drinking in a future pregnancy and to offer health care. It can also inform community education programmes. In one study, women at significantly increased risk of using alcohol during pregnancy were those who regularly drank at risky levels, drank during a previous pregnancy (adjusted OR (aOR) 43.9; 95 per cent confidence interval (CI) 27.0 to 71.4); smoked cigarettes, or had a partner who drank alcohol (Peadon *et al.* 2011). In this group a tolerant attitude to alcohol use in pregnancy was highly predictive of intention to use alcohol in a future pregnancy (aOR 5.1; 95 per cent CI 3.6 to 7.1) but the woman's educational level or knowledge of the potential harms of alcohol to the unborn child were not related to attitude. Thus, education alone will not prevent drinking behaviour in pregnancy. Our challenge, which is far more difficult than simply providing information, is to change community attitudes to alcohol, in particular during pregnancy.

Clinicians – both at the primary care and specialist level – have a crucial role in identifying individual women with alcohol dependency or 'binge' drinking behaviour and referring them to the appropriate service. Ideally this will be done *before* the woman is pregnant. Unless these women are identified there will be missed opportunities for treating women themselves, identifying exposed children who are at risk of and require assessment for FASDs, and preventing FASDs.

Much has been written about the challenge of asking about alcohol use and various tools have been validated for use in pregnancy (Muggli *et al.* 2010). The most important thing is that health professionals ask! If questions about alcohol are asked routinely in the context of lifestyle and dietary behaviours, most women are happy to provide information. Regrettably, many clinicians fear that by asking pregnant women about alcohol use they might cause undue maternal stress and anxiety: only 23 per cent of pediatricians (Elliott *et al.* 2006) and 45 per cent of health professionals (Payne *et al.* 2005) routinely ask pregnant patients about their alcohol use in pregnancy and 12 per cent of health professionals never ask (Payne *et al.* 2005). In contrast, 96 per cent of women said they wanted their doctor to ask about alcohol use and to provide clear advice to avoid alcohol (Peadon *et al.* 2011).

In recording alcohol use in pregnancy one challenge is to 'standardize' the meaning of a standard drink. This would facilitate comparison of alcohol policy, alcohol use and study results. A standard drink is defined as *a drink containing a specified amount of pure alcohol (ethanol), regardless of its type (wine, beer, spirits) or volume*. In the UK one standard drink is equivalent to eight grams of pure alcohol, whereas in Australia it is ten grams and in Japan 19.75 grams (International Center for Alcohol Policies 2009). Another challenge is to routinely document alcohol use in pregnancy. In Australia for example, midwives record its use in only three of eight States and Territories thus the National Perinatal Data Collection is incomplete, illustrating a crucial missed opportunity for identifying pregnancies at risk.

Establishing FASDs prevalence

Unless we have current data on the prevalence of FASDs in our local settings it is difficult to persuade governments that the problem exists, let alone to commit funding for diagnostic and clinical services, prevention programmes and support for care-givers. However, establishing prevalence is a challenge because diagnosis is a complex, time-consuming and costly process requiring multidisciplinary assessment by health professionals and input from parents and teachers. Also, diagnostic criteria differ from one continent to another. Not surprisingly, published rates of FASDs prevalence vary widely, both internationally and within countries, reflecting the use of different diagnostic criteria and study methods and variable alcohol use. Clinic-based data may overestimate and passive surveillance data underestimate prevalence and there are few high quality, population-based data available. Most studies do not use active case-finding. Most report on FAS and partial FAS but few include children across the entire FASD spectrum, namely with neurodevelopmental disorder. Some report birth prevalence, some population prevalence and some incidence. All these factors make comparisons between countries difficult. Nevertheless there are some consistent messages: most authors acknowledge that prevalence/incidence rates are underestimates; that rates are consistently higher in high-risk Indigenous than non-Indigenous groups; and that prevalence is increasing.

In a 2009 review, May and colleagues reported findings from active case ascertainment studies using in-school screening and diagnosis in primary school-aged children (May *et al.* 2009). The prevalence of FAS was estimated at 2–7 per 1,000 in mixed-race, mixed-socio-economic populations in the US and the prevalence of FASDs at about 2–5 per cent in the US and some Western European countries (May *et al.* 2009). Using similar methods, the prevalence estimate for FAS in Italy is 4–12 per 1,000, partial FAS 18–46 per 1,000 and FASDs 2.3–6.3 per cent (May *et al.* 2011).

The highest rates of FAS and partial FAS reported internationally are from studies of Grade I children in communities in the Western Cape (68–89 per 1,000) (May *et al.* 2007) and Northern Cape (74–119 per 1,000) Provinces (Urban *et al.* 2008) of South Africa. In population-based studies the prevalence of FASDs was also high in First Nations people in British Columbia (25 per 1,000) and Yukon (46 per 1,000) (May *et al.* 2009) and the North West (189 per 1,000) (Robinson *et al.* 1987). In the North West study FAS was identified in as many as 120 per 1,000 children. Data from the 1980s and early 1990s show a FAS prevalence rate of 2–8 per 1,000 American Indians, although more recent data are not available. Prevalence data from the Lililwan study in primary school-aged Australian

Aboriginals are not yet published; however, 50 per cent of the population studied was exposed to high levels of alcohol *in utero* (Elliott *et al.* 2012; Fitzpatrick *et al.* 2012).

Making an early diagnosis

Early diagnosis is important because it allows for early intervention, which is associated with improved long-term outcomes in FASDs. Diagnosis allows families and schools to have realistic expectations for the child and to provide remediation or consider alternative education pathways. Diagnosis is also a key to enabling families to apply to government support schemes such as 'disability' and 'carers' allowances. Early diagnosis of a child with an FASD also identifies mothers at risk of drinking during future pregnancies and provides an opportunity for interventions to manage their alcohol use and prevent damage to subsequent children. An Australian study, in which 51 per cent of children reported with FAS also had a sibling with FAS, highlights the tragedy of missed opportunities for prevention (Elliott *et al.* 2008).

Ideally, diagnosis is made by a multidisciplinary team which can identify a child's strengths and weaknesses and thus inform their management plan. However, few diagnostic services for FASDs exist outside North America and many existing clinics are not sustainable, relying on short-term or research funding (Peadon *et al.* 2008). Making a diagnosis of an FASD is a costly and time-consuming process and requires trained medical professionals who, in many countries, are few and far between. Significant challenges to diagnosis include lack of clinician knowledge about FASDs (in Australia only 12 per cent of health professionals and 19 per cent of pediatricians knew the four essential diagnostic features of FAS) and entrenched clinician attitudes (53 per cent of health professionals and 70 per cent of pediatricians believe that the diagnosis of FAS is stigmatizing). Many health professionals feel very ill-equipped to deal with FAS, many are unsure where to refer for a definitive diagnosis, and most want information for themselves and their patients (Elliott *et al.* 2006; Payne *et al.* 2005). This mirrors the experience of teachers, who, through the observable student response in the learning environment, see a pattern of FASDs emerge, but do not know where to make a referral to (Carpenter, Chapter 11, this publication). Their traditional assessment services in educational psychology are also only just refining their assessment response to children and young people with FASDs, and many of the traditional assessment tools and approaches need careful revisiting to ensure that they accurately profile the needs of this complex population.

Providing evidence-based health care and education

There will never be a 'magic bullet' for the treatment of FASDs. The benefit of identifying specific areas of dysfunction during a multidisciplinary assessment is that a child's needs can be specifically addressed by relevant allied health, pharmacological, behavioural, and school-based treatments that have been successfully used in other developmental disorders. Of the treatments proposed for use in FASDs, few have been tested in randomized controlled trials (RCTs). In one systematic review of interventions for FASDs, only seven from over 6,000 publications were RCTs (Peadon *et al.* 2009). Most were poorly designed studies with a small sample size and inconclusive results. Caregivers and teachers often provide anecdotal evidence for strategies for dealing with children with FASDs at home and in school. Before these can be adopted and funded by service providers there is an urgent need for proof of effect. A number of large-scale RCTs funded by the Centers for Disease Control in the USA are in progress and may help address the challenge of providing the high-level evidence of efficacy that is required for government funding of therapies.

Educating and upskilling professional groups

FASDs are complex disorders. Thus, in addition to medical and allied health professionals, there is an urgent need to educate the wide range of professional groups who are likely to encounter individuals with FASDs during their work, including teachers and those working in legal, community, foster care, and drug and alcohol services. There is good evidence that education can change clinician knowledge, attitudes and clinical practice (Payne *et al.* 2011a, 2011b). The US Department of Health and Services offers free online training for health professionals[1] and the University of Washington offers online training in the FASD 4-Digit Diagnostic Code and workshops for FASD Diagnostic Training for Interdisciplinary Clinical Teams.[2] NOFAS-UK regularly distributes an electronic *FASD Forum* containing original articles and listing recent publications about FASDs.[3] Resources for schools, service providers and key workers are available on numerous reputable sites.[4] Blackburn and colleagues' recent book is invaluable, providing resources and practical strategies to enable teachers to deal with the range of learning difficulties associated with FASDs (Blackburn *et al.* 2012). As suggested in its title, personalized individual educational plans are promoted for children. NOFAS-UK has developed a set of videos and fact sheets for teachers and provides details of primary curricula, information for midwives, and workshops for professional training.[5] Increasingly, information about FASDs for the legal profession (Killingley, Chapter 16, this publication), is being made available, for example from the American Bar Association.[6]

Supporting parents and care-givers

For many families, living with FASDs is an isolating and stressful experience. Delays in diagnosis, lack of professional expertise, absence of diagnostic services and lack of specific therapies lead to feelings of neglect and despair. These feelings are exacerbated by unrealistic expectations of children in the education system, the inability of many adults with FASDs to live and work independently, and the increased long-term risk of drug and alcohol abuse, contact with the law and mental health disorders. Many children with FASDs are placed in out-of-home care – as many as 60 per cent in some settings – because their mother is alcohol dependent and deemed unable to care for the child. It is particularly important to screen all children identified for foster placement for both alcohol exposure in pregnancy and FASDs (Williams, Chapter 8, this publication). As early as possible care-givers need to be given information about FASDs and put in contact with parent-support groups. A Google search reveals many sites providing information about parent-support services, including: the FASD Ontario Network of Expertise,[7] Government of British Columbia Canada,[8] National Organisation for Fetal Alcohol Syndrome and Related Disorders (NOFASARD) Australia[9] and the National Organizations on Fetal Alcohol Syndrome in the USA[10] and UK.[11] Several books, listed at the FAS Book Store at Amazon.

com provide insightful parent perspectives.[12] Professionals, and parents themselves, can be powerful advocates, for the rights of children with disability including access to services, financial and educational support.

Developing and disseminating consistent, evidence-based alcohol policy for pregnancy

Most countries have developed a health policy regarding alcohol use in pregnancy (International Center for Alcohol Policies 2009). Advice varies internationally and by jurisdiction within countries and has evolved – generally for the better – as new scientific evidence has become available. The Public Health Agency of Canada[13] warns 'There is no safe amount or safe time to drink alcohol during pregnancy'. In 2005, the US Surgeon General 'warned pregnant women and women who may become pregnant to abstain from alcohol consumption in order to eliminate the chance of giving birth to a baby with any of the harmful effects of the Fetal Alcohol Spectrum Disorders (FASD)'.[14] This updated the more lenient 1981 advice that 'pregnant women should limit the amount of alcohol they drink.' Similarly, in Australia the recent guideline advises that:

> for women who are pregnant or planning a pregnancy, not drinking is the safest option
> *(Commonwealth of Australia 2009: 67)*

This provides a clear, concise, and more conservative message than the previous (2001) national guideline, which equivocated. It advised that: 'women who are pregnant or might soon become pregnant: *may* consider not drinking; should never become intoxicated; and if they choose to drink, over one week, should have less than seven standard drinks *and*, on any one day, no more than two standard drinks (spread over at least two hours)' (Commonwealth of Australia 2001: 16, Guideline 11).

This message is complex, confusing and was open to misinterpretation by health professionals and women.

Importantly, policy should be evidence-based and widely disseminated to health professionals and the general public. Yet, in Australia for example, only 13 per cent of health professionals surveyed gave advice to women consistent with the 2002 Australian guideline (Elliott *et al.* 2006; Payne *et al.* 2005). Regarding the 2009 Australian guideline, the correct public health message has failed to reach the general public. When women aged 14–27 years were asked what they considered to be a 'safe' amount for a single drinking session the average was 6.5 drinks – considerably higher than the recommended four standard drinks (FARE 2012a). If policy is truly evidence-based, then the messages about alcohol consumption should be consistent worldwide – a worthy challenge.

Prevention of FASDs

Our most important challenge is prevention of FASDs. Primary prevention – to eliminate exposure to alcohol *in utero* – will take commitment, funding and time and, just as with tobacco, requires a multi-pronged, national approach. It requires an understanding about why pregnant women drink and an undertaking to address the social disadvantage underpinning alcohol use. It should include development and dissemination of alcohol policy, public health campaigns to increase community awareness of the harms of alcohol to mother and child, school-based education programmes, and labelling of alcoholic beverages. Alcohol use in pregnancy is strongly associated with tolerant attitudes to alcohol use in pregnancy; however education (knowledge of harms) does not influence attitude. Thus, education alone will not change drinking behaviour and other strategies will be important.

The most effective way to decrease excessive drinking is to restrict access to and promotion of alcohol. This can be achieved through legislation, including increasing the price of alcohol through increased taxation, minimum pricing, and volumetric taxation. In some high-risk communities access has been restricted by legislation for 'dry communities', restrictions on the 'take-away' of full-strength alcohol, restrictions on the purchase of excessive alcohol, and laws to prevent serving alcohol to pregnant women. The number of alcohol outlets and their opening hours can also be restricted. Restricting the 'visibility' of alcohol can be achieved by preventing advertising, including controlling the placement of alcohol on supermarket shelves, use of plain packaging and prohibition of alcohol sponsorship of sporting and other events. Prevention must have the support of governments and evaluation of prevention policy – a previous omission – is an imperative. Our biggest challenge is to stand up to the alcohol industry, to which profit is king. Prevention of FASDs will require unpopular decisions but is an achievable challenge.

A coordinated national approach for FASDs

The Australian government's House of Representatives recently conducted and published an inquiry into the prevention, diagnosis and management of FASDs (House of Representatives 2012) in which one of the recommendations was development of a national coordinated plan to address FASDs, such as that proposed by the Foundation of Alcohol Research and Education (FARE 2012b). There is a crucial need for governments to acknowledge the challenge of FASDs and to progress the agenda. A national plan provides a framework for addressing the challenges we face in the prevention, diagnosis and management of FASDs and in supporting research and advocating for people living with FASDs and their families.

Notes

1 http://fasdcenter.samhsa.gov/educationTraining/courses/FASDTheCourse
2 See: http://depts.washington.edu/fasdpn/htmls/team-train.htm.
3 info@nofas-uk.org
4 www.mcf.gov.bc.ca/fasd/kw_support.htm
5 www.nofas-uk.org
6 www.americanbar.org/groups/child_law/what_we_do/projects/child_and_adolescent_health/fasd.htm
7 www.fasdontario.ca/cms/resources/support-groups
8 www.mcf.gov.bc.ca/fasd/kw_support.htm
9 www.nofasard.org
10 www.nofas.org
11 www.nofas-uk.org
12 www.come-over.to/FAS/store/
13 www.phac-aspc.gc.ca/hp-gs/guide/03_ap-ag-eng.php
14 www.surgeongeneral.gov/news/2005/02/sg02222005.html

References

Blackburn, C., Carpenter, B. and Egerton, J. (2012) *Educating Children and Young People with Fetal Alcohol Spectrum Disorders: Constructing personalised pathways to learning*, Abingdon: Routledge.

Centers for Disease Control and Prevention (2010) 'State-specific weighted prevalence estimates of alcohol use among women 18–44 years of age, behavioral risk factor surveillance system', Atlanta, GA: CDC [online at: www.cdc.gov/ncbddd/fasd/monitor_table.html; accessed: 14 January 2013].

Colvin, L., Payne, J., Parsons, D., Kurinczuk, J. and Bower, C. (2007) 'Alcohol consumption during pregnancy in non-Indigenous West Australian women', *Alcoholism: Clinical and Experimental Research*, 32(2): 276–84.

Commonwealth of Australia (2001) *Australian Alcohol Guidelines: Health risks and benefits*, Canberra, ACT: National Health and Medical Research Council.

Commonwealth of Australia (2009) *Australian Guidelines to Reduce Health Risks from Drinking Alcohol*, Canberra, ACT: National Health and Medical Research Council.

Denny, C.H., Tsai, J., Floyd, R.L. and Green, P.P./National Center on Birth Defects and Developmental Disabilities, CDC (2009) 'Alcohol use among pregnant and non-pregnant women of childbearing age – United States, 1991–2005', *Morbidity and Mortality Weekly Report*, 58 (19): 529–32.

Elliott, E. and Peadon, E. (2011) 'Fetal alcohol spectrum disorders', *BMJ Best Practice* [online at: http://bestpractice.bmj.com/best-practice/monograph/1141/resources/credits.html; accessed: 14 January 2013].

Elliott, E., Latimer, J., Fitzpatrick, J., Oscar, J. and Carter, M. (2012) 'There's hope in the valley', *Journal of Paediatrics and Child Health*, 48(3): 190–2.

Elliott, E.J. and Bower, C. (2004) 'FAS in Australia: fact or fiction?', *Journal of Pediatrics and Child Health*, 40(1/2): 8–10.

Elliott, E.J., Payne, J., Haan, E., Bower, C. (2006) 'Diagnosis of fetal alcohol syndrome and alcohol use in pregnancy: a survey of paediatricians' knowledge, attitudes and practice', *Journal of Pediatrics and Child Health*, 42(11): 698–703.

Elliott, E.J., Payne, J., Morris, A., Haan, E. and Bower, C. (2008) 'Fetal alcohol syndrome: a prospective national surveillance study', *Archives of Disease in Childhood*, 93(9): 732–7.

Fitzpatrick, J.P, Elliott, E.J., Latimer, J., Carter, M., Oscar, J., Ferreira, M., Carmichael Olson, H., Lucas, B., Doney, R., Salter, C., Peadon, E., Hawkes, G. and Hand, M. (2012) 'The Lililwan Project: study protocol for a population based, active case ascertainment study of the prevalence of Fetal Alcohol Spectrum Disorders (FASD) in remote Australian Aboriginal communities', *BMJ Open*, 2: 1–12 [online at: http://bmjopen.bmj.com/content/2/3/e000968.full.pdf+html; accessed: 14 January 2013].

Foundation for Alcohol Research and Education (FARE) (2012a) 'Three years on: alcohol guidelines invisible and unknown', media release, 6 March [online at: www.fare.org.au/wp-content/uploads/2011/07/Media-release-060312-Three-years-on-alcohol-guidelines-invisible-and-unknown.pdf; accessed: 14 January 2013].

Foundation for Alcohol Research and Education (FARE) (2012b) 'The Australian Fetal Alcohol Spectrum Disorders Action Plan 2013–2016' [online at: www.fare.org.au/wp-content/uploads/2011/07/FARE-FASD-Plan.pdf; accessed: 14 January 2013].

Fryer, S.L., Mattson, S.N., Jernigan, T.L., Archibald, S.L., Jones, K.L. and Riley, E.P. (2012) 'Caudate volume predicts neurocognitive performance in youth with heavy prenatal alcohol exposure', *Alcoholism: Clinical and Experimental Research*, 36(11): 1932–41.

Ho, R. and Jacquemard, R. (2009) 'Maternal alcohol use before and during pregnancy among women in Taranaki, New Zealand', *Journal of the New Zealand Medical Association*, 122 (1306) [online at: http://journal.nzma.org.nz/journal/122-1306/3883/; accessed: 14 January 2013].

House of Representatives (2012) *FASD: the hidden harm. Inquiry into the prevention, diagnosis and management of Fetal Alcohol Spectrum Disorders*, Standing Committee on Social Policy and Legal Affairs, Canberra, ACT: Commonwealth of Australia 2012 [online at: www.aph.gov.au/Parliamentary_Business/Committees/House_of_Representatives_Committees?url=spla/fasd/index.htm; accessed: 14 January 2013].

International Center for Alcohol Policies (2009) 'International guidelines on drinking and pregnancy', Washington, DC: International Center for Alcohol Policies [online at: www.icap.org/Table/InternationalGuidelinesOnDrinkingAndPregnancy; accessed: 14 January 2013].

Jones, K.L. and Smith, D.W. (1973) 'Recognition of the fetal alcohol syndrome in early infancy', *Lancet*, 302(7836): 999–1001.

Jones, K.L., Smith, D.W., Ulleland, C.N. and Streissguth, P. (1973) 'Pattern of malformation in offspring of chronic alcoholic mothers', *Lancet*, 1(7815): 1267–71.

Lemoine, P., Harousseau, H., Borteyru, J.P. and Andmenuet, J.C. (1968) 'Les enfants de parents alcooliques: anomalies observees a proposos de 127 cas' [Children of alcoholic parents: abnormalities observed in 127 cases], *Ouest Medecine*, 21(6): 476–82.

Marchetta, C.M., Denny, C.H., Floyd, R.L., Cheal, N.E., Sniezek, J.E. and McKnight-Eily, L.R./ Centres for Disease Control (2012) 'Alcohol use and binge drinking among women of childbearing age: United States, 2006–2010', *Morbidity and Mortality Weekly Report*, 61(28): 534–8.

May, P.A., Fiorentino, D., Coriale, G., Kalberg, W.O., Hoyme, H.E., Aragón, A.S., Buckley, D., Stellavato, C., Gossage, J.P., Robinson, L.K., Jones, K.L., Manning, M. and Ceccanti, M. (2011) 'Prevalence of children with severe fetal alcohol spectrum disorders in communities near Rome, Italy: new estimated rates are higher than previous estimates', *International Journal of Environmental Research and Public Health*, 8(6): 2331–51.

May, P.A., Gossage, J.P., Marais, A.S., Adnams, C.M., Hoyme, H.E., Jones, K.L., Robinson, L.K., Khaole, N.C., Snell, C., Kalberg, W.O., Hendricks, L., Brooke, L., Stellavato, C. and Viljoen, D.L. (2007) 'The epidemiology of fetal alcohol syndrome and partial FAS in a South African community', *Drug and Alcohol Dependence*, 88(2/3): 259–71.

May, P.A., Gossage, J.P., Kalberg, W.O., Robinson, L.K., Buckley, D., Manning, M. and Hoyme, H.E. (2009) 'Prevalence and epidemiologic characteristics of FASD from various research methods with an emphasis on recent in-school studies', *Mental Retardation and Developmental Disabilities Research Reviews*, 15(3): 176–92.

Muggli, E., Cook, B., O'Leary, C., Forster, D. and Halliday, J. (2010) *Alcohol in Pregnancy: What questions should we be asking? Report to the Commonwealth Department of Health and Ageing*, Parkville, Victoria: Murdoch Children's Research Institute.

NHMRC (National Health and Medical Research Council) (2009) *Australian Guidelines to Reduce Health Risks from Drinking Alcohol*, Canberra, ACT: Commonwealth of Australia.

Payne, J., Elliott, E., D'Antoine, H., O'Leary, C., Mahony, A., Haan, E. and Bower, C. (2005) 'Health professionals' knowledge, practice and opinions about fetal alcohol syndrome and alcohol consumption in pregnancy', *Australian and New Zealand Journal of Public Health*, 29(6): 558–64.

Payne, J., France, K., Henley, N., D'Antoine, H., Bartu, A., O'Leary, C., Elliott, E. and Bower, C. (2011a) 'Changes in health professionals' knowledge, attitudes and practice following provision of educational resources about prevention of prenatal alcohol exposure and fetal alcohol spectrum disorder', *Paediatric and Perinatal Epidemiology*, 25(4): 316–27.

Payne, J.M., France, K.E., Henley, N., D'Antoine, H.A., Bartu, A.E., Mutch, R.C., Elliott, E.J. and Bower, C.(2011b) 'Paediatricians' knowledge, attitudes and practice following provision of educational resources about prevention of prenatal alcohol exposure and fetal alcohol spectrum disorder', *Journal of Paediatrics and Child Health*, 47(10): 704–10.

Peadon, E., Fremantle, E., Bower, C. and Elliott, E.J. (2008) 'International survey of diagnostic services for children with FASD', *BMC Pediatrics*, 8: 12 [online at: http://dx.doi.org/10.1186/1471-2431-8-12; accessed: 13 January 2013].

Peadon, E., Payne, J., Henley, N., D'Antoine, H., Bartu, A., O'Leary, C., Bower, C., Elliott, E. (2010) 'Women's knowledge and attitudes regarding alcohol consumption in pregnancy: a national survey', *BMC Public Health*, 10: 510 [online at: http://dx.doi.org/10.1186/1471-2458-10-510; accessed: 13 January 2013].

Peadon, E., Payne, J., Henley, N., D'Antoine, H., Bartu, A., O'Leary, C., Bower, C. and Elliott, E.J. (2011) 'Attitudes and behaviour predict women's intention to drink alcohol during pregnancy: the challenge for health professionals', *BMC Public Health*, 11: 584 [online at: www.biomedcentral.com/1471-2458/11/584/; accessed 5 June 2013].

Peadon, E., Rhys-Jones, B., Bower, C. and Elliott, E.J. (2009) 'Systematic review of interventions for children with FASD', *BMC Pediatrics*, 9(1): 35 [online at: http://dx.doi.org/10.1186/1471-2431-9-35; accessed: 13 January 2013].

Robinson, G.C., Conry, J.L. and Conry, R.F. (1987) 'Clinical profile and prevalence of fetal alcohol syndrome in an isolated community in British Columbia', *Canadian Medical Association Journal*, 137(3): 203–7.

Streissguth, A.P. and O'Malley, K. (2000) 'Neuropsychiatric implications and long-term consequences of fetal alcohol spectrum disorders', *Seminars in Clinical Neuropsychiatry*, 5(3): 177–90.

Urban, M., Chersich, M.F., Fourie, L.A., Chetty, C., Olivier, L. and Viljoen, D. (2008) 'Fetal alcohol syndrome among grade 1 schoolchildren in Northern Cape Province: prevalence and risk factors', *South African Medical Journal*, 98(11): 877–82.

US Department of Health and Human Services, FASD Center for Excellence, Substance Abuse and Mental Health Services Administration (SAMHSA) (2012) 'Module 1: Historical Perspectives on Alcohol and Pregnancy', *FASD: The course* [online at: http://fasdcenter.samhsa.gov/educationTraining/courses/FASDTheCourse; accessed November 2012].

Yang, Y., Roussotte, F., Kan, E., Sulik, K.K., Mattson, S.N., Riley, E.P., Jones, K.L., Adnams, C.M., May, P.A., O'Connor, M.J., Narr, K.L. and Sowell, E.R. (2012) 'Abnormal cortical thickness alterations in fetal alcohol spectrum disorders and their relationships with facial dysmorphology', *Cerebral Cortex*, 22(5): 1170–9.

3

FETAL ALCOHOL SYNDROME

The causal web from disadvantage to birth defect

Ron Gray

> [T]he prevalence of this disorder seems to be high anywhere in the world where alcohol consumption is present in the culture, where poverty is common, and where hope for the future is almost nonexistent. In those situations people have looked for ways to escape from their situation. Alcohol has been one way to do so. Wherever and whenever that occurs, the prevalence of FASD will be high.
>
> *(Jones 2011: 3)*

Key points

- It is useful and productive to take a population health perspective on fetal alcohol syndrome (FAS).
- We know that alcohol is the cause of FAS but for prevention what we really want to know is why, in some populations, do more women drink heavily or binge drink during pregnancy than in others?
- Heavy drinking during pregnancy is a result of a complex interplay of social, cultural and political factors known as 'social determinants' or the 'causes of the causes'.
- Three populations known to be at increased risk of FAS are: the inner city African-American populations in the United States; the mixed ethnicity population of the Western South Africa Cape and the Indigenous Australian population.
- In these populations, social injustice affecting rates of FAS is causing considerable childhood disability and is destroying the lives of children and their families on a major scale.
- The role of intimate partner violence in leading to excessive female alcohol consumption has been relatively neglected and is an important area for future research.

Introduction

This chapter outlines a *population perspective* on FAS. Let me explain why this might be helpful. Just as individuals can be unwell we can also have 'sick' populations (Rose 1985). For example, populations undergoing famine, populations plagued by infectious disease or, of more recent interest, populations with high rates of obesity. Now a consistent finding on FAS is that the condition occurs much more frequently (is more prevalent) in some populations rather than others. More specifically, FAS is more prevalent in socially disadvantaged and politically disenfranchised populations (Jones 2011). These, then, will be our 'sick' populations of interest. So the fundamental issue for those working in public health is how do we improve the health of 'sick' populations? This is what we mean by prevention. But we can't make any headway with prevention until we know the causes which are making the populations 'sick': any successful attempt at FAS prevention would need to address them. Of course we know that for any particular child with FAS, exposure to alcohol during intra-uterine life is a necessary precursor. So this simplifies our search for causes somewhat: we really want to know why, in some populations, do more women drink heavily or binge drink during pregnancy than in others? The answer comprises a set of inter-related social, cultural and political factors which are currently styled 'social determinants' or sometimes the 'causes of the causes' (Marmot 2007).

So what are the social determinants or causes of heavy/binge drinking in populations with high FAS prevalence? In this chapter I will try to make a start on answering this question in relation to three specific disadvantaged populations with a high FAS prevalence: African-American populations living in the United States, Cape Coloured populations living in South Africa and the Indigenous population of Australia. I chose these populations for three reasons. First, the levels of FAS in these populations are at such high levels that they are unlikely to be explained away as artefacts of research. Second, the histories and cultures of these populations and their geographical locations are sufficiently different to illustrate the uniqueness of context and place in determining high levels of FAS but with sufficient commonality to show how social and political forces can penetrate different communities with similar devastating effects. Finally, they are populations in which there has been a lot of clinical and research interest (see, for example, the relevant chapters in this publication) and hence they are well-documented. For clarity, I will consider these populations separately, but close with some unifying observations on high FAS prevalence level as a socially determined inequality in health.

I write for a general audience with an interest in alcohol research in order to make the case for taking a population perspective on FAS. Accordingly, I have cited literature selectively and not attempted to comprehensively and systematically document all the literature in this area. That would require a book-length treatment in itself. For more comprehensive and detailed information on FAS in the US, South Africa and Australia readers are referred to Chapters 20, 22 and 23 in this publication. Also, I do not cover prevention in this chapter although my firm belief is that effective preventative strategies will take into account the social and political determinants of FAS prevalence (Rosenthal *et al.* 2005). Surely scientific advances in neuro-protection and improvements in health services will be important in FAS prevention, but on their own are likely to be insufficient.

FAS: the causal web

Causation of disease is often presented as following a chain or sequence of events, but this is almost certainly a misleading oversimplification. In the case of FAS there are a number of influences at different levels involved in the causation. It is their interplay which eventually converges on and promotes the use of alcohol during pregnancy which then leads to FAS. So perhaps the picture of a spider's web (MacMahon *et al.* 1960) and the added complexity which that involves is more appropriate than the metaphor of a chain.

Of course not all children exposed to alcohol in the uterus will go on to develop FAS. Hence varying individual susceptibility operating through genetic and epigenetic factors is also important in causation. In particular, evidence has accumulated on the effects of genetic polymorphisms of alcohol metabolizing enzymes on FAS risk and these effects are important in determining individual responses (Green and Stoler 2007; Warren and Li 2005). However, at the population level genetic effects are unlikely to account for much of the high prevalence noted in the populations I consider and hence are not considered further in this chapter.

At one level drinking during pregnancy (or choosing not to) involves a health choice. However, this choice may be constrained by addiction, culture, education and material circumstances. In addition, the pathways to problem drinking are extremely complex (Moussas *et al.* 2009) incorporating neurobiological, genetic, family, social and political influences. Furthermore, in addition to social disadvantage, inequitable gender relationships and threat or commission of violence against women may lead to hopelessness and use of alcohol as a means of escape. These are all part of what I termed, above, the web of causation. So there are important implications here for prevention. If we want women to be able to make healthy choices in their lives then we need to empower them by helping to remove these barriers.

Another implication of the causal web is that social determinants could act at a number of points in the web to influence the final outcome. To give an example, poverty could increase FAS risk by increasing risk of being a heavy/binge drinker during pregnancy. We say this is an effect of poverty mediated through alcohol use. But it could also act in other ways such constraining dietary choices leading to poor nutrition in pregnancy or increasing risk of being a cigarette smoker during pregnancy both of which are thought be co-factors in the occurrence of FAS. So these would be effects of poverty mediated through poor nutrition and through cigarette toxicity to the fetus respectively.

We now turn to the three populations of interest.

Inner city African-American populations in the United States

After the initial descriptions of FAS in the medical literature, establishing how common the condition was became of great interest in the United States and elsewhere. A number of studies were funded to examine alcohol consumption in pregnancy and then to follow-up the children to assess them for the presence of clinical signs of FAS. Many of these studies, showed a much higher rate in African-American populations than in white populations. Abel prepared summary estimates of rates using many of these studies up to the mid-1990s finding that FAS occurs ten times more frequently in African-American/low socioeconomic status populations than Caucasian middle socioeconomic status populations (Abel 1995). He also makes the point that ethnicity is strongly confounded by socioeconomic status. In the paper where he presents the summary estimates, he concludes by saying:

> FAS is more common among minorities in the inner cities of the United States, not because some minorities are genetically at-risk for FAS but because a high percentage of minority women eke out an existence at incomes below the poverty line ... Poverty, not genotype, provides the kind of host environment that exacerbates alcohol's toxic actions.
>
> *(Abel 1995: 441)*

This finding might seem surprising at first because, in general terms, there are relatively high rates of abstention and relatively low rates of heavy drinking among African-American women (Collins and McNair 2002). However, in the minority of African-Americans who do develop problem drinking, the consequences are more severe than for the white population. For example, although African-Americans are less likely to develop alcohol dependence than those in the white population, once they become dependent the risk of persistent or recurrent dependence is greater (Chartier and Caetano 2010).

With specific regard to drinking during pregnancy there is little evidence to suggest that African-American women are more likely to drink during pregnancy than white women. However, they are less likely to reduce their level of consumption during pregnancy (Morris *et al.* 2008). Moreover it seems that the group where this finding is most marked is the group of African-American women who are heavy or binge drinkers (Tenkku *et al.* 2009).

So why should this group of problem drinkers be less likely to reduce consumption or stop? Well, at the level of the individual woman there has been interest in the concept of stress/distress as a mediator of the effects of social disadvantage on problem drinking. Mulia and colleagues (2008a) have investigated the effect of psychological distress as a mediator of ethnic disparities in problem drinking in the United States. They postulated a 'stress process model' in which psychological distress and problem drinking arise from exposure to severe economic hardship, stressful life events and living in disadvantaged neighbourhoods. In a prospective study of 392 American mothers receiving a welfare benefit scheme known as Temporary Assistance for Needy Families, they found that the degree of neighbourhood disorder and stressful life events increased the risk for problem drinking, largely through an effect on a measure of psychological distress. Interestingly, social support had no protective effect (Mulia *et al.* 2008a). In a second study analysing data from the 2005 US National Alcohol Survey they assessed the mediating role of psychological distress between social disadvantage and problem drinking for three ethnic groups – white, Hispanic and African-Americans. While African-Americans were in general exposed to greater disadvantage the experience of disadvantage had similar effects on problem drinking in all groups (Mulia *et al.* 2008b). So experience of disadvantage and the degree of disadvantage might in part explain the reduced likelihood of reducing consumption when pregnant.

The pervasive effects of racism have been postulated to contribute to stress in the African-American population and to lead to using alcohol as an 'escape' in turn leading to an increased risk of alcohol problems. This hypothesis was put to the test by Martin *et al.* (2003) who found that personal reports of discriminatory experiences had a direct impact on problem drinking in the 1999–2000 National Survey of Black Workers. Furthermore, this association was independent of socioeconomic status and partly mediated by the idea that alcohol provides an escape. The idea that perceived racism could have such an important impact on health is borne out by a meta-analysis of 134 studies which indicated that perceived discrimination may be related to both mental and physical health outcomes and that this association may occur through the mechanisms of stress responses and through health behaviours (Pascoe and Smart Richman 2009). Hence the role of stress caused by disadvantage and by perceived racism may well have an important explanatory role and further investigation of these proposed mechanisms would seem useful.

The level of problem drinking in a population can be related both to advertising and availability of alcohol. There is a considerable evidence base that the highly segregated, poor neighbourhoods in which many African-American women live have higher densities of alcohol outlets including bars and liquor outlets than comparable white neighbourhoods (Hay *et al.* 2009; LaVeist and Wallace 2000; Romley *et al.* 2007). Furthermore billboard advertisements for alcohol products are more common in African-American neighbourhoods (Alaniz 1998; Hackbarth *et al.* 1995; Kwate and Lee 2007). So targeted advertising combined with increased availability are also likely to be important in determining the higher risk in this group.

Finally, the history of the African-American population in the United States has been one characterized by oppression, inequity and racial discrimination. This has constrained wealth and hence opportunity for African-Americans and resulted in social deprivation on a vast scale (Oliver and Shapiro 2006).

To summarize the key research findings in this population then we can say the following:

- African-American women are not more likely to drink or to drink during pregnancy than the white population.
- However, if they drink heavily or binge drink then they are less likely to change behaviour when pregnant than the white population.
- Social disadvantage does not in itself lead to heavy drinking but it can exacerbate heavy drinking and its consequences.
- Stress/distress may mediate the effects of social disadvantage on problem drinking but this effect seems to be present in all ethnic groups studied.
- The increased availability and targeted advertising of alcohol in segregated African-American neighbourhoods are likely to be in part responsible for the problem use of alcohol in these neighbourhoods.
- The effects of racism across the lifetime of an individual are associated with escapist drinking.
- The experience of racism, particularly institutionalized racism, across the entire history of the African-American population in the United States has structured ethnic and socioeconomic inequalities in health in that population.

Cape Coloured (mixed ancestry) population of South Africa

Although FAS was described first in South Africa in 1985 (Palmer 1985), the first epidemiological surveys on alcohol and pregnancy were conducted in the 1990s by Denis Viljoen, a geneticist working at the University of Cape Town, and his collaborators from the United States. Since then there has been a considerable amount of work in South Africa to establish prevalence, risk factors for drinking while pregnant and preventative measures (May *et al.* 2007) (see Chapter 22 in this publication for further details). I confine myself here to examining some of the 'causes of the causes' in the Cape Coloured population. Although FAS has been shown to be particularly prevalent in other groups, particularly those living in rural areas, it is the Cape Coloured population where most is known about social determinants.

The Cape Coloured population now consists of the descendants of White European colonists (mainly British and Dutch), the South Asian indentured labourers and slaves they brought with them to South Africa, and the descendants of the indigenous populations of the Cape region. Under the old apartheid system this group also known as 'Bruin Afrikaners' comprised the Afrikaans-speaking working-class population of the Western Cape.

Farming has always been central to the South African economy; large areas of the Western Cape have been used for wine production for over 300 years. Wine was historically used in part payment for labour of the impoverished labour force – the so-called *dop* system (London 1999) or 'tot' system. This reduced the cost of wages for farmers and also gave them an outlet for poor quality wine which they might not be able to sell commercially. Although the *dop* system was outlawed 40 years ago, the legacy of the *dop* system remains, with many farm workers, including pregnant women, drinking frequently, episodically and heavily (ibid.).

Heavy alcohol consumption is pervasive in this society and a binge pattern of drinking, concentrated on the weekends, is common in women (May *et al.* 2005, 2008). The traditional use of *papsak* low-quality wine sold in foil bags was banned in 2007 although drinking homemade wine is still common.

Farm workers drink more than urban South Africans, have high levels of alcohol dependence, and have generally poorer health; domestic violence is particularly prevalent. Furthermore, they live in very impoverished conditions with low pay, poor quality housing, little recreational opportunity and exposure to agricultural chemicals (London 1999). The women, who make up around 30 per cent of the workforce, face difficult challenges in their lives and as a result drink heavily including during pregnancy.

So in this population of farm workers alcohol started as an exploitative means of exchange, and went on to become an important outlet for recreation in an impoverished society and a means to escape from a desperate and at times hazardous existence.

In a revealing ethnographic study of eight farms in the Western Cape, du Toit showed how paternalism is the means by which order is maintained, exploitation is permitted and dissent is dealt with (du Toit 1993). Each farm is a little community headed by the farmer (manager). The central concept is that of *mekaar verstaan* (understanding one another). For the worker, as long as you and the farmer understand one another then you are part of the farm – part of the symbolic 'family'. However, if you and the farmer no longer understand one another then it is time to go – to be cast out of the 'family'.

As du Toit puts it:

> This brings us to the second (very obvious) feature: the way power functions on the farm. The farm is, after all, a profoundly unequal community – and in the Western Cape, paternalism is not only a discourse about the farm, but also about race. On the farm, racial and social identities are virtually interchangeable: In the parlance of the workers, the most common term for the farmer is simply *ons witman* (our white man), while farmers, in their turn, often refer to *ons kleurlinge* (our coloureds). And to be coloured, in terms of paternalist discourse, is to be child-like, unable to take responsibility for yourself, dependent on white masters for protection.
>
> *(du Toit 1993: 322)*

In such a paternalistic system there can be no antagonism between the 'father' and his 'children', only between the farm and the outside world. Du Toit again:

> Paternalism conceives the farm as a crucially threatened community. It denies systematic antagonism within the farm, but asserts an antagonism between the potentially harmonious farm as community and that which threatens its harmony: the lazy, irresponsible, or drunken worker, with the thief, with the city lawyer, the trade unionist.
>
> *(du Toit 1993: 322)*

So in a way *dop* was something 'father' gave you and to be seen to reject this would be indicative of not understanding one another and could potentially lead to being outcast from the farm and made destitute.

Wine production and consumption is now a global affair and although we are currently focused on the Western Cape of South Africa, the social determinants in this case illustrate well the geographical span of the causal web. The British have a taste for South African wines: the UK accounts for around a third of all South African wine exports. Between the wine producers of South Africa and the retailers in the UK – mainly the large supermarket chains – are positioned a group of intermediaries: the wine brokers. This group, numbering only a dozen or so, exert a huge influence and have great power to make or break a supplier. In turn the supermarkets want to sell wine as cheaply as possible to their customers and so the overall effect is to put the squeeze on the suppliers who must therefore reduce their costs. Hence employment for farm workers is now less secure with many more employed now as seasonal workers than on permanent contracts, with correspondingly reduced rights, terms and conditions of employment (Human Rights Watch 2011; War on Want 2009). Such pressures are likely to intensify pressures and potentially increase problem drinking.

So to summarize:

- The Cape Coloured population has the highest measured prevalence of FAS in the world.
- Drinking during pregnancy is part of the culture of heavy drinking which has become entrenched over a 300-year period.
- The micropolitics of paternalism on the farm were critical to the survival of the *dop* practice.
- Although *dop* is now banned in law the legacy of this system continues.
- Global export markets may bring pressures to bear on the supply chain for South African wine with negative effects on the workers.

Indigenous Australian population

Unlike the two previous populations, the Indigenous Australian population (comprising the Aboriginal and Torres Strait Islander Australians) were all there before colonization by Europeans. Currently this group comprise around 2.5 per cent of the Australian population. In general terms the health of Indigenous Australians is far worse than that of the total population with alcohol a major contributory factor to the health gap (Vos *et al.* 2009). With regard to FAS, a prospective national surveillance study in Australia found that the prevalence in the Indigenous population was over 100 times the non-Indigenous rate (Elliott *et al.* 2008). Higher Indigenous rates were also found in a study of FAS in North Queensland (Harris and Bucens 2003).

When discussing determinants of health for Indigenous Australians one has to be careful about generalization. As Hunter points out in the context of Indigenous mental health:

> Differences by ethnic group (only the most obvious of which is Aboriginal versus Torres Strait Islander), language, custom, postcolonial history and involvement with the mainstream economy are substantial. Summarising mental health status, then, is fraught with the twin dangers of generalisation and decontextualisation.
>
> *(Hunter 2007: 88)*

Nevertheless, with that caveat in mind, what social and political factors could be important in this group?

In a recent comprehensive review of alcohol misuse by Indigenous Australians the historical determinants of colonialism and dispossession are seen as fairly central to understanding the present position (Wilson *et al.* 2010). Following colonization, many Indigenous Australians developed a taste for alcohol and the European settlers used it with them as a means of exchange for sex or labour. Furthermore, the oppression and dispossession led to may Indigenous Australians using alcohol as a means of escape (Saggers and Gray 1998).

Another important factor contributing to alcohol misuse and compounding the historical determinants was the effect of national (or state-level) formulated alcohol policies to try to reduce consumption and harm in Indigenous populations. As Brady describes, initial restriction on sales then prohibition of sale to Indigenous Australians may have promoted secretive binge-pattern drinking and, following the repeal of prohibition, matters became worse rather than better. Furthermore, the tension between viewing Indigenous Australians as a special population with specific needs and the desire to see them integrated into the general population and treated equally has led to lack of clarity and direction in recent alcohol policy (Brady 2007).

One policy which has been highlighted as having a major effect on mental health in Indigenous populations was the policy of taking children away from their families (National Inquiry into the Separation of Aboriginal and Torres Strait Islander Children from their Families Australia 1997). As part of a policy called 'assimilation' there was widespread forced removal of children from their families, particularly those of mixed ethnicity. This practice continued from the early twentieth century up to the 1960s. In part this was motivated by a belief that the Indigenous Australians were a 'doomed race' who would in due course die out.

In recent years civil rights have improved for Indigenous Australians; for example they gained the same voting rights as the white population in 1984. However, their health, education and educational outcomes, employment prospects and hence income still lag considerably behind the rest of the population (Department of Families, Housing, Community Services and Indigenous Affairs 2008).

However, a 2007 report called *Little Children are Sacred* (Wild and Anderson 2007) highlighted the extent of alcohol-related harm and child abuse in the Indigenous communities leading to a radical and intrusive response by the then government which included suspending the Racial Discrimination Act in order to target these communities. Fortunately this act was reinstated by the Rudd government and the 'intervention' as it came to be known has ended.

One does not want to romanticize the notion of a long-lost golden age where the Indigenous Australians lived a life free of social division and exploitation; however, it seems inescapable that their civilization was largely destroyed and brutalized as a result of colonialism. Alcohol became a means of escape to some degree and consequent harms, one of which was an increased prevalence of FAS, have blighted the community.

To summarize:

- Colonialism and dispossession are seen as fairly central to understanding the present health status of Indigenous Australians with many Indigenous Australians using alcohol as a means of escape (Saggers and Gray 1998).
- National (or state-level) formulated alcohol policies to try to reduce consumption and harm in Indigenous populations have been poorly thought through and may have worsened the problem rather than improved matters.

Intimate partner violence and alcohol

In addition to high prevalence of FAS, both Cape Coloured and Indigenous Australian women have a high prevalence of assault from intimate partner violence (Berry *et al.* 2009; Eaton *et al.* 2012). The situation is less clear for African-American women; however a study from Massachusetts demonstrated that intimate partner violence resulting in female homicide disproportionately affected African-American and Hispanic women (Azziz-Baumgartner *et al.* 2011). There are well-documented and complex interconnections between alcohol use and violence, particularly in the context of unequal gender relations within populations. However, the use of alcohol and the phenomenon of cultural patriarchy should in no way be used to excuse or diminish individual responsibility for such violent acts. The determinants of intimate partner violence in the three populations are likely to be extremely complex and are beyond the scope of this chapter. Nevertheless, it seems plausible that intimate partner violence or the threat of it can lead to hazardous drinking by women, a consequence of which could be FAS.

Of course intimate partner violence is but the most graphic illustration of the abuse of power and unequal gender relations in a society. There are other insidious and subtle consequences which can fuel feelings of hopelessness and exacerbate alcohol problems. However, the effects of addressing gender inequality (desirable in themselves) should not necessarily be assumed to automatically have positive effects on either women's alcohol consumption or reducing prevalence of violence against women. The research on this is equivocal and hence the impact of addressing gender inequalities on alcohol consumption and interpersonal violence should be an important research priority (Roberts 2011).

Implications: FAS as a social inequality

That inequalities in FAS prevalence exist between and within countries has been repeatedly demonstrated. The three populations examined above demonstrate that these inequalities are socially and politically driven. Hence we can rightly refer to them as social inequalities. Krieger defines social inequalities as:

> Social inequalities (or inequities) in health refer to health disparities, within and between countries, that are judged to be unfair, unjust, avoidable, and unnecessary (meaning: are neither inevitable nor irremediable) and that systematically burden

populations rendered vulnerable by underlying social structures and political, economic, and legal institutions.

(Krieger 2001: 698)

The publication in 2008 of an influential report by the World Health Organization's Commission on Social Determinants of Health (CSDH 2008) brought health inequalities to the fore of political thinking once again and highlighted the differences in life-expectancy, disability and disease between and within countries. The Commission pointed out that:

Where systematic differences in health are judged to be avoidable by reasonable action they are, quite simply, unfair. It is this that we label health inequity. Putting right these inequities – the huge and remediable differences in health between and within countries – is a matter of social justice. Reducing health inequities is, for the Commission on Social Determinants of Health (hereafter, the Commission), an ethical imperative. Social injustice is killing people on a grand scale.

(CSDH 2008: 1)

If we consider FAS in this light, although it may not be killing people, one could certainly argue that through FAS, social injustice is causing considerable childhood disability and is destroying the lives of children and their families on a major scale. Thus apart from educating and exhorting women not to drink during pregnancy, preventative approaches should engage with the social determinants of problem drinking and FAS within 'sick' populations.

References

Abel, E.L. (1995) 'An update on incidence of FAS: FAS is not an equal opportunity birth defect', *Neurotoxicology and Teratology*, 17(4): 437–43.
Alaniz, M.L. (1998) 'Alcohol availability and targeted advertising in racial/ethnic minority communities', *Alcohol Health and Research World*, 22(4): 286–9.
Azziz-Baumgartner, E., McKeown, L., Melvin, P., Dang, Q. and Reed, J. (2011) 'Rates of femicide in women of different races, ethnicities, and places of birth: Massachusetts, 1993–2007', *Journal of Interpersonal Violence*, 26(5): 1077–90.
Berry, J.G., Harrison, J.E. and Ryan, P. (2009) 'Hospital admissions of indigenous and non-indigenous Australians due to interpersonal violence, July 1999 to June 2004', *Australian and New Zealand Journal of Public Health*, 33(3): 215–22.
Brady, M. (2007) 'Equality and difference: persisting historical themes in health and alcohol policies affecting Indigenous Australians', *Journal of Epidemiology and Community Health*, 61(9): 759–63.
Chartier, K. and Caetano, R. (2010) 'Ethnicity and health disparities in alcohol research', *Alcohol Research and Health*, 33(1/2): 152–60.
Collins, R.L. and McNair, L.D. (2002) 'Minority women and alcohol use', *Alcohol and Research Health*, 26(4): 251–6.
CSDH (Commission on Social Determinants of Health) (2008) *Closing the Gap in a Generation: Health equity through action on the social determinants of health. Final report of the Commission on Social Determinants of Health*, Geneva: World Health Organization.
Department of Families, Housing, Community Services and Indigenous Affairs (2008) *Closing the Gap on Indigenous Disadvantage: The challenge for Australia*, Greenway, ACT: Commonwealth of Australia (online at: www.fahcsia.gov.au/our-responsibilities/indigenous-australians/publications-articles/closing-the-gap/closing-the-gap-on-indigenous-disadvantage-the-challenge-for-australia-2009; accessed: 7 June 2013).
du Toit, A. (1993) 'The micro-politics of paternalism: the discourses of management and resistance on South African fruit and wine farms', *Journal of Southern African Studies*, 19(2): 314–36.

Eaton, L.A., Kalichman, S.C., Sikkema, K.J., Skinner, D., Watt, M.H., Pieterse, D. and Pitpitan, E.V. (2012) 'Pregnancy, alcohol intake, and intimate partner violence among men and women attending drinking establishments in a Cape Town, South Africa township', *Journal of Community Health*, 37(1): 208–16.

Elliott, E.J., Payne, J., Morris, A., Haan, E. and Bower, C. (2008) 'Fetal alcohol syndrome: a prospective national surveillance study', *Archives of Disease in Childhood*, 93(9): 732–7.

Green, R.F. and Stoler, J.M. (2007) 'Alcohol dehydrogenase 1B genotype and fetal alcohol syndrome: a HuGE minireview', *American Journal of Obstetrics and Gynecology*, 197(1): 12–25.

Hackbarth, D.P., Silvestri, B. and Cosper, W. (1995) 'Tobacco and alcohol billboards in 50 Chicago neighborhoods: market segmentation to sell dangerous products to the poor', *Journal of Public Health Policy*, 16(2): 213–30.

Harris, K. and Bucens, I. (2003) 'Prevalence of fetal alcohol syndrome in the Top End of the Northern Territory', *Journal of Paediatrics and Child Health*, 39(7): 528–33.

Hay, G.C., Whigham, P.A., Kypri, K. and Langley, J.D. (2009) 'Neighbourhood deprivation and access to alcohol outlets: a national study', *Health Place*, 15(4): 1086–93.

Human Rights Watch (2011) *Ripe with Abuse: Human rights conditions in South Africa's fruit and wine industries*. New York, NY: Human Rights Watch [online at: www.hrw.org/sites/default/files/reports/safarm0811webwcover.pdf; accessed: 15 September 2011].

Hunter, E. (2007) 'Disadvantage and discontent: a review of issues relevant to the mental health of rural and remote Indigenous Australians', *Australian Journal of Rural Health*, 15(2): 88–93.

Jones, K.L. (2011) 'The effects of alcohol on fetal development', *Birth Defects Research Part C: Embryo Today*, 93(1): 3–11.

Krieger, N. (2001) 'A glossary for social epidemiology', *Journal of Epidemiology and Community Health*, 55(10): 693–700.

Kwate, N.O. and Lee, T.H. (2007) 'Ghettoizing outdoor advertising: disadvantage and ad panel density in black neighborhoods', *Journal of Urban Health*, 84(1): 21–31.

LaVeist, T.A. and Wallace, J.M. Jr. (2000) 'Health risk and inequitable distribution of liquor stores in African American neighborhoods', *Social Science and Medicine*, 51(4): 613–17.

London, L. (1999) 'The "dop" system, alcohol abuse and social control amongst farm workers in South Africa: a public health challenge', *Social Science and Medicine*, 48(10): 1407–14.

MacMahon, B., Pugh, T.F. and Ipsen, J. (1960) *Epidemiologic Methods*, Boston, MA: Little Brown and Co.

Marmot, M. (2007) 'Commission on Social Determinants of Health. Achieving health equity: from root causes to fair outcomes', *Lancet*, 370(9593): 1153–63.

Martin, J.K., Tuch, S.A. and Roman, P.M. (2003) 'Problem drinking patterns among African Americans: the impacts of reports of discrimination, perceptions of prejudice, and "risky" coping strategies', *Journal of Health and Social Behaviour*, 4(3): 408–25.

May, P.A., Gossage, J.P., Brooke, L.E., Snell, C.L., Marais, A.S., Hendricks, L.S., Croxford, J.A. and Viljoen, D.L. (2005) Maternal risk factors for fetal alcohol syndrome in the Western Cape Province of South Africa: a population-based study', *American Journal of Public Health*, 95(7): 1190–9.

May, P.A., Gossage, J.P., Marais, A.S., Adnams, C.M., Hoyme, H.E., Jones, K.L., Robinson, L.K., Khaole, N.C.O., Snell, C., Kalberg, W.O., Hendricks, L., Brooke, L., Stellavato, C. and Viljoen, D.L. (2007) 'The epidemiology of fetal alcohol syndrome and partial FAS in a South African Community', *Drug and Alcohol Dependency*, 88(2/3): 259–71.

May, P.A., Gossage, J.P., Marais, A.S., Hendricks, L.S., Snell, C.L., Tabachnick, B.G., Stellavato, C., Buckley, D.G., Brooke, L.E. and Viljoen, D.L. (2008) 'Maternal risk factors for fetal alcohol syndrome and partial fetal alcohol syndrome in South Africa: a third study', *Alcoholism: Clinical and Experimental Research*, 32(5): 738–53.

Morris, D.S., Tenkku, L.E., Salas, J., Xaverius, P.K. and Mengel, M.B. (2008) 'Exploring pregnancy-related changes in alcohol consumption between black and white women', *Alcoholism: Clinical and Experimental Research*, 32(3): 505–12.

Moussas, G., Christodoulou, C. and Douzenis, A. (2009) 'A short review on the aetiology and pathophysiology of alcoholism', *Annals of General Psychiatry*, 8: 10.

Mulia, N., Schmidt, L., Bond, J., Jacobs, L. and Korcha, R. (2008a) 'Stress, social support and problem drinking among women in poverty', *Addiction*, 103(8): 1283–93.

Mulia, N., Ye, Y., Zemore, S.E. and Greenfield, T.K. (2008b) 'Social disadvantage, stress, and alcohol use among black, Hispanic, and white Americans: findings from the 2005 U.S. National Alcohol Survey', *Journal of Studies on Alcohol and Drugs*, 69(6): 824–33.

National Inquiry into the Separation of Aboriginal and Torres Strait Islander Children from their Families Australia (1997) *Bringing Them Home: Report of the National Inquiry into the Separation of Aboriginal and Torres Strait Islander Children from their Families*, Sydney, NSW: Human Rights and Equal Opportunities Commission.

Oliver, M.L. and Shapiro, T.M. (2006) *Black Wealth/White Wealth: A new perspective on racial inequality*, 2nd edition, New York, NY: Routledge.

Palmer, C. (1985) 'Fetal alcohol effects: incidence and understanding in the Cape', *South African Medical Journal*, 68(11): 779–80.

Pascoe, E.A. and Smart Richman, L. (2009) 'Perceived discrimination and health: a meta-analytic review', *Psychological Bulletin*, 135(4): 531–54.

Roberts, S.C. (2011) 'What can alcohol researchers learn from research about the relationship between macro-level gender equality and violence against women?', *Alcohol and Alcoholism*, 46(2): 95–104.

Romley, J.A., Cohen, D., Ringel, J. and Sturm, R. (2007) 'Alcohol and environmental justice: the density of liquor stores and bars in urban neighborhoods in the United States', *Journal of Studies on Alcohol and Drugs*, 68(1): 48–55.

Rose, G. (1985) 'Sick individuals and sick populations', *International Journal of Epidemiology*, 14(1): 32–8.

Rosenthal, J., Christianson, A. and Cordero, J. (2005) 'Fetal alcohol syndrome prevention in South Africa and other low resource countries', *American Journal of Public Health*, 95(7): 1099–101.

Saggers, S. and Gray, D. (1998) *Dealing with Alcohol: Indigenous usage in Australia, New Zealand and Canada*. Melbourne, VIC: Cambridge University Press.

Tenkku, L.E., Morris, D.S., Salas, J. and Xaverius, P.K. (2009) 'Racial disparities in pregnancy-related drinking reduction', *Maternal and Child Health Journal*, 13(5): 604–13.

Vos, T., Barker, B., Begg, S., Stanley, L. and Lopez, A.D. (2009) 'Burden of disease and injury in Aboriginal and Torres Strait Islander Peoples: the indigenous health gap', *International Journal of Epidemiology*, 38 (2): 470–7.

War on Want (2009) *South African Wine Workers and British Supermarket Power*, London: War on Want (online at: www.waronwant.org/attachments/Sour%20Grapes%20wine%20report.pdf; accessed: 18 August 2011).

Warren, K.R. and Li, T.K. (2005) 'Genetic polymorphisms: impact on the risk of fetal alcohol spectrum disorders', *Birth Defects Research Part A, Clinical and Molecular Teratology*, 73(4): 195–203.

Wild, R. and Anderson, P. (2007) *Ampe Akelyernemane Meke Mekarle 'Little Children are Sacred': Report of the Northern Territory Board of Inquiry into the Protection of Aboriginal Children from Sexual Abuse* (online at: www.inquirysaac.nt.gov.au; accessed: 18 August 2011).

Wilson, M., Stearne, A., Gray, D. and Sherry, S. (2010) 'The harmful use of alcohol amongst Indigenous Australians', *Australian Indigenous HealthInfoNet* (online at: www.healthinfonet.ecu.edu.au/alcoholuse_review; accessed: 5 May 2011).

4
WOMEN'S ALCOHOL CONSUMPTION IN THE UK

Moira Plant

Introduction

The pattern of drinking in the UK, one of heavy episodic weekend drinking, is the well-recognized Northern European pattern. More recently, although the pattern of drinking has remained the same, the amount drunk on each occasion has increased. The Cabinet Office Prime Minister's Strategy Group was the first to define a 'binge' as twice the daily limit; therefore six or more units for women or eight or more units for a man. A UK unit contains eight grams of alcohol, the amount of alcohol contained in a small glass of wine, half a pint of ordinary strength beer, lager or cider, or a small glass of spirits. This definition of binge has often led to misunderstanding, and in some ways implies that the pattern of drinking in the UK has changed. The fact is this pattern of consumption has remained unchanged for centuries. What has changed is the amount being drunk on each occasion. A recent survey by the British Liver Trust and *Prima* magazine notes one woman saying 'I was shocked to discover I was a binge drinker' (Prima 2009). This misleading idea that being a binge drinker, however defined, is more important and serious than the amount being drunk is now common in the UK. This pattern of heavy episodic drinking is pertinent to this book as what is now being called binge drinking is recognized as the most risky for the unborn child. However, it is important to note that fewer women drink than men and women generally drink less than men (Plant and Plant 2006; Wilsnack *et al.* 2000). For this reason men are more likely to experience, cause or inflict alcohol-related harm (Plant 2008).

In 2001 a survey of women in Britain revealed that 8 per cent of woman aged 18–24 years had consumed at least 35 units of alcohol in the past week (Plant and Plant 2001; Plant *et al.* 2002). This is defined as 'harmful drinking' by the Department of Health and the Home Office (2007). High levels of heavy drinking by young women have been noted by other investigators (NHS Information Centre 2011; NHS Information Centre Scotland 2011; ONS 2004, 2006; Scottish Government 2007, 2008; Williamson *et al.* 2003).

It is reasonable to suggest that due to these higher levels of consumption by some young British women may have led to an increase in the number of babies born with some degree of alcohol-related birth harm. Evidence from a number of sources suggests that women will continue to drink at pre-pregnancy levels until the pregnancy is confirmed. This is particularly true if the pregnancy was unplanned (Tough *et al.* 2006). In a national UK study approximately 84 per cent of UK mothers under the age of 24 years reported their pregnancies were unplanned (Dex and Joshi 2005; Hanson *et al.* 2010). Therefore, at the most vulnerable time for the fetus, the mother may still be drinking at pre-pregnancy level. However, the lack of recent UK evidence on alcohol-related birth defects leaves the scale of this problem unknown. The UK has the one of the highest rates of teenage pregnancy in Europe. Such pregnancies are especially commonplace among young women living in socially deprived areas (ONS 2005; Social Exclusion Unit 1999; Youth Information 2007). Teenagers and other young people who engage in unprotected sex are likely to be heavy drinkers (Alcohol Concern 2002; Bullock 2001; Cooper 2002; Karshin 2002; Leigh and Miller 1995; Leigh *et al.* 2008).

The UK government has tried to change the UK pattern of drinking (Slack 2007) and transform it into a Mediterranean pattern with weekly alcohol consumption being spread over five or six days of the week rather than concentrated into the weekend. However the Office for National Statistics surveys would suggest that people in the UK are now less likely to spread their drinking over five days or more than they were in 1998 (Plant 2008). As regards what is known as the Mediterranean pattern, countries like France and Spain are becoming concerned as more and more of their young people start mimicking the drinking pattern and beverage choices of their UK counterparts rather than the other way round.

Social context of drinking

The social context of women's drinking in the UK has changed dramatically over the past 50 years. We have moved from the situation where pubs were the man's domain and women were only accepted if they were accompanied by a man. Now women, due to their increased spending power, are encouraged, and drinks promotions in some clubs will advertise that women will be allowed in free of charge or that their first drink is free. The rationale behind this is that if you encourage the women into the clubs the men will simply follow. A further change in the drinking milieu in the UK is the changed face of many city centres. Pubs and clubs are now open longer and later. The majority of these establishments cater to the under-thirties. The other change in drinking habits which until recently was seen only in young women, but is now beginning to become a pattern for young men also, is the pre-drinking or front-loading which occurs every Friday and Saturday night. This consists of groups of women arranging to meet in a friend's house to get prepared for an evening out. Each young woman will bring alcohol which she has purchased, usually very cheaply, in the local supermarket. This alcohol will be drunk, often with many different types of alcohol mixed together. Then the young women, dressed and ready to enjoy themselves, will go out to the pubs and clubs in the city centres. In this way they save money on the alcohol bought later in the evening in clubs. The dynamic of this is interesting; they are going from a single gender private (safe) environment into a mixed gender public (less safe?) environment. The sense of 'we are the champions' and can do anything is carried with them. Of course this also means that they are away from the 'prying eyes' of parents or other adults who know them and who may then 'spoil their fun'. There is no simple answer to this although there is clear evidence to suggest that legislating to ensure there is a minimum price on alcohol particularly that sold in supermarkets does have an effect on reducing consumption. This has not been seen as a popular move by many politicians (Meier *et al.* 2010; Purshouse *et al.* 2010). Sadly the debate has deteriorated into a party political rather than a public health issue. A visit to many city centres on any weekend shows how women's behaviour has changed in relation to drinking. In the past young women were far less likely to drink to the point of drunkenness and, if they did, it was certainly not something they bragged about to their friends. Just as young women's drinking has changed so has their attitude to drunken behaviour. In the UK at this point in time we are in a situation where young women are as likely as young men to boast about their risky behaviour when drunk almost as a badge of honour.

Heavy drinking among UK women

Between 1980 and 2006 overall per capita alcohol consumption in the UK rose by 21 per cent (British Beer and Pub Association, pers. comm.). The early 1990s showed a marked increase in women's overall weekly alcohol consumption (Goddard 2001). More recently there has been a stabilization then a slight decrease in consumption. There are a number of factors which could explain this: first and most obviously, a true reduction in consumption. Other factors are likely to include a longer time interval between surveys in the early 2000s and in 2006 a revised method of recording and analysing these data collected. This revision included an acknowledgement that drinks within the same category could be of widely varying strengths. Thus from 2006 onwards, beers lagers and ciders were recorded as either 'normal strength' or 'strong'. Furthermore, and of greater importance to women than men, the number of units in a glass of wine was changed to take into account the larger glass sizes that are being served in many clubs and pubs. This is particularly relevant because in the UK wine is a much more popular drink among women than men (for further details see Goddard 2007). As noted in the Office for National Statistics *General Lifestyle Survey* 2009: 'approximately 60 per cent of the units of alcohol consumed by women come from wine whereas only around 25 per cent of men's units do so' (ONS 2011: 47).

Some study findings have now been reanalysed to take account of this (Scottish Government 2008). This suggests that alcohol consumption among women has recently been 40–45 per cent higher than previously assumed (Goddard 2007, 2008; Scottish Government 2008).

A recent report from the Office for National Statistics (ONS) taking a longer view reports that in the decade between 1998 and 2008 the percentage of women aged 16–24 who drank more than six units on one day changed little from 23 per cent to 25 per cent. Although the major focus on UK women's drinking has related to the younger women, it is important to remember that women in their thirties are now drinking more than in the past and are in some cases out-drinking their younger sisters (Prima 2009). The importance of this is that women in their thirties and older are still in the childbearing age range. It is unwise to try to predict a woman's drinking career; evidence suggests that people's drinking changes over the lifespan often related to changing life events such as full time work, stable relationships and family. However if women in their thirties have been drinking heavily in the typical binge drinking pattern since their teen years, then they may well have developed some harm to psychological and physical health. Noting this issue of women in their thirties the ONS report mentioned above which took a longer view (from 1998 to 2008) reported that the corresponding figures for the 25–44 year age group were 11 per cent in 1998 and by 2008 this had risen to 20 per cent (ONS 2010). We must be cautious therefore of constantly focusing on the younger age group when the 25–44 year old women, who have been drinking for longer may be the ones who are more likely to be putting their unborn children at risk of alcohol-related harm.

In relation to the binge pattern of drinking the most recent national statistics in England report about half of women aged 16–24 years report drinking on between one and three days in the past week. The corresponding percentage for those aged 25–44 years is 44 per cent (ONS 2010). Another interesting difference among those who drink in these two age groups of childbearing women is their beverage choice. The younger group drink mainly spirits (37 per cent), with wine being the next most popular choice, at 22 per cent, whereas the older group more commonly drink wine (58 per cent), with ordinary strength beer, lager or cider being the next most popular choice at 18 per cent (op. cit.). Although the majority of drinkers (females and males) of all ages now report having heard of measuring alcohol consumption in 'units', few report they keep a weekly check on their consumption. Interestingly the heavier drinkers (15 units and over) are more likely to report doing this but even in this group only 10 per cent report doing so. Not surprisingly women are far more likely to do so than their male counterparts (op cit.).

Reasons for changes in drinking

There are many explanations put forward as the reasons for the change in women's drinking. Examples of these are gender empowerment, being married versus cohabiting, the different roles women have during their lives, the impact of feminism and social inequality (Grittner *et al.* 2012, 2013; Plant 2008). The issue of gender empowerment is being explored by such international measures as the Gender-Empowerment scale developed by the United Nations (United Nations Development Programme 2005). This scale includes factors such as economic participation and opportunity, political empowerment, educational attainment, and health and well-being. However, the UK ranks below countries such as the Scandinavian countries, Canada and New Zealand on this scale and per capita consumption in women is lower in these countries than in the UK (Lopez-Claros and Zahidi 2005). Many more people are choosing to live together but not getting married and evidence suggests that, regardless of education or the presence of children, women who cohabit with partners drink more than those who are married (Plant *et al.* 2008). The multiple roles that many women often have to play have also been explored in relation to alcohol and related problems (Kuntsche *et al.* 2011). Yet another debate surrounds the issue of feminism and its impact on female drinking. In a 2008 review this author wrote:

> Twenty years ago Morrissey (1986) speculated that women cannot win with alcohol. Women who cannot adjust to a traditional feminine (patriarchal) role are at risk of developing alcohol problems; women who can adjust to this role of domestic wife/mother but find it disrupted for any reason are at risk of developing alcohol problems; women who work full time may adopt traditionally masculine behaviours through contact in the workforce, so this group are at risk of developing alcohol problems; and women who attempt the stressful combination of work and motherhood are at risk, not only of developing alcohol problems, but of potentially damaging their unborn child.
>
> *(Plant 2008: 164)*

Whatever the debate and conflicting views on women's roles, one role that women played in the past has certainly changed. Historically the other role women had was that of informal social controllers of drinking behaviour in men. Male behaviour when drinking in mixed groups has always been more restrained. More recently, young women are not taking on the role of informal social controllers; in fact they are behaving in the same way as their male counterparts. This may be one of the reasons for the increase in risky behaviour which we are now seeing in the UK.

Not all people in the UK drink. Many of the people who abstain from alcohol do so for ethnic or religious reasons. As noted by the North West Public Health Observatory (NWPHO 2011: 1) 'There are now more than six million individuals over the age of 16 in England who do not drink alcohol'. Is it possible that we will reach a tipping point in the UK where this increase in abstainers begins to balance what many young people see as the norm: i.e. getting so drunk on Friday and Saturday nights that they have difficulty remembering what they did? The view that this drunken behaviour is almost expected does put pressure on the many young people who do not wish to behave in this way.

Alcohol-related health damage

In general the pattern of drinking predicts the related problems. Due to the pattern of high-dose drinking in the UK, alcohol-related problems tend to be related to accidents, arguments and assaults, including sexual assault or rape (Plant 2008). Harm associated with childbearing includes miscarriage and prenatal alcohol exposure (Henriksen *et al.* 2004). Nationally and locally recorded statistics on the negative consequences of drinking can be seen as reasonably reliable. Hospital admissions data recording physical and psychological harm related to alcohol appear to be robust given there are routine and accepted measures used across most countries. However self-reports of alcohol-related harm are to some extent culturally defined. For example as noted by Kuendig *et al.*: 'The reporting of adverse consequences is not only influenced by alcohol consumption, but also by attributional processes related to demographic and socioeconomic statuses' (Kuendig *et al.* 2008: 150).

In relation to recently published data (NWPHO 2011) there has been a 24.6 per cent increase in alcohol-related hospital admissions with some geographical areas in England showing much higher increases than others.

The organ in the body that bears the weight of breaking down alcohol to enable the body to excrete it is the liver. Even in experienced drinkers the liver can only break down about one unit of alcohol an hour. Therefore if a women drinks two large glasses of wine in one hour it will take approximately six hours for her Blood Alcohol Level (BAL) to return to zero. Any harm to the liver means that it will take even longer for the alcohol to leave her system and during this time alcohol will be circulating round her body. If she is pregnant this also means alcohol will be circulating round the body of the fetus. Over the past three decades there has been a sharp rise in the number of deaths from liver disease in the UK. Since the 1970s this has shown a clear upward trend. By the early 2000s another change in these figures occurred. Prior to this time the most common age for both women and men to die from liver disease was between 55 and 64 years. The beginning of the 2000s showed that this age group, although still rising in numbers, was being overtaken by the age group of 45 to 54 year olds (Donaldson 2001, 2009). Many deaths from liver disease are alcohol-related. There has also been an upsurge in the numbers of younger women developing and dying from alcohol-related liver disease (Gilmour 2004). The relevance to this book is that if a pregnant woman with liver disease continues to drink during her pregnancy the fetus will have alcohol circulating through its system for longer than normal because the mother's liver does not work effectively to break down the alcohol she has consumed. The significance of this is in the increased severity of harm to the unborn child (Majewski 1993; Palmer 2004). Heavy alcohol consumption continues to be a huge chronic health problem, probably involving over 22,000 deaths each year (British Medical Association 2008). A number of these chronic health problems have been described in the literature.

The impact of age

This idea of heavy drinking in adolescence being associated with harm in later life is not new; what is new is that 'later life' does not appear to be that much later, leaving the possibility of a longer period of life being lived with some serious health problems.

Recent research carried out into a group of adolescents who had started to drink in a binge-type pattern by the time they reached 13 years of age and maintained this pattern during the rest of their teen years found that they were: 'nearly 4 times as likely to be overweight or obese and almost 3.5 times as likely to have high blood pressure when they were 24 years old than were people who never or rarely drank heavily during adolescence' (Oesterle et al. 2004).

The emotional/psychological aspects of harm related to heavy drinking are also well established. Levels of depression and anxiety related to heavy alcohol consumption appear to be increasing. There has been a significant increase in young women being admitted to hospital in England for alcohol-related psychiatric problems (British Medical Association 2008; Williams et al. 2005).

It is unwise and potentially very misleading to try to predict people's future drinking consumption levels from their present behaviour. Even so the increase in heavy drinking in young people is well documented (Hibell et al. 2009; Plant et al. 2005). This, associated with the rise in these alcohol-related chronic conditions, should not be ignored. There are a number of different ways in which young people start, continue or stop drinking and this area of trajectories of alcohol use is becoming increasingly relevant to the prediction of health service provision (Sher et al. 2004, 2011; Schulenberg et al. 1996; Schulenberg and Maggs 2002; Tucker et al. 2003). Even so, history shows us that what is today posited as 'the truth' in any field will change with the discovery of new knowledge. As so eloquently noted by the playwright Oscar Wilde 'the truth is rarely pure and seldom simple' (2007: Act I). As with many areas in the alcohol field, care needs to be taken not to become blinkered to one way of thinking; examples include general myths about women's drinking (Wilsnack and Wilsnack 2003), the prediction of drinking patterns in young people (Bachman et al. 2002), even whether a binge is indeed a binge (Gmel et al. 2011).

To use one of the now in vogue examples of this complexity, the evidence is that 'age of first drink' may be predictive of future alcohol-related problems (York et al. 2004). This may not be as simple as it at first appears. The majority of people, female and male, are more likely to remember their first drink as not necessarily the true (remember Oscar Wilde) first time they ever drank alcohol but rather the earliest one which was associated with some kind of emotional arousal. Therefore what they report as their first drink may not be an accurate recollection. As noted by Kuntsche (pers. comm.) the more relevant marker may be first experience of being drunk rather than first drink. Some studies such as that carried out by Pitkänen et al. (2005) in Finland suggest that a delay in the initiation of drinking may be a way of preventing harm in this group. However it is important to explore these data a little further. There are a lot of questions that need to be asked and more work is needed to find the answers. Some of these questions are uncomfortable ones. For example, is it early onset drinking which predicts future problem drinking? Is it early trauma which predicts early onset drinking? Is it early trauma which predicts future problem drinking? Is it more likely to be a combination of different factors? (Plant et al. 2004).

To emphasize this aspect a recent study by Shin and colleagues analysing data from the US National Longitudinal Study of Adolescent Health noted:

> all types of or combinations of types of maltreatment were strongly associated with adolescent binge drinking, controlling for age, gender, race, parental alcoholism, ... the effect of childhood maltreatment on later alcohol abuse needs to recognise the clustering effects of multiple types of childhood maltreatment on alcohol problems.
>
> *(Shin et al. 2009: 277)*

Another relevant example in the context of this book is the evidence suggesting that alcohol consumption patterns (both daily and weekly intake) remain the same between pre-conception and the time when pregnancy is confirmed (Tough et al. 2006). Note that this is not the same as when the woman actually becomes pregnant; many women are pregnant for a number of weeks before their pregnancies are confirmed. This occurs frequently in adolescents who are at particular risk in relation to their health and that of their babies during pregnancy. This group is vulnerable in many ways. A major issue is around the acknowledgement of being pregnant.

Again the reasons for this may be complex: many young women have irregular menstrual cycles and may well not realize they are pregnant; they may be drinking, having an active sexual life but not using regular contraception; the pregnancy may be an unwelcome and terrifying thing which they want to deny; they may not wish to stop drinking as it will make their friends suspicious that they are pregnant, a fact they do not wish to acknowledge even to themselves. The repercussions of this defence mechanism of denial of pregnancy means a delayed change from pre-pregnancy to pregnancy drinking patterns and worryingly less likelihood of attending routine ante-natal appointments. Other factors include issues around weight gain and nutritional status with teen mums experiencing lower weight gain. With the maternal body at a stage when it needs more nutrients for its own growth and development, the mother and fetus are in even greater competition for nutrients than occurs normally. There may also be a reduced flow of nutrients to the fetus due to immature placental development. The issue of eating disorders in this group is also relevant with eating disorders associated with higher risks of neural tube defects. Others factors include increased risk of miscarriage and low birth weight. After the birth it is not surprising to note that many of these teen mums experience a degree of post-partum depression. As with other age groups alcohol may be used to self-medicate for this depression. On the positive side, teenagers who plan pregnancy often use it as an opportunity to change their lifestyle reducing alcohol and other drug consumption and improving their diet.

Conclusions

Women's drinking in the UK, particularly when of childbearing age, has changed over the past decades. Evidence suggests that the increase in consumption noted in the UK is levelling out and the most recent surveys suggest that the trend may be a reduction in the per capita consumption. This is the good news. The bad news is that women in the UK are drinking more than women in countries viewed as heavy drinking such as France and Spain. Heavy alcohol use is associated with a number of physical and psychological health problems which are beginning to appear in women at a younger age than previously found. This means a longer period of life with some of the chronic harm associated with heavy alcohol use. This may also mean a greater risk of alcohol-related harm to the unborn child. The typical UK heavy episodic drinking now named binge drinking is known to be the most risky for the unborn child.

Bibliography

Alcohol Concern (2002) *Alcohol and Teenage Pregnancy*. London: Alcohol Concern.
Bachman, J.G., O'Malley, P.M., Schulenberg J.E., Johnston, L.D., Bryant, A.L. and Merline, A.C. (2002) *The Decline of Substance Use in Young Adulthood: Changes in Social Activities, Roles, and Beliefs*, Mahwah, NJ: Lawrence Erlbaum Associates.
British Medical Association (2008) *Alcohol Misuse: Tackling the UK Epidemic*, London: British Medical Association.
Bullock, S.L. (2001) 'About last night: dates, drinks and sex. A study of the association between alcohol use and sexual activity among heterosexuals, including sexual behavior at high risk for the transmission of STDs and HIV', *Dissertation Abstracts International*, 62(4): 1823B.
Cooper, M.L. (2002) 'Alcohol use and risky sexual behavior among college students and youth: evaluating the evidence,' *Journal of Studies on Alcohol*, Suppl.14: 101–17.
Department of Health and the Home Office (2007) *Safe, Sensible, Social: The Next Steps in the National Alcohol Strategy*, London: Department of Health and the Home Office.
Dex, S. and Joshi, H. (eds) (2005) *Children of the 21st Century: From birth to nine months*, Bristol: Policy Press.
Donaldson L. (2001) *Annual Report of the Chief Medical Officer*, London: Department of Health.
Donaldson, L. (2009) *Annual Report of the Chief Medical Officer*, London: Department of Health [online at: http://webarchive.nationalarchives.gov.uk/20130107105354/http://www.dh.gov.uk/en/Publicationsandstatistics/Publications/AnnualReports/DH_096206; accessed: 10 January 2013].
Gilmour, I. (2004) 'The medical effects of heavy drinking', presentation at International Conference *Binge Drinking: Problems and Responses*, Bristol, 26 November.
Gmel, G., Kuntsche, E. and Rehm, J. (2011) 'Risky single-occasion drinking: bingeing is *not bingeing*', *Addiction*, 106(6): 1037–45.
Goddard E. (2001) *Obtaining Information about Drinking through Surveys of the General Population (National Statistics Methodology Series NSM 24)*, London: Office for National Statistics.
Goddard, E. (2007) *Estimating Alcohol Consumption from Survey Data: Updated method of converting volumes to units (National Statistics Methodology Series NSM 37)*, Newport: Office for National Statistics.
Goddard, E. (2008) *Smoking and Drinking among Adults, 2006*, London: Office for National Statistics.
Grittner, U., Kuntsche S., Graham K. and Bloomfield K. (2012) 'Social inequalities and gender differences in the experience of alcohol problems' *Alcohol and Alcoholism*, 47(5): 597–605.
Grittner, U., Kuntsche, S., Gmel, G. and Bloomfield, K. (2013) 'Alcohol consumption and social inequality at individual and country levels: results from an international study', *European Journal of Public* Health, 23(2): 332–9.
Hanson, K., Joshi, H. and Dex, S. (2010) *Children of the 21st Century: First five years*, Bristol: The Policy Press.
Hawkins, J.D., Catalano, R.F. and Miller, J. (1992) 'Risk and protective factors for alcohol and other drug problems in adolescence and early adulthood: implications for substance abuse prevention', *Psychological Bulletin*, 112: 64–105.

Henriksen, T.B., Hjollund, N.H., Jensen, T.K., Bonde, J.P., Andersson, M., Kolstad, H., Ernst, E., Giwercman, A., Skakkebæk, N.E. and Olsen, J. (2004) 'Alcohol consumption at the time of conception and spontaneous abortion', *American Journal of Epidemiology*, 160(7), 661–7.

Hibell, B., Guttomsson, U., Ahlström, S., Balakireva, O., Bjarnasson, T., Kokkevi, A. and Kraus, L. (2009) The 2007 ESPAD Report: Alcohol and other drug use among students in 35 European countries. Stockholm: Swedish Council for Information on Alcohol and Other Drugs.

Hill, K.G., White, H.R., Chung, I.J., Hawkins, J.D. and Catalano, R.F. (2000) 'Early adult outcomes of adolescent binge drinking: person- and variable-centered analyses of binge drinking trajectories', *Alcoholism: Clinical and Experimental Research*, 24(6): 892–901.

Huizink, A.C. and Mulder, E.J. (2006) 'Maternal smoking, drinking or cannabis use during pregnancy and neurobehavioral and cognitive functioning in human offspring,' *Neuroscience and Biobehavioral Reviews*, 30: 24–41.

Karshin, C.M. (2002) 'Examination of the relationship between alcohol consumption and risky sexual behavior among college students,' *Dissertation Abstracts International*, 62(7): 3155B.

Kuendig, H., Plant, M.L., Plant, M.A., Kuntsche, S., Miller, P., Gmel, G., Ahlström, S., Bergmark, K.H., Olafsdóttir, H., Elekes, Z., Csemy, L. and Knibbe, R. (2008) 'Beyond drinking: differential effects of demographic and socioeconomic factors on alcohol-related adverse consequences across European countries', *European Addiction Research*, 14(3): 150–60.

Kuntsche, S., Knibbe, R.A., Kuntsche, E. and Gmel, G. (2011) 'Housewife or working mum – each to her own? The relevance of societal factors in the association between social roles and alcohol use among mothers in 16 industrialized countries', *Addiction*, 106(11): 1925–32.

Leigh, B.C. and Miller, P. (1995) 'The relationship of substance use with sex to the use of condoms and other contraceptives among young adults in two urban areas of Scotland', *AIDS Education and Prevention*, 7(3): 278–84.

Leigh, B.C., Gaylord, J., Hoppe, M.J., Rainey, D., Morrison, D.M. and Gillmore, M.R. (2008) 'Drinking and condom use: results from an event-based daily diary,' *AIDS and Behavior*, 12(1): 104–12.

Lopez-Claros, A. and Zahidi, S. (2005) *Women's Empowerment: Measuring the global gender gap*, Geneva: World Economic Forum.

Majewski, F. (1993) 'Alcohol embryopathy: experience in 200 patients', *Developmental Brain Dysfunction*, 6: 248–65.

Meier, P., Brennan, A. and Purshouse, P. (2010) 'Policy options for alcohol price regulation: the importance of modeling population heterogeneity', *Addiction*, 105(3): 383–93.

Naimi, T.S., Brewer, R.D., Mokdad, A., Denny, C., Serdula, K. and Marks, J.S. (2003) 'Binge drinking among US adults,' *Journal of the American Medical Association*, 289(1): 70–5.

National Centre for Social Research/National Foundation for Educational Research (2005) Smoking, Drinking and Drug Use among Young People in England in 2004. London: National Centre for Social Research/National Foundation for Educational Research.

NHS Information Centre (2011) *Statistics on Alcohol: England, 2011*, London: Health and Social Care Information Centre.

NHS Information Centre Scotland (2011) *Statistics on Alcohol: Scotland, 2011*, Edinburgh: ISD Scotland Publications.

NWPHO (North West Public Health Observatory) (2011) *Local Alcohol Profiles for England*, Health e-news, October, Liverpool: Centre for Public Health, Liverpool John Moores University.

Oesterle, S., Hill, K.G., Hawkins, J.D., Guo, J., Catalano, R.F. and Abbott, R.D. (2004) 'Adolescent heavy episodic drinking trajectories and health in young adulthood', *Journal of Studies on Alcohol*, 65(2): 204–12.

ONS (Office for National Statistics) (2004) *Results from the 2003 General Household Survey*, London: Office for National Statistics.

ONS (Office for National Statistics) (2005) *Teenage Conception Statistics for England 1998–2005*, London: Office for National Statistics, Teen Pregnancy Unit.

ONS (Office for National Statistics) (2006) *Statistics on Alcohol: England 2006*, London: Office for National Statistics.

ONS (Office for National Statistics) (2010) *Statistics on Alcohol: England, 2010* [online at: www.statistics.gov.uk/hub/index.html; accessed: 10 January 2013].

ONS (Office for National Statistics) (2011) *General Lifestyle Survey London*, London. Office for National Statistics.

Office for Standards in Education, Children's Services and Skills (2007) *TellUs2: Children and Young People Survey*, London: Office for Standards in Education, Children's Services and Skills.

Palmer, M. (2004) *Dr Melissa Palmer's Guide to Hepatitis and Liver Disease: What you need to know*, New York, NY: Penguin Putnam.

Pitkänen T., Lyyra A.-L. and Pulkkinen L. (2005) 'Age of onset of drinking and the use of alcohol in adulthood: a follow-up study from age 8–42 for females and males', *Addiction*, 100(5): 652–61.

Plant, M., Miller, P., Plant, M., Kuntsche, S., Gmel, G., Ahlström, W., Allamani, A., Beck, F., Bergmark, K., Bloomfield, K., Csémy, L., Elekes, Z., Knibbe, R., Kraus, L., Ólafsdóttir, H., Rossow, I. and Vidal, A. (2008) 'Marriage, cohabitation, and alcohol consumption in young adults: an international exploration', *Journal of Substance Use*, 13(2): 83–98.

Plant, M.A. and Plant, M.L. (2006) *Binge Britain: Alcohol and the national response*, Oxford: Oxford University Press.

Plant, M.A., Miller, P. and Plant, M.L. (2005) 'Trends in drinking, smoking and illicit drug use among 15 and 16 year olds in the United Kingdom (1995–2003)', *Journal of Substance Use*, 10(6): 331–9.

Plant, M.L. (2008) 'The role of alcohol in women's lives: a review of issues and responses', *Journal of Substance Use*, 13(3): 155–91.

Plant M.L. and Plant M.A. (2001) 'Heavy drinking by young British women gives cause for concern', *British Medical Journal*, 323(7322): 1183.

Plant, M.L., Miller, P. and Plant, M.A. (2004) 'Childhood and adult sexual abuse: relationships with alcohol and other drug use', Child Abuse Review, 13(3): 200–14.

Plant, M.L., Plant, M.A. and Mason, W. (2002) 'Drinking, smoking and illicit drug use amongst British adults: gender differences explored', Journal of Substance Use, 7(1): 24–33.

Prima (2009) 'If you are drinking this much every evening you're drinking too much', *Prima Magazine*, November: 51–4.

Purshouse, R., Meier, P., Brennan, A., Taylor, K. and Rafia, R. (2010) 'Estimated effect of alcohol pricing policies on health and health economic outcomes in England: an epidemiological model', Lancet, 375(9723): 1355–64.

Schulenberg, J., Wadsworth, K.N., O'Malley, P.M., Bachman, J.G. and Johnston, L.D. (1996) 'Adolescent risk factors for binge drinking during the transition to young adulthood: variable-and pattern-centered approaches to change', *Developmental Psychology*, 32(4): 659–79.

Schulenberg, J.E. and Maggs, J.L. (2002) 'A developmental perspective on alcohol use and heavy drinking during adolescence and the transition to young adulthood', *Journal of Studies on Alcohol*, Suppl. 14: 54–70.

Scottish Government (2007) Alcohol Information Scotland [online at: www.alcoholinformation.isdscotland.org; accessed: 11 January 2013].

Scottish Government (2008) *Scottish Health Survey 2003: Revised consumption figures*, Edinburgh: Scottish Government.

Sher, K.J., Gotham, H.J. and Watson, A.L. (2004) 'Trajectories of dynamic predictors of disorder: their meanings and implications', *Development and Psychopathology*, 16(4): 825–56.

Sher, K.J., Jackson, K.M. and Steinley, D. (2011) 'Alcohol use trajectories and the ubiquitous cat's cradle: cause for concern?', *Journal of Abnormal Psychology*, 120(2): 322–35.

Shin, S.H., Edwards, E.M. and Heeren, T. (2009) 'Child abuse and neglect: relations to adolescent binge drinking in the National Study of Adolescent Health (ADDHealth Study)' *Addictive Behaviors*, 34(3): 277–80.

Slack, J. (2007) 'Cabinet minister admits: "We can't curb the binge drinkers"', *Daily Mail*, 1 January.

Social Exclusion Unit (1999) *Teenage Pregnancy*, London: Social Exclusion Unit.

Tough, S., Tofflemire, K., Clarke, M. and Newburn-Cook, C. (2006) 'Do women change their drinking behaviors while trying to conceive? An opportunity for pre-conceptual counseling', *Clinical Medicine and Research*, 4(2): 97–105.

Tucker, J.S., Orlando, M. and Ellickson, P.L. (2003) 'Patterns and correlates of binge drinking trajectories from early adolescence to young adulthood', *Health Psychology*, 22(1): 79–87.

United Nations Development Programme (2005) *Human Development Report*, New York, NY: United Nations.

Walker, A., Maher, J., Coulthard, M., Goddard, E. and Thomas, M. (2001) *Living in Britain: Results of the 2000 General Household Survey*, London: The Stationery Office.

Wilde, O. (2007) *The Importance of Being Earnest*, London: Penguin Popular Classics.

Williams, S., Hickman, M., Bottle, A. and Aylin, P. (2005) 'Hospital admissions for drug and alcohol use in people aged under 45,' *British Medical Journal*, 330: 115.

Williamson, J., Sham, P. and Ball D. (2003) 'Binge drinking trends in a UK community based sample,' *Journal of Substance Use*, 8: 234–7.

Wilsnack R.W., Vogeltanz, N.D., Wilsnack, S.C., Harris, T.R., Ahlström, S., Bondy, S., Csémy, L., Ferrence, R., Ferris, J., Fleming, J., Graham, K., Greenfield, T., Guyon, L., Haavio-Mannila, E., Kellner, F., Knibbe, R., Kubicka, L., Loukomskaia, M., Mustonen, H., Nadeau, L., Narusk, A., Neve, R., Rahav, G., Spak, F., Teichman, M., Trocki, K., Webster, I. and Weiss, S. (2000) 'Gender differences in alcohol consumption and adverse drinking consequences: cross-cultural patterns', *Addiction*, 95(2): 251–65.

Wilsnack, S. and Wilsnack, R.W. (2003) 'International Gender and Alcohol Research: recent findings and future directions', Bethesda, MD: NIAAA [online at: http://pubs.niaaa.nih.gov/publications/arh26-4/245-250.htm; accessed: 11 January 2013].

York, J.L., Welte, J., Hirsch, J., Hoffman, J.H. and Barnes, G. (2004) 'Association of age of first drink with current alcohol drinking variables in a national general population sample', *Alcohol: Clinical and Experimental Research*, 28(9): 1379–87.

Youth Information (2007) [online at: www.youthinformation.com, click 'alcohol; accessed: 6 June 2013].

PART II
Families – living with FASDs

5

FETAL BEHAVIOUR AND THE EFFECT OF MATERNAL ALCOHOL CONSUMPTION

Peter G. Hepper

Introduction

The prenatal period is the most rapid stage of development in our lives. It begins with a single cell and ends, roughly nine months later, with the birth of a baby. It is often considered that birth marks the start of our lives, supported by giving the age of zero to individuals when born. The prevailing view, for many years, regarding prenatal development was that it was simply one of growth. Development was viewed as being passive, following a pre-determined plan, and was undertaken in the safe, protective custody of the mother's womb. Both these facts are now known to be incorrect.

The illusion of safety in the womb was removed by the tragedy involving the drug thalidomide (Lenz 1988). Mothers who took the drug (marketed as Distaval in the UK) had a significant risk of having a baby born with structural abnormalities. A spectrum of abnormalities resulting from exposure to the drug was identified, including gross limb malformations, abnormalities of the musculature of the face and eye, and malformations of the heart. Here was a clear and unambiguous signal that the fetus was susceptible to factors in its environment that could cause it long-term permanent damage.

Research examining the mechanisms of neurobehavioural development found that it did not simply proceed according to an in-built blueprint, but rather was dependent upon external input and interactions with the environment (Greenough 1986). It is now recognized that development is an interactive process, with experiences and interactions with internal and external stimuli playing a crucial role in development, sculpting neural structures (Blakemore and Cooper 1970), physical form (Moessinger 1988) and organ function (Nathanielsz 1999).

The prenatal period is now characterized as a period of active development in which the fetus is a driver of its own progression, its experiences being central to shaping developmental processes and outcomes. However, it is also susceptible to adverse effects arising from exposure to substances that may impact negatively on these developmental processes. One such substance is alcohol. It is the aim of this review to examine the effects of alcohol on the behaviour of the human fetus and the implications of this for its development.

Prenatal alcohol, fetal alcohol syndrome and fetal alcohol spectrum disorders

Lemoine and colleagues (1968) observed that mothers who consumed large amounts of alcohol during their pregnancy gave birth to children who displayed three characteristic features: central nervous system dysfunction; growth retardation; and a particular facial appearance. This constellation of features was subsequently termed fetal alcohol syndrome (FAS) (Jones and Smith 1973). Further research revealed that prenatal exposure to alcohol resulted in a range of effects that included deficits in physical form, growth, organ structure, and behavioural, psychological and social functioning. These effects, found in combination or in isolation, are captured by the umbrella term fetal alcohol spectrum disorders (FASDs) (Riley et al. 2011).

One of the most commonly occurring impacts of prenatal alcohol exposure is the neurobehavioural effects it exerts on the fetus (British Medical Association 2007). These effects may be wide-ranging, influencing a variety of basic psychological processes including learning, cognition, emotion, perception and motor performance (Mattson et al. 2011; Riley and McGee 2005), which, in turn, lead to more general behavioural, social, sexual and educational problems (Kelly et al. 2000; Streissguth 1997).

While the effects of prenatal alcohol exposure have been explored after birth, there has been little research to explore its effects before birth. Given the importance of the prenatal period for development, such information may be vital for a comprehensive understanding of the effects of alcohol on developmental processes and outcomes.

The behaviour of the human fetus

Fetal behaviour can be defined as any observable action or reaction (to an external stimulus) by the fetus (Hepper 1992). Early studies of the fetus used reports based on maternal perception (Neldam 1986) or by measuring the physical displacement of the mother's abdomen (Sontag and Wallace 1934) as indications of movement and responsiveness; these measures, however, were indirect at best. The development of ultrasound enabled the behaviour of fetus to be visualized directly (Reinold 1971) and documented in detail (e.g. de Vries et al. 1985). So acute is the resolution of these machines that the opening and closing of the pupil of the fetus's eye can be observed (Horimoto et al. 1993).

It is not intended to provide a comprehensive review of all aspects of the behaviour of the fetus here, and readers are referred elsewhere (Lecanuet et al. 1995; Nijhuis 1992) for more detail. Rather, an overview of fetal behaviour is provided, with the focus being to illustrate two key points regarding the development of the behaviour of the fetus. First, that behaviour becomes increasingly complex during development, reflecting brain maturation and, second, that the fetus is responsive to external stimuli.

Developing complexity and organization

The first spontaneous movements of the fetus appear at around seven to eight weeks gestation. These first movements originate in the fetus's spine and are slow and may result in passive movement of the fetus's arms and legs. Over the next few weeks, individual limb and other movements emerge (see Table 5.1), and by 20 weeks gestation the vast majority of individual

TABLE 5.1 The gestational age at which movements are first observed

Movement patterns	Gestational age (weeks)
First movements	7
Startle	8
General movement	8–9
Hiccup	9
Single arm movements	9
Head movements	9–10
Single leg movement	10
Stretch	10
Body rotation	10
Breathing	10–12
Mouth movement	10–11
Tongue movements	11
Yawn	11
Finger movements	12
Sucking and swallowing	12

Source: compiled from Nijhuis 1992 and Lecanuet *et al.* 1995.

movements that the fetus will exhibit *in utero* can be observed (de Vries *et al.* 1982, 1985). Initially, movements are independent and occur in isolation, but with advancing gestation movements become more coordinated and the fetus begins to exhibit bouts of activity and inactivity (James *et al.* 1995). The coordination and integration of movements reaches its peak at the end of gestation, when fetal behavioural states emerge (Nijhuis *et al.* 1982a, 1982b).

Four states are recognized in the human fetus – quiet sleep, active sleep, quiet awake, active awake (Nijhuis *et al.* 1982b). These states are defined by three variables: heart rate pattern (A:B:C:D); the presence or absence of eye movements; and the presence or absence of body movements. These combine together in a stable pattern from 36 weeks gestation to delineate the four states (see Table 5.2). The fetus remains in a particular state for a relatively long period of time and moves from one state to the next in a very rapid fashion. After 36 weeks gestation, the fetus spends very little time in 'no state'. It is argued that the appearance of behavioural states reflects a significant advance in brain integration and function (Nijhuis *et al.* 1982b).

TABLE 5.2 The behavioural parameters and their combination in the four fetal behavioural states

Fetal state	Descriptor	Eye movements	Body movements	Heart-rate pattern
1F	quiet sleep	absent	absent	A
2F	active sleep	present	present	B
3F	quiet	present	absent	C
4F	active	present	present	D

Responding to external stimuli

The first response exhibited by the fetus to an external stimulus is in reaction to tactile stimuli presented around the lips at eight weeks gestation. The whole body (with the possible exception of the back) is responsive to touch by 14 weeks gestation (Humphrey and Hooker 1959). The first response to an auditory stimulus is observed at around 24–26 weeks gestation (Hepper and Shahidullah 1994a) and to visual stimulus at 26–28 weeks gestation (Polishuk *et al.* 1975). Most attention has been paid to the fetus's response to auditory stimuli, largely due to their ease of presentation (Hepper and Shahidullah 1994a). As the fetus matures, the range of frequencies that it responds to widens, and the intensity of the stimulus required to elicit a response decreases (Hepper and Shahidullah 1994b). These elicited movements are a result of the coordinated action of different parts of the brain, and thus examine in more detail higher and integrated functions of the brain than spontaneous movements (Leader 1995). For example, responding to a sound stimulus requires not only the exhibition of response, e.g. movement, but also the detection of the stimulus (the sound) and some, possibly central, registration of the stimulus in order to elicit any movement (Hepper 1992).

Fetal behaviour and brain function

A central goal of observing and documenting the behaviour of the human fetus has been to use these observations to provide information about the functioning of its brain (Hepper 1995a; Krasnegor *et al.* 1998). Two approaches have been used to demonstrate the link between brain and behaviour in the fetus.

First, developments in brain function may be evidenced through changes in behaviour. For example, the increased sensitivity of the fetus to quieter sounds suggests underlying changes in the neural system responsible for detecting and responding to these sounds (Hepper and Shahidullah 1994a). The emergence of behavioural states is linked to the greater interconnectivity between different parts of the brain (Nijhuis *et al.* 1982a). Thus, as the brain develops, corresponding changes in behaviour are observed.

The second approach has examined the behaviour of the fetus when its health has been compromised. Many studies have found atypical behaviour in fetuses whose well-being is under threat; for example, those suffering from chromosomal or genetic disorders (Hepper and Shahidullah 1992), structural deficits (Visser *et al.* 1985), growth retardation (Sival and Prechtl 1992) or maternal illness (e.g. diabetes, Doherty and Hepper 2000). Thus, abnormalities of brain function are reflected in the behaviour of the fetus.

Observing how alcohol affects the behaviour of the fetus will provide evidence of how alcohol influences the brain of the fetus, during the period when exposure is occurring. Studies that have examined the behaviour of the human fetus in response to exposure to alcohol are now reviewed.

Maternal alcohol consumption and human fetal behaviour

There have been very few studies that have examined the effects of maternal consumption of alcohol on the fetus. Three types of studies have been reported:

1. those which have examined the behaviour of the fetus of mothers who drink when there is no alcohol in the mother's system;
2. studies that have examined the behaviour of the fetus when there is alcohol present in the mother's system; and
3. case studies.

The effect of alcohol on fetal behaviour when there is no alcohol in the mother's system

Only a few studies of this type have been conducted examining the startle response of the fetus (n = 3) and its habituation response (n = 1).

The spontaneous startle is perhaps the most basic movement of the fetus and reflects the functioning of the nervous system in its most primitive state. The first spontaneous startles are observed at approximately eight weeks gestation, peak at around nine weeks gestation and then decline in occurrence, until they are rarely observed after mid-gestation (de Vries *et al.* 1982, 1985). The startle response may be defined as a rapid movement, which lasts about one second, initiated in the limbs and spreading through the body (de Vries *et al.* 1985). The progressive disappearance of the startle response during gestation is thought to reflect the development of integration of the fetus's nervous system and its consequent organization into more complex, coordinated and sophisticated patterns of movement. Of particular importance for this is the development of inhibitory pathways which act to limit the excitatory pathway controlled startle movement.

The 'elicited' startle is similar in appearance to the spontaneous startle described above, i.e. it is a sudden, rapid movement of the whole body and limbs, but is observed immediately following the presentation of an external stimulus. Beginning at 24–26 weeks gestation, the fetus is observed to startle following the presentation of a loud sound (Hepper and Shahidullah 1994b). The elicited startle response also develops with advancing gestation, becoming elicited by less intense sounds. However, its overall structure, a rapid whole body movement, remains consistent across gestation. As noted above, elicited responses require three elements: the sensory detection of the stimulus; a 'central' registration of the stimulus; and a motor response. Changes in the neural system underlying any of these three components may be responsible for the changes observed with advancing gestation.

Little and colleagues (2002) examined 70 fetuses at 18–20 weeks gestation, when they observed spontaneous startles, and at 25 weeks gestation, when they observed elicited startles – in response to a loud sound. Fetuses of mothers who did not drink were compared with those of mothers who did drink (an average of 2.5 units of alcohol/week). There was no alcohol in the blood of women when tested. Fetuses of mothers who drank exhibited significantly more spontaneous startles than fetuses of mothers who did not drink. The opposite finding was found when examining elicited startles; fetuses of mothers who drank exhibited fewer startles than fetuses of mothers who did not drink. One interesting observation from both experiments was that there was no correlation between the amount the mother drank and the effect on the fetus. This supports previous observations that individual differences in mothers and fetuses play a significant role in determining the effects of alcohol on the individual. It was argued that the results indicated that alcohol retards normal neural maturation, preserving the primitive response of spontaneous startles and delaying the emergence of the elicited startle.

A second study (Hepper et al. 2005) followed the development of spontaneous startle behaviour across gestation in fetuses of mothers who did not drink and mothers who did drink (an average of 4.2 units of alcohol/week). Spontaneous startles were observed in the same fetuses at 20, 25, 30 and 35 weeks gestation. The study found that, when exposed to alcohol, fetuses exhibited a greater number of spontaneous startles at all gestational ages. Interestingly, the difference in startle behaviour between fetuses of mothers who drank, and those who did not drink, decreased as gestation advanced. There was a 'catch up' by those fetuses exposed to alcohol, i.e. they exhibited increasingly fewer spontaneous startles as gestation progressed. The difference, however, remained significant at 35 weeks gestation (when the observations ceased), and so whether the 'catch-up' continues beyond this time, or if there remains a permanent difference, is unknown.

In a more recent study (Hepper et al. 2012), the effect of alcohol on the elicited startle was examined longitudinally in two groups of fetuses. In one group (n = 21) the mothers did not drink alcohol; in the other (n = 18) mothers consumed approximately ten units of alcohol per week. Fetuses were examined at 29 weeks gestation and again at 32 and 35 weeks and their elicited startle response recorded in response to the presentation of a loud sound. At 29 weeks gestation fetuses exposed to alcohol exhibited a weaker startle response than did fetuses not exposed to alcohol. However at 32 and 35 weeks gestation there was no difference between the groups. Thus, for elicited startles, these observations indicate that prenatal exposure to alcohol delays the emergence of the elicited startle response in the fetus but this response 'catches-up' to fetuses not exposed to alcohol by 32 weeks of gestation.

Most recently one study has examined the habituation performance of the fetus (Hepper et al. 2012). Habituation is defined as the decrement in response to repeated presentation of the same stimulus and is considered a form of learning (Hepper and Leader 1996). The normal habituation process requires an intact and functioning central nervous system, including the cortices (Hepper 1995a), and thus provides a useful tool to examine brain function in the fetus (Hepper and Leader 1996). Adverse maternal conditions (e.g. diabetes, Doherty and Hepper 2000; epilepsy, Lynch et al. 2008), fetal conditions (e.g. Down syndrome, Hepper and Shahidullah 1992) and environmental conditions (e.g. maternal smoking, Leader 1987) have all been demonstrated to alter the fetus's habituation response.

Habituation was examined longitudinally in fetuses at 35, 36 and 37 weeks of gestation. The study examined mothers who drank heavily (20+ units per week) and those who drank moderately (5–10 units/week) as well as mothers who drank as a binge (their drinking was confined to two to three days per week) or mothers who drank evenly across the week. The habituation responses of these fetuses were compared to those of fetuses with mothers who did not drink alcohol. Both drinking pattern and the amount of alcohol consumed influenced the fetal habituation response. Fetuses took longer to habituate (i.e. required more stimulus presentations) if their mothers binge drank and if their mothers drank heavily. These results demonstrate that prenatal alcohol exposure affects the functioning of the brain before birth. Habituation is a measure of basic information processing (Hepper et al. 2012); the slower habituation performance observed in this study indicates that alcohol has reduced the efficiency of the fetal brain to process information. This may be a result of alcohol-induced structural damage to the brain and/or the effects of acute exposure.

Fetal behaviour immediately following the mother's consumption of alcohol

A number of studies have examined the behaviour of the fetus immediately following the consumption of alcohol by its mother. These studies, conducted after 36 weeks of gestation, have focused on two aspects of behaviour: fetal breathing movements and behavioural states.

The fetus exhibits breathing movements from around 10–12 weeks gestation, although they are infrequent. Their incidence increases from 26 weeks gestation until about 36 weeks gestation, with the most rapid increase between 26–30 weeks gestation (James et al. 1995). They become organized into bouts of breathing movements and no breathing movements from around 28 weeks gestation (Cosmi et al. 2003).

Studies examining breathing movements have observed the fetus after the maternal consumption of: two glasses of white wine at 37–40 weeks of pregnancy (Akay and Mulder 1996); a drink of one ounce of 80 per cent proof vodka in 90 ml of ginger ale when 37–39 weeks pregnant (Fox et al. 1978); and a drink of ethanol (1.9 ounces) diluted in soda water between 37–40 weeks of pregnancy (McLeod et al. 1983). All studies reported that fetal breathing movements declined immediately upon consumption of alcohol and had disappeared 30–40 minutes after consumption (the time of peak maternal ethanol concentrations). Breathing movements remained suppressed for at least 3.5 hours after consumption (the observation ended here), at which time maternal blood ethanol levels were zero (McLeod et al. 1983). There appeared to be a dose-related effect as the breathing movements of fetuses of mothers given one ounce of alcohol (Fox et al. 1978) were supressed for a shorter period than those given 1.9 ounces of alcohol (McLeod et al. 1983).

The behavioural states of the fetus observed at 37–40 weeks gestation were disrupted immediately following maternal consumption of two glasses of white wine (Mulder et al. 1998). Both the occurrence of fetal breathing movements and eye movements were reduced, and thus the behavioural state organization of the fetus was effectively abolished.

These studies indicate that alcohol, when consumed by the mother, immediately begins to suppress the behaviour of the fetus, before abolishing it completely within 30–40 minutes. This effect continues long after the time alcohol has been removed from the mother's body.

Case studies

Case studies often report instances of unusual, unique or extreme factors involved in the subject. With regard to those examining the behaviour of the fetus in response to maternal alcohol consumption they involve levels of consumption unable to be explored in controlled experimental situations. However, despite the limitations of case studies, they can provide information on the effects of high levels of alcohol exposure on the fetus.

Mulder and colleagues (1986) reported an observation of behavioural states in a fetus exposed to high levels of daily alcohol consumption throughout pregnancy. During the first trimester, the mother consumed a minimum of ten glasses of beer per day, and for the remainder of her pregnancy, consumed between 2–10 glasses per day. The mother was admitted to hospital at 36 weeks gestation and the behavioural states of her fetus were documented at 38 and 40 weeks gestation. At these ages, the fetus should move very quickly from one state to the next and spend very little time in 'no state' (Nijhuis et al. 1982b). Moreover, the transition between states usually follows an orderly transition from quiet sleep to active sleep to active (Nijhuis *et al.* 1982b). In this case, the fetus spent a considerable amount of time in the 'no state' condition, and exhibited unusual state transitions, moving directly from quiet sleep to active.

A second study (Castillo *et al.* 1989) reported an observation of the breathing and body movements of the fetus of a mother when heavily intoxicated and subsequently later, when not intoxicated. The mother had a history of heavy drinking during pregnancy. At the first observation, at 37 weeks gestation, the mother had a blood alcohol level of 322 mg/dL (the legal limit for driving in the UK is 80 mg) at the start of the 60-minute observation. Twenty-four hours later, the behaviour of the fetus was observed again when the mother's blood alcohol level was less than 10 mg/dL. Both body movements and breathing movements were significantly less frequent when the fetus was observed while the mother was intoxicated than when not intoxicated.

The case studies reveal that alcohol suppresses behaviour and affects the coordination of the brain, as evidenced through its disruption of fetal behavioural states.

Summary

The few studies that have been reported indicate that maternal consumption of alcohol influences the behaviour of the fetus. Immediately following the consumption of alcohol by the mother, the behaviour of the fetus is suppressed and, within a short period of time, movements are abolished. Following exposure to alcohol during pregnancy, the neuro-behavioural development of the fetus is delayed, although there is some catch-up in later stages of pregnancy. One study indicates impaired information processing before birth which may have long-term consequences for the ability of the individual to learn after birth.

These studies demonstrate, among others, two important points. First, the effects observed occur at relatively low levels of alcohol consumption. Indeed, even one glass of wine suppresses the behaviour of the fetus. Second, the observed suppression of behaviour persists even after there is no alcohol present in the mother's blood stream. This raises the important consideration that the length of time the fetus is exposed to alcohol is not the same as that determined from the presence of alcohol in its mother's blood, but is likely to be much longer.

Alcohol readily crosses the placenta to enter the fetal blood stream. However, the fetus's ability to clear alcohol from its blood is poor due to the immaturity of its liver function (Brien *et al.* 1983). Alcohol may therefore persist in the fetal system after alcohol has been removed from its mother's system (Nava-Ocampo *et al.* 2004, Pikkarainen and Raiha 1967). Moreover, alcohol may pool in the amniotic fluid and provide a secondary route for transmission to the fetus through its swallowing of amniotic fluid. The fetus swallows amniotic fluid from 15 weeks gestation (Hepper 1992), and may therefore also experience alcohol via this route.

The consequences of behavioural suppression

The disruption of behaviour caused by exposure to alcohol may adversely affect the neurobehavioural development of the fetus. Neural development is partly experience dependent and hence disruptions to normal 'experiences', movements, etc. may exert an adverse effect on the development and functioning of the fetus's brain and body (Hepper

1992). Movement of the joints is essential for the normal formation of the limbs (e.g. Drachman and Coulombre 1962) and specific sensory experience is necessary for the development of the brain (e.g. Blakemore and Cooper 1970). Whether the prolonged suppression of behaviour as elicited by maternal alcohol consumption contributes to the adverse consequences of prenatal alcohol exposure is unknown but remains a significant possibility and is in need of exploration.

Learning to drink

Prenatal exposure to alcohol may have one further consequence: it may prime the individual to have a preference for alcohol after birth.

There is much evidence to indicate that the human fetus learns before birth (DeCasper and Fifer 1980; Dirix *et al.* 2009; Hepper 1991). Of relevance here, is the ability of the fetus to learn about chemosensory stimuli present in its environment. Studies have demonstrated that the newborns of mothers who eat garlic (Hepper 1995b), carrots (Mennella *et al.* 2001) and anise (Schaal *et al.* 2000) during pregnancy exhibit a differential response to this smell/flavour after birth as newborns. In general terms, prenatal exposure leads to an increased preference for the chemosensory stimulus experienced before birth. The same process appears to operate for prenatal experience of alcohol. Newborns of mothers who drank during pregnancy exhibited more 'pleasurable' responses as assessed by the Facial Action Coding system when presented with the odour of ethanol than newborns of mothers who did not drink (Faas 2001). The longevity of prenatal chemosensory learning has yet to be fully explored, but animal studies (e.g. Hepper and Waldman 1992; Hepper and Wells 2006; Simitzis *et al.* 2008; Smotherman 1982) indicate these preferences are maintained well beyond the new-born period and influence feeding and drinking behaviour in later life.

Conclusion

The behaviour of the fetus is influenced by exposure to alcohol. The effects on behaviour may exert an adverse effect on normal neurobehavioural processes, contributing to the adverse consequences seen after birth arising from prenatal alcohol exposure. Furthermore, prenatal exposure may prime the individual to prefer alcohol after birth. The fact that even one glass of alcohol suppresses behaviour indicates that alcohol may influence the fetus's brain at very low levels of exposure. Moreover, alcohol remains active in the fetal system for much longer than in its mother.

The use of behavioural observations of the fetus may enable the early identification of problems arising from prenatal alcohol exposure and may facilitate new understandings of the effect of alcohol on the fetus. Although, at present, damage caused by alcohol exposure prenatally is untreatable, the identification of the existence of problems when the brain is at its most plastic may, in future years, enable the development of treatments to address the damage caused.

Acknowledgements

This work was partially funded by a grant (RRG3.7) from the R&D Office, Dept. of Health and Social Services and Public Safety, NI, and a grant (5 U24 AA014828) from the National

Institute on Alcohol and Alcohol Abuse (NIAAA) and done in conjunction with the Collaborative Initiative on Fetal Alcohol Spectrum Disorders (CIFASD). Additional information about CIFASD can be found at www.cifasd.org.

References

Akay, M. and Mulder, E.J.H. (1996) 'Investigating the effect of maternal alcohol intake on human fetal breathing rate using adaptive time-frequency analysis methods', *Early Human Development*, 6: 153–64.

British Medical Association (2007) *Fetal Alcohol Spectrum Disorders: A guide for healthcare professionals*, London: BMA.

Blakemore, C. and Cooper, G.F. (1970) 'Development of the brain depends on the visual environment', *Nature*, 228: 477–8.

Brien, J.F., Loomis, C.W., Tranmer, J. and McGrath, M. (1983) 'Disposition of ethanol in human maternal venous blood and amniotic fluid', *American Journal of Obstetrics and Gynecology*, 146: 181–6.

Castillo, R.A., Devoe, L.D., Ruedrich, D.A. and Gardner, P. (1989) 'The effects of acute alcohol intoxication on biophysical activities: a case report', *American Journal of Obstetrics and Gynecology*, 160: 692–3.

Cosmi, E.V., Anceschi, M.M., Cosmi, E., Piazze, J.J. and La Torre, R. (2003) 'Ultrasonographic patterns of fetal breathing movements in normal pregnancy', *International Journal of Gynaecology and Obstetrics*, 80: 285–90.

DeCasper, A.J. and Fifer, W.P. (1980) 'Of human bonding – newborns prefer their mothers' voices', *Science*, 208: 1174–6.

de Vries, J.P.P., Visser, G.H.A. and Prechtl, H.F.R. (1982) 'The emergence of fetal behaviour: I. qualitative aspects' *Early Human Development*, 7: 301–22.

de Vries, J.P.P., Visser, G.H.A. and Prechtl, H.F.R. (1985) 'The emergence of fetal behaviour: II. quantitative aspects', *Early Human Development*, 12: 99–120.

Dirix, C.E.H., Nijhuis, J.G., Jongsma, H.W. and Hornstra, G. (2009) 'Aspects of fetal learning and memory', *Child Development*, 80: 1251–8.

Doherty, N.N. and Hepper, P.G. (2000) 'Habituation in fetuses of diabetic mothers', *Early Human Development*, 59: 85–93.

Drachman, D.B. and Coulombre, A.J. (1962) 'Experimental clubfoot and arthrogyposis multiplex congenita', *Lancet*, 2: 523–6.

Faas, A.E. (2001) 'Estudios Funcionales del Sistema Nervioso Central del Recién Nacido: Aplicaciones del aprendizaje no asociativo en la evaluación neonatal' (PhD thesis), Córdoba, Argentina: Universidad Nacional de Cordoba.

Fox, H.E., Steinbrecher, M., Pessel, D., Inglis, J., Medvid, L. and Angel, E. (1978) 'Maternal ethanol ingestion and the occurrence of human fetal breathing movements', *American Journal of Obstetrics and Gynecology*, 132: 354–8.

Greenough, W.T. (1986) 'What's special about development? Thoughts on the bases of experience-sensitive synaptic plasticity', in W.T. Greenough and J.M. Juraska (eds) *Developmental Neuropsychology*, New York: Academic Press.

Hepper, P.G. (1991) 'An examination of fetal learning before and after birth', *Irish Journal of Psychology*, 12: 95–107.

Hepper, P.G. (1992) 'Fetal psychology: an embryonic science', in J.G. Nijhuis (ed.) *Fetal Behaviour: Developmental and perinatal aspects*, Oxford: Oxford University Press.

Hepper, P.G. (1995a) 'The behaviour of the foetus as an indicator of neural functioning', in J.-P. Lecanuet, W. Fifer, N. Krasnegor and W.P. Smotherman (eds) *Fetal Development: A psychobiological perspective*, Hillsdale, NJ: Lawrence Erlbaum.

Hepper, P.G. (1995b) 'Human fetal "olfactory" learning', *International Journal of Prenatal and Perinatal Psychology and Medicine*, 7: 147–51.

Hepper, P.G., Dornan, J.C. and Little, J.F. (2005) 'Maternal alcohol consumption during pregnancy may delay the development of spontaneous fetal startle behavior', *Physiology and Behaviour*, 83: 711–14.

Hepper, P.G., Dornan, J.C. and Lynch, C. (2012) 'Fetal brain function in response to maternal alcohol consumption: early evidence of damage', *Alcoholism: Clinical and Experimental Research*, 36: 168–75.

Hepper, P.G., Dornan, J.C., Lynch, C. and Maguire, J.F. (2012) 'Alcohol delays the emergence of the fetal elicited startle response, but only transiently', *Physiology and Behavior*, 107: 76–81.
Hepper, P.G. and Leader, L.R. (1996) 'Fetal habituation', *Fetal and Maternal Medicine Reviews*, 8: 109–23.
Hepper, P.G. and Shahidullah, S. (1992) 'Trisomy 18: behavioral and structural abnormalities. An ultrasonographic case study', *Ultrasound in Obstetrics and Gynecology*, 2: 48–50.
Hepper, P.G. and Shahidullah, S. (1994a) 'The development of fetal hearing', *Fetal and Maternal Medicine Review*, 6: 167–79.
Hepper, P.G. and Shahidullah, S. (1994b) 'Development of fetal hearing', *Archives of Disease in Childhood*, 71, F81–7.
Hepper, P.G. and Waldman, B. (1992) 'Embryonic olfactory learning in frogs', *Quarterly Journal of Experimental Psychology B*, 44B: 179–97.
Hepper, P.G. and Wells, D.L. (2006) 'Perinatal olfactory learning in the domestic dog', *Chemical Senses*, 31: 207–12.
Horimoto, N., Hepper, P.G., Shahidullah, S. and Koyanagi, T. (1993) 'Fetal eye movements', *Ultrasound in Obstetrics and Gynecology*, 3: 362–9.
Humphrey, T. and Hooker, D. (1959) 'Double simultaneous stimulation of human fetuses and the anatomical patterns underlying the reflexes elicited', *Journal of Comparative Neurology*, 112: 75–102.
James, D., Pillai, M. and Smoleniec, J. (1995) 'Neurobehavioural development in the human fetus', in J.-P. Lecanuet, W. Fifer, N. Krasnegor, and W.P. Smotherman (eds) *Fetal Development: A psychobiological perspective*, Hillsdale, NJ: Lawrence Erlbaum.
Jones, K.L. and Smith, D.W. (1973) 'Recognition of the fetal alcohol syndrome in early infancy', *Lancet*, 2: 999–1001.
Kelly, S.J., Day, N. and Streissguth, A.P. (2000) 'Effects of prenatal alcohol exposure on social behaviour in humans and other species', *Neurotoxicology and Teratology*, 22: 143–9.
Krasnegor, N.A., Fifer, W., Maulik, D., McNellis, D., Romero, R. and Smotherman, W.P. (1998) 'Fetal behavioural development: measurement of habituation, state transitions, and movement to assess fetal well-being and to predict outcome', *Journal of Maternal and Fetal Investigations*, 8: 51–7.
Leader, L.R. (1987) 'The effects of cigarette smoking and maternal hypoxia on fetal habituation', in K. Maeda (ed.) *The Fetus as a Patient*, Amsterdam: Elsevier.
Leader, L.R. (1995) 'The potential value of habituation in the prenate', in, J.-P. Lecanuet, W. Fifer, N. Krasnegor and W.P. Smotherman (eds) *Fetal Development: A psychobiological perspective*, Hillsdale, NJ: Lawrence Erlbaum.
Lecanuet, J.-P., Fifer, W., Krasnegor, N. and Smotherman, W.P. (eds) (1995) *Fetal Development: A Psychobiological Perspective*, Hillsdale, NJ: LEA.
Lemoine, P., Harousseau, H., Borteyru, J.P. and Menuet, J.C. (1968) 'Les enfants de parents alcooliques: anomalies observes; à propos de 127 cas', *Quest Médical*, 21: 476–82.
Lenz, W. (1988) 'A short history of thalidomide embryopathy', *Teratology*: 38, 203–15.
Little, J.F., Hepper, P.G. and Dornan, J.C. (2002) 'Maternal alcohol consumption during pregnancy and fetal startle behaviour', *Physiology and Behaviour*, 76: 691–4.
Lynch, C., Hepper, P.G. and Morrow, J. (2008) 'Habituation in fetuses exposed to antiepileptic drugs', *Epilepsia*, 50: 202.
Mattson, S.N., Crocker, N. and Nguyen, T.T. (2011) 'Fetal alcohol spectrum disorders: neuropsychological and behavioural features', *Neuropsychology Review*, 21: 81–101.
McLeod, W., Brien, J.F., Loomis, C., Carmichael, L., Probert, C. and Patrick, J. (1983) 'Effects of maternal ethanol ingestion on fetal breathing movements gross body movements and heart rate at 37 to 40 weeks gestational age', *American Journal of Obstetrics and Gynecology*, 145: 251–7.
Mennella, J.A., Jagnow, C.P. and Beauchamp, G.K. (2001) 'Prenatal and postnatal flavor learning by human infants', *Pediatrics*, 107: E88 [online at: www.ncbi.nlm.nih.gov/pmc/articles/PMC1351272/pdf/nihms-5608.pdf; accessed: 11 January 2013].
Moessinger, A.C. (1988) 'Morphological consequences of depressed or impaired fetal activity', in W.P. Smotherman and S.R. Robinson (eds) *Behavior of the Fetus*, Caldwell, NJ: Telford.
Mulder, E.J.H., Kamstra, A., O'Brien, M.J., Visser, G.H.A. and Prechtl, H.F.R. (1986) 'Abnormal fetal behavioural state regulation in a case of high maternal alcohol intake during pregnancy', *Early Human Development*, 14: 321–6.

Mulder, E.J.H., Morssink, L.P., van der Schee, T. and Visser, G.H.A. (1998) 'Acute maternal alcohol consumption disrupts behavioral state organization in the near-term fetus', *Pediatric Research*, 44: 774–9.

Nathanielsz, P.W. (1999) *Life in the Womb: The origin of health and disease*, New York, NY: Promethean Press.

Nava-Ocampo, A.A., Velázquez-Armenta, Y., Brien, J.F. and Koren, G. (2004) 'Elimination kinetics of ethanol in pregnant women', *Reproductive Toxicology*, 18: 613–17.

Neldam, S. (1986) 'Fetal movements as an indicator of fetal well-being', *Danish Medical Bulletin*, 33: 212–20.

Nijhuis, J.G. (ed.) (1992) *Fetal Behaviour: Developmental and perinatal aspects*, Oxford: Oxford University Press.

Nijhuis, J.G., Martin, C.B. and Prechtl, H.F.R. (1982a) 'Behavioural states of the human fetus', in H.F.R. Prechtl (ed.) *Continuity of Neural Functions from Prenatal to Postnatal Life: Clinics in developmental medicine*, London: Blackwell.

Nijhuis, J.G., Prechtl, H.F.R., Martin, C.B. and Bots, R.S.G.M. (1982b) 'Are there behavioural states in the human fetus?' *Early Human Development*, 6: 177–95.

Pikkarainen, P.H. and Raiha, N.C. (1967) 'Development of alcohol dehydrogenase activity in the human liver', *Pediatric Research*, 1: 165–8.

Polishuk, W.Z., Laufer, N. and Sadovsky, E. (1975) 'Fetal reaction to external light', *Harefuah*, 89: 395–7.

Reinold, E. (1971) 'Beobachtung foetaler Aktivitat in der ersten Halfte der graviditat mit dem ultraschall', *Padiatrie und Padologie*, 6: 274–9.

Riley, E.P., Infante, M.A. and Warren, K.R. (2011) 'Fetal Alcohol spectrum disorders: an overview', *Neuropsychology Review*, 2: 73–80.

Riley, E.P. and McGee, C.L. (2005) 'Fetal alcohol spectrum disorders: an overview with emphasis on changes in brain and behaviour', *Experimental Biology and Medicine*, 230: 357–65.

Schaal, B., Marlier, L. and Soussignan, R. (2000) 'Human foetuses learn odours from their pregnant mother's diet', *Chemical Senses*, 25: 729–37.

Simitzis, P.E., Deligeorgis, S.G., Bizelis, J.A. and Fegeros K. (2008) 'Feeding preferences in lambs influenced by prenatal flavour exposure', *Physiology and Behavior*, 93: 529–36.

Sival, D.A. and Prechtl, H.F.R. (1992) 'The relation between the quantity and quality of prenatal movements in pregnancies complicated by IUGR and premature rupture of membranes', *Early Human Development*, 30: 193–209.

Sontag, L.W. and Wallace, R.F. (1934) 'Preliminary report of the Fels Fund Study of foetal activity', *American Journal of Diseases of Children*, 48: 1050–7.

Smotherman, W.P. (1982) 'In utero chemosensory experience alters taste preferences and corticosterone responsiveness', *Behavioral and Neural Biology*, 36: 61–8.

Streissguth, A.P. (1997) *Fetal Alcohol Syndrome: A guide for families and communities*, Baltimore, MD: Paul H. Brooks.

Visser, G.H.A., Laurini, R.N., deVries, J.I.P., Bekedam, D.J. and Prechtl, H.F.R. (1985) 'Abnormal motor behaviour in anencephalic fetuses', *Early Human Development*, 12: 173–82.

6

PARENTING IN THE EARLY YEARS

Simon Brown and Julia Brown

Introduction

The main purpose of this book is to expand the knowledge about fetal alcohol spectrum disorders (FASDs) among those who work in a professional capacity with children and young people. In 1999 when our daughter was five years old and diagnosed with an FASD no such textbook or reference point existed. As parents we did lots of the 'right things' purely by accident and by following our instinct as to what seemed to work.

We rapidly realized we were the professional experts as we lived with our daughter, we knew her and we understood her difficulties and the root causes more thoroughly than those who were supposed to be advising us. This resulted in the slightly ludicrous position whereby we were teaching them and advising them on how best to help us.

This chapter describes our parenting journey in the context of this paucity of professional knowledge, insufficient support and lack of appropriate information about FASDs in our daughter's earliest years.

Supporting other families

One of the most common scenarios we come across in our work supporting other families/carers looking after those affected by FASDs is that which we call the 'tennis game of help', with the parent/carer requesting help and the professional service, be it school, medical or social services often responding, 'What help do you want?', followed by the desperate carer replying, 'Just help.' Matters can often continue in this unsatisfactory state, with increasing frustration on both sides for many months! So, what 'help' do parents need in those early years?

For many parents, especially first time parents, the first few years of parenting can be a bewildering move into an alien world. Many adults, even those who would perhaps perceive themselves to be successful, intelligent, articulate and well informed, find themselves completely stumped as they enter the world of an 18-month-old toddler. The added complexity of caring for a child with special needs leaves many families totally lost.

Young children with FASDs

For us personally, initially, it did not seem so difficult. Our daughter arrived in our lives when she was a year old. Like many children who have been involved in the care system, it had been suggested that her global developmental delay was possibly partly a result of her premature birth but was more likely due to other subsequent circumstances which resulted in her being placed in the care of the local authority. However, we were assured all would be well once she was in a loving, stable, secure, nurturing home.

Physical/health issues

We can look back now, with the wisdom of hindsight, and see that our daughter was a 'textbook example' of a child with an FASD. She was small and underweight. She had an amazing appetite, and would – if allowed – happily demolish an adult-sized portion of dessert, with extra cream. Despite this her weight gain was painfully slow. We consistently had to dress her in clothes that were a size – or more – smaller than her chronological age; finding school uniform that fitted was a challenge. In addition, we discovered she was long-sighted and had a squint which was corrected by glasses, and her hair was unusually fine and took a long time to grow.

Motor coordination

She walked at 19 months and, having 'furniture walked' for months before that, was very unstable on her feet and had no spatial awareness; we became expert at rearranging furniture in friends' houses, especially glass-topped coffee tables. She enjoyed music and dancing, was fascinated by *Teletubbies*, liked toys suitable for a baby – anything bright, chunky and if it made a noise, especially a musical one, then she would be fascinated with it for hours, repeatedly pushing the button to make it 'sing'. However, she could not operate each side of her body independently, which made riding a bike impossible. She had severe difficulties with her fine motor skills which impacted on her ability to get dressed independently and to hold a pencil to draw and write.

Communication issues

When she first arrived, her vocabulary consisted of one word, 'ooh'. We taught her to talk, with an especially concentrated effort at meal times, beginning with single sounds, such as 'p-p-p', then moved on to 'Dada'. Her speech came slowly, and at first it was not clear; she was hard to understand. Then, with a rush, the words came – and have never stopped since. She once talked in the car non-stop for 45 minutes until Grandma finally asked her to stop. There was silence for a few seconds, then a little voice said, 'Grandma, aren't I doing good being quiet?'

When she was five and commencing compulsory education, a speech and language therapy assessment reported that her expressive vocabulary was at a seven-year level, while her receptive language was scored at just a little below that of an average three-year-old.

Social difficulties

She was bright, friendly and had no sense of 'stranger danger', wanting to be friends with everyone. She was a beautiful, affectionate, lively, determined, engaging child.

Parenting a young child with FASDs – the challenges

People commented that we must be exhausted as our daughter was 'on the go' all the time. At night, it was difficult to get her to sleep; we had to cuddle her, stay with her or sometimes put her in the back of the car and drive around the local housing estate. However, once she was finally settled she would sleep through – most of the time – until five o'clock the next morning.

As this was our first experience of parenting, we enjoyed having her, and we simply assumed the many difficulties were a result of her being 'a bit behind'. We noticed she did master certain skills, eventually, but later than other children. It was not until she was three years old and of an age to enter the education system, beginning with play groups and nursery, that the sheer breadth of the developmental gap between her and her peers became fully apparent. It was at this point that professional help was first offered on a more formal basis to us and our daughter.

However, our search for help was motivated by our daughter being refused places at local nurseries and playgroups. We visited our GP who referred us to the community paediatrician who, after an assessment, referred us to physiotherapy, occupational therapy, speech and language therapy and the local authority's special education team. It was this latter team that assigned our daughter a nursery place in a unit for children with learning difficulties and referred us to the educational psychologist.

The waiting times for speech and language therapy and occupational therapy were quite long, but we were fortunate to be in a position to pay for private assessments so we had something to begin with in terms of defining our daughter's difficulties and the help we could give her to enable progress. We were finally referred to the genetics team at Guy's and St Thomas' Hospital in London who identified that our daughter had fetal alcohol syndrome (FAS). She was five years old.

Identifying the support needs of families of young children with FASDs

Practical help

Returning once more to our opening question of what 'help' parents need – including us and many others we have encountered – one useful 'help' in those early years would have been respite care. We were never offered any such service, nor did we ask for it, as we were unaware such services existed. Children with FASDs are often are described as being hyperactive and may also be diagnosed with attention deficit hyperactivity disorder (ADHD) (see Blackburn *et al.* 2012). This is accompanied by a total lack of awareness of danger, spatial awareness deficits, poor social and personal self-care skills. This means these children require a higher, constant level of supervision and practical assistance. This can be physically and emotionally tiring for the carers. The respite offered does not need to be huge chunks of time – a couple of hours can make a major difference.

We were fortunate in that we were able to give our daughter one-to-one assistance, but when families have more than one child, especially more than one child with an FASD, the demands on carers increase. In such circumstances respite care can enable them to focus on another child, as well as have time for themselves.

Finances and financial support is another area where many parents of a child with an FASD struggle. Many do not realize they may be entitled to claim disability benefits for their child or to access various grants. We often find with the parents whom we support that one or both parents have had to give up paid employment outside the home to cope with the demands of caring for their child affected by an FASD. Again, information and signposting to other organizations provide a vital lifeline of support. Disability Living Allowance (DLA) was an entitlement we discovered through a chance conversation with another parent at the school gate; we were aware of DLA, but thought it was a benefit for adults and did not realize that it could be claimed for children.

Understanding

Another issue we commonly hear about and even, to some degree, experienced ourselves, is that parental deficits are cited as the reason for a child's difficulties, rather than a biological cause such as an FASD. Parenting classes may be offered as part of the solution. Unfortunately, many 'traditional' parenting techniques, such as consequences, reward charts and time out do not work for children with FASDs, especially younger ones.

Therefore problems can escalate as parents feel even more of a failure, or the child is deemed to be oppositional defiant because of his or her failure to comply with a set of instructions they do not understand.

It is helpful if parents understand their child's condition and the areas in which they are likely to have difficulties, and if they can gain advice from others who have FASDs parenting experience in relation to practical daily strategies. We still remember the medical and school staff who gently pointed out to us our daughter's needs were significant and would be lifelong, and supported us as we came to a realistic place where we accepted this. We sought to achieve a right balance of knowing her limitations, but ensuring she was given every appropriate opportunity to fulfil her potential.

Emotional support

Another area where parents need support is on an emotional level. From our experience of managing The FASD Trust,[1] we have found that birth parents, especially mothers, often experience guilt. Other carers feel angry. For many adopters and long-term foster carers, there is a sense of loss, a grieving process about what might have been and will not be in terms of the child's abilities and future life outcomes. In the early years, as they struggle on a daily basis with the physical demands of caring for their child with an FASD, many carers have a tortuous search to find the root cause of the difficulties, before launching on an exhausting quest to 'cure' their child.

Signposting

In addition, many carers are unaware of the existence of support agencies, both voluntary and statutory. One of the most supportive things that professionals working with families can do is inform them about or refer them to such groups and organizations. It can be exceedingly isolating for any parent or carer to be at home with a young child, let alone a child with significant additional needs. Such isolation can extend socially as parents feel unsure or unable to venture out with their 'badly behaved' child. Attendance at support groups or other activities can enable them to gain confidence, knowledge and friends.

Support from professionals

Another kind of help relates to schooling. When children with FASDs begin more formal attendance at nursery or pre-school, an opportunity arises for them to be constantly compared with other children, which means that their difficulties are highlighted. It is often, as in our case, at this stage that referrals begin to be made to various agencies for diagnosis and support. However, for many parents, even those who are experienced parents of non-disabled children, the world of special educational needs (SEN) is a foray into another alien world. We learnt as we went through the system, but the ideal scenario would have been for someone to have provided explanations, information and advice earlier. Such support, information and advice is available (for example from the Parent Partnership[2]) for those with children with SEN, but parents or carers are unaware, until they are informed, about the guidance available to them.

When we work in a particular field, its systems, processes and acronyms all become familiar, and we forget that for a parent or carer encountering our area for the first time, it can initially be a confusing, overwhelming experience. This is where expert knowledge and ability to patiently and clearly explain systems is an invaluable support to parents and carers.

The four Rs – golden rules for parents

Finally in terms of giving practical guidance and support to parents in those early years, it must be borne in mind that our children with FASDs do not 'fit in the box'. Consequently, our Golden Rules for those early years for parents are not the '3 Rs' but the '4 Rs' – Routines, Rules, Repetition and Relax. It is important to establish clear routines, to have simple rules that you ensure the child adheres to constantly and to repeat everything, many times over. This is all laying the solid foundations which will make life easier for the child as he or she gets older. The earlier the child's condition is diagnosed, the earlier professional therapy and intervention is given, the more the child has a stable, consistent home life and routines, the more people around the child are aware of their condition, the more the chances of the child having positive outcomes as a young person and adult increase.

The fourth 'R' is 'relax'. So many parents and carers become caught up in the stress and anxiety of addressing their child's needs – worrying because they are not reaching their 'milestones', or because they are not doing what it says in the parental manual; concerned about lack of money, schooling or the future – that they can forget to enjoy their child. It must not be forgotten that our children can be friendly, affectionate, happy, helpful, and good at music, art or horse-riding.

When our daughter was small, we laughed a lot and would take time just to enjoy being together as a family. She is slowly acquiring the skills she needs for life, not when her peers do, but at her own individual pace. We can look back now and say, 'Yes – it is exhausting hard work at times, and continues to be', but as we are sitting writing this, our beautiful daughter is in the room next door, and we can hear her laughing.

Notes

1   www.fasdtrust.co.uk
2   www.parentpartnership.org.uk

Reference

Blackburn, C., Carpenter, B. and Egerton, J. (2012) *Educating Children and Young People with FASD*, Abingdon: Routledge.

7

LIFE AS WE KNOW IT

A perfectly normal family

Sarah Muir-Timmins and John Timmins

Introduction

When people learn that our children have fetal alcohol spectrum disorder (FASDs), it triggers a range of questions. When we explain they have FASDs and are also adopted, there are even more questions. Quite often people end their questioning by telling us how good we are to have 'taken on the children', or how good we are and how 'lucky the children are'. Lucky is not a word that readily springs to my mind when I think of our children. Good is not how I feel most days when I am struggling to stay calm, and trying to understand what has sparked the latest tantrum or fight.

This chapter describes our family life with two adopted children who have FASDs. Brief glimpses of 'normal family life' are overshadowed by the need for rigid routine, structure and clarity in order to support the needs of two children with disrupted early experiences and FASDs. Despite this, changing our perspective and expectations of family life has enabled us to enjoy our children, celebrate their achievements and appreciate the positive changes they have brought to our lives.

Assumptions and expectations

To start at the beginning, John and I spent years on the fertility/IVF cycle without success. To feel like a failure at what everyone else seemed to manage naturally was difficult, and really rocked our confidence.

The decision to adopt seemed like the answer for us to be parents. We had been told by the social workers that the likelihood of us being able to adopt a baby was remote, and there was a strong possibility that any child placed with us would have some difficulties relating to their disruptive family backgrounds. It was stressed that many children placed for adoption may have attachment issues and behavioural problems. However, we felt we were prepared and that we would be able to overcome most difficulties, once the children settled into a new family and had time to adjust. John came from a large family and I had a background in social work. We were prepared; we could manage – or so we thought!

The whole process of adoption, once approved, set us up for a belief that we could manage; surely we could manage. We spent a long time looking at possible matches, considering the possibilities of various children becoming 'our' children. At first we thought that the 'right' child would be there for us, and we would recognize the right match instantly. We were wrong. We looked through the advertisements of children needing families, never quite seeing the 'perfect' match.

After several months we saw two young siblings waiting for a family. The eldest was a two-year-old girl with an FASD. Her younger brother was aged one year. The social worker confidently said that he was not affected by an FASD, even though the birth mother continued to drink through the first stages of the pregnancy. We agonized over whether we could manage; we spent hours talking about what FASDs really meant on a day-to-day level, and what family life might be like with children who had special needs. We read the information relating to the children; we searched the internet about FASDs. We were told that this kind of information describes the worst case scenario. We wanted to manage; our friends told us that we would be fine. We wanted to believe it would be okay. So we said yes. Before we knew it, we had two very active children aged 13 months and 25 months. And so began family life; but not as most people know it.

Early days

Looking back now, I think that I spent the first year like a rabbit caught in the headlights. I went through the motions of parenting, trying to develop bonds and build attachment with the children. But I was completely shell-shocked and exhausted.

Early days with our son

Our son was 13 months old when he came to us and, as already stated, we were told he was not affected by FASDs. However, he experienced a hearing loss and difficulties sleeping. He still has a slight hearing loss and continues to suffer from ear infections. Much of his disrupted sleeping, I now feel, related to his difficulties attaching to me in particular. He would scream when held, go stiff and arch his back when lifted out of his cot. His hearing loss meant his speech was delayed. He has had two operations to correct his hearing problems, and now he manages quite well, except for the ear infections. His speech is great now – in fact he never stops talking; he is incessant.

Early days with our daughter

Our daughter, who was 25 months when she joined our family, equally did not seem to sleep much. Feeding her was so difficult. We quickly realized that our daughter did not feel pain very much or for very long; she could fall, bang, trip without it causing her any alarm. Again we learnt that we had to watch her more than others; we had to anticipate her actions because she could not see the dangers or consequences. During an assessment with a therapist at the Child and Adolescent Mental Health Services (CAMHS) we were advised that our daughter was a risk to herself, and potentially to other children, because of her impulsive nature. We were advised she needed close supervision; how much was left for us to work out ourselves.

Early medical and health issues

Both children took so long to feed, we felt as if we were spending most of the day trying to get them to eat anything at all. Both children were tiny. They suffered with reflux and found eating soft wet foods difficult. Both refused to eat anything that was warm, and always had cold foods. They still much prefer dry foods. We regularly went to the hospital to see the speech and language therapist, dieticians and paediatricians. We were lucky that we received speech and language therapy once a week, and were supported by the paediatrician. However, the children remained small. I could hold both children in one arm even when they were at nursery.

Neither of the children seemed to need much sleep or be able to sleep through the night. At times our son would wake up to 10 or 12 times in one night. Our daughter often had night terrors and still does now. There were days when I was so tired that I felt nauseous. Our tiredness was never helped by social workers telling us that they would settle eventually. However, after six years, the bags under my eyes are more like a sign of membership to some exclusive club – those who parent hyperactive children. This is not a club I would recommend joining if you don't have to!

Early practical safety issues

We were also just not prepared for how quick they were, and how destructive two such tiny children could be. The logistics of getting them in and out of the car were one of my first challenges. I watched the other mothers with two young children take one toddler out of the car and ensure that the first child would stand still on the pavement while they took the second child out. Not so for me. I learnt to take one child out of the car, and clamp them securely between my legs as I struggled to get the next one out. If I let the standing child free they would be off in a shot. Neither child responded to calls of 'Stop. Wait for me.' They were off!

During a trip out with another mum to a park which, unbeknown to me had a fishing lake in it, our daughter, who was three years old, decided to race off. Even though she was so small, she ran very quickly, paying absolutely no attention to anything or anyone. She raced away from me straight out to the lake, out along a jetty with no apparent inclination to stop. That horrid sick feeling of impending danger filled me as I ran after her shouting her name. Thankfully a scream to 'Sit now!' stopped her in her tracks (along with every dog in a 100 yard radius), and I got to her before she took off again. I had learnt my lesson.

Much as I wanted to treat our daughter the same as other little girls her age and be a mother just like the others at toddler group we could not. Our daughter just never saw the danger. She never sought reassurance that she could do something. She never asked for help to do anything. She just went ahead and did what she wanted regardless of whether she sent other children flying or whether she hurt herself.

Becoming 'experts' on our children

We were really lucky to find a brilliant nursery/pre-school for our daughter that helped. They recognized that there was something different about her early development. For example, she did not play with other children. She was incredibly sociable, and adults thought she was very sweet and endearing, but she just could not get along with children her age. So began what we anticipate will be a long and challenging involvement with the Education Department at the local authority. An appointment with a clinical psychologist at CAMHS helped. The outcome of this appointment was that the psychologist stated that without one-to-one adult support our daughter was a risk to herself and to other children. This forced the Education Department to assess her needs and consequently support her with a Statement of Special Educational Needs (SEN).

It was a sad reflection that we were pleased to have a written record of the risk our three-year-old posed to herself and others. However, it did open up the options of access to special support units for her. Her needs can be summarized as needing support with attention, listening and concentration (a particular barrier to learning), holding conversations, turn taking, social and emotional development, developmental immaturity, and a lack of understanding of the needs of others.

What most people see when they meet our daughter is a cute little girl with beautiful red hair, who is talkative, busy and very agile. Adults humour her slightly strange behaviour and her slightly strange repetitive questioning. Children pull away from her invading their space and her intense stare and irrelevant questions.

Our daughter asks so many questions that at best it is irritating. As you are trying to get on with preparing the tea or unpacking the shopping a typical dialogue will be:

OUR DAUGHTER: 'Where did you get this from?'
MUM: 'The supermarket.'
OUR DAUGHTER: 'Did you get it from a shop?'
MUM: 'Yes, from the supermarket.'
OUR DAUGHTER: 'Which shop did you get it from?'

…and so it goes on.

Either she is not able to listen to the answers, rushing to think of her next question, or I am not giving her the answer she is wanting. Communication and misunderstanding is often really difficult and a source of arguments, tantrums and tears.

Our daughter's difficulty in concentrating means that games or tasks are rarely completed. She rushes from one activity to another. No sooner have you got the paints out than she wants to do something else. She cannot settle to anything unless our son is with her. She has a need to know what everyone is doing for fear she is missing out on something. The impact is that our son gets little chance to do anything on his own. In addition, neither John nor I can go to the toilet or have any conversation without her needing to know where we are, what we are doing or what we said.

Our daughter's inability to concentrate also has implications for her learning and seems to be one of the major obstructions. It feels to us that she is living on a rush of adrenaline; consequently, she tires quickly and becomes irritable if she is tired or hungry.

Any trip out, whether to family or the hospital or the doctors requires a bag full of games, toys, books and colouring, all of which will be skirted over and discarded within the first 10–15 minutes. Then boredom sets in, and that is when things get hard work and at times embarrassing. What is now seen is an eight-year-old girl having a three-year-old tantrum or rolling around the floor making noises.

Our daughter is incredibly immature for her age. She is eight years old, and now out of nappies. She does not really know how to play games. She watches CBeebies, preferring the preschool programmes. She takes everything literally, so many programmes are far too scary for her.

She does not understand emotions, either her own or other people's. She does not recognize when she is hungry or tired. She often laughs when someone else is upset. She does not always recognize when we are cross. Until we realized this, it caused great problems when she would laugh at us while we were telling her off. Needless to say this just made us more cross!

The reality of how different we are

We quickly recognized that the traditional methods for behaviour management such as the naughty step did not work. Our children just do not understand what they are being punished for. All they hear is that they are bad; they have little sense of what it is you are unhappy about.

Limited concentration and inability to pick up on emotions or social cues make it very difficult for our children to learn appropriate social behaviour. Our daughter often hits or bites when she is cross or frustrated at something. We can say to her that it is not okay to bite; she will say sorry straight away, then go and do it again, saying, 'Sorry, sorry. I forgot.' While this seems just plain naughty, it is actually true for her. Knowing this, however, does not always stop us getting cross with her. How do you teach a child who cannot remember and just does not get the idea of social niceties?

Once you start writing about your children it feels very hard to get the balance right while giving a realistic picture of what the difficulties are for John and me. And I really do mean John and me, not for the children. We have to learn how to parent our children to get the best from them and be able to give them the best of us. That is hard. It means putting up with a lot of things that go against the grain. At times this means walking away from rudeness, walking away from hits and shouts, walking away from soiling when they were too 'busy' to go to the toilet.

If we tell them off every time that they shout in anger, use their fingers to eat, forget to use the toilet, break their toys, hit out at each other, all we are doing is exhausting ourselves, making parenting a horrid 'policing' job and instilling in them they are always wrong, naughty or stupid. So we have learnt to choose which behaviour to focus on and which to try to ignore. Supernanny would be pulling her hair out at us I'm sure! I hate noise and shouting – I always have done so. For me, the level of shouting and yelling really grates and some days it is just too much. I also feel for our neighbours!

It is very difficult to predict what is going to cause difficulty or upset for our daughter. Sometimes it will be having a bath; other times she loves it. Sometimes it will be getting dressed or brushing her hair. Asking her to stop playing to eat a meal, to get into the bath, to get into bed or go to the toilet nearly always cause an upset. This is despite the fact that meal times, bath time and bed time follow the same routines daily. Sometimes she will get cross if she thinks our son has more sausages, fish, chips or peas than her, so it is always best to give her more, or cut them into more pieces – although I draw the line at counting how many peas I have given them each!

Daily routines such as getting dressed in the mornings, bath time and getting into pyjamas, especially for our son, means you need to be an octopus! It is like trying to catch hold of and dress a cross between a slippery eel and a jumping bean; he is all over the place. You need to catch him and hold on as best you can!

Our daughter is always keen to please and desperately wants to be included and be part of everything. I think that is why other children find her so irritating and why adults find her sweet. She is always asking people questions and wants to know things from them. While this *seems* endearing, it also makes her very vulnerable.

On their own the children are easy. It is much easier to be able to give them the attention they need, thus avoiding tantrums. There is not the constant need for them to know what the other is doing. Maybe we should be pleased that they like being with each other – mostly. At times though, they have to be separated. We found quite early on that while it was great to bath them together, it soon became dangerous.

The reality is they are always jumping on top of, pulling or pushing each other – rough and tumble to the extreme. If given a chance they will extend this to other unsuspecting children who are not used to it. In our parenting experience, children with FASDs seem to see the landscape in an entirely different way; they miss out on vital social cues as they dash off to explore/climb/fall/bash.

Although I have given a picture of mayhem and madness in our lives, we have managed to install some order.

Molehills into mountains – simple events become challenges

We have mishaps, which thankfully have not resulted in serious accidents.

For example, one weekend, while John was away having a well-deserved golfing break with his brothers, I was just congratulating myself on a very successful Sunday lunch when the positive atmosphere changed. I told the children to wait five minutes before going on the trampoline after lunch; they agreed and went to play in our son's room. Ten minutes later, on hearing a very loud bang coming from the attic room, I rushed upstairs as the children came flying down (all intact, thankfully). They had climbed on the radiator and managed to pull it off the wall, pipes broken, water flowing! As I rushed around trying to find towels, buckets and emergency plumbers, I shouted for our daughter to get out of the way before the whole house flooded. She followed me again straightaway asking if she should put her swimming costume on. 'Why?' I yelled. 'Because if the house floods I can swim in it,' she replied.

At the time I did not see the funny side. Once I had calmed down and stopped panicking, her propensity to take everything literally made me cry and laugh. The whole incident made me realize what a balance we live on. No real damage was done. The carpet is damaged, and we now have to do that long put-off decorating job. We had said to the children so many times, 'Don't climb or pull on the radiators, otherwise…'

What kept going through my mind that night was the what ifs. What if they had pulled the radiator on to themselves; what if the water had been hot? We have been so lucky to avoid serious incidents. Again another lesson re-learnt. We cannot forget that they forget and get distracted so easily, regardless of how old they are, how many times we have told them something, or how well they seem to be doing two minutes earlier.

In addition, simple events such as attending medical appointments can be a challenge. On one occasion, I took our daughter into hospital for an operation to correct her squint. We had prepared her, as any parent would. I took her into the hospital, having phoned first, spoken to the play therapist on the ward, explained our situation. Our daughter happily came into the ward; she enjoyed seeing the playroom, looking at the book showing what happens to a little boy who has day surgery.

We had rehearsed on a doll getting into the gown, having 'magic cream' put on your hand, going to the theatre, having a special sleep, etc. On the day, she and I set off. She seemed fine, but I was a little apprehensive that any play room was going to occupy her for more than five minutes. I had managed to get her moved up the operating list so we were the first appointment of the day.

None of this made any difference. Even thinking about it now, I find it upsetting. Rehearsing and showing through stories and dolls what is going to happen is great – in theory – but they were stories and dolls. She had not grasped literally what was going to happen to her. Maybe it was the fear of the unknown. The lasting image for me is of the tears and the panic on her face. It took three of us to hold her in order to administer the anaesthetic. I nearly got more of it than her as she jerked and pulled her head around so much. It also took two of us to steady her as she came out of it still panicking.

I am sure other parents will have similar stories of their children and horrible hospital experiences. I am not saying this is unique to children with special needs or FASDs. But it is yet another thing they have to struggle to make sense of and cope with. Children with FASDs are at times so vulnerable, so immature, so limited in what they can understand that, regardless of their age, we have to think for them, and anticipate needs and risks. The need for adults to 'be the external brain' is a phrase often used.

Glimpses of normal family life

As already described, parenting a child with an FASD is hard, as is parenting any child. There are days when we say to ourselves, 'We got that so wrong today.' Mostly these days are when we are both extra tired or worried or stressed about other things. Managing FASDs is okay most of the time. It can be unpredictable and fun. It is when you also have to cope with other things such as illness, money worries and work issues that managing children's additional needs can be just too much to handle; I have cried, 'Why me? Why couldn't I have had normal children who don't need so much of me?'

The children need routines; they need order, although this can be hard to maintain, as in any house with young children. There are days when things go well: the right sandwiches are given for lunchtime; the shoes are on the right feet; the right school top and coat is on – the right way round; and the socks have been put on so the seams do not hurt the toes. In this sense our household is no different to any other. Then our daughter goes off to school in a taxi 20 miles away, and I take our son into his school, which is five miles in the opposite direction.

At times I look at them when they are asleep, at peace and relaxed, and kick myself for making such a fuss. Be grateful; they want me. We have times when John and I can sit back and think, we have had a really good day – that was fun. This is usually following a day where we have been busy the whole time, either a day trip out or holidays. The best ones are when we go back to the same place, same holiday cottage; we have not tried a trip abroad yet. If I am honest we are hesitant about managing the flight.

The children have swimming lessons, play tennis, have just started hockey, and our daughter goes to Brownies. Just like a normal family. They are both doing better than we hoped at school, and most of the time I would say they are happy children. They play together sometimes, and at other times they fight and try to kill each other. Just like a normal family. There are times when we go to visit extended family, and they are perfectly behaved.

They play and say 'thank you' and only argue over which of them had the most chocolate – just like a normal family. Other times we go out for a play, they rush around and fight over whose turn it is to go down the slide backwards or upside down – just like a normal family.

John and I are used now to not being left alone, to having children who need attention *all* the time. We do have a 'normal family', this is our norm.

Giving the children a perspective on their disability

We have told our daughter and our son that they are adopted; that daddy and I chose them. We tell them that we saw a photo of them, fell in love with them, and wanted to have them with us as a family. We have also said that they could not live with their birth parents as their birth mother was not well enough to look after them, and their father looked after her. We have begun to tell them that the reason they are 'fizzy' (our word for hyperactive/overactive) is because their birth mother drank things that were not good for her when they were in her tummy and that is why they get fizzy.

They know they are special. They are special because we chose them; special because they need help for some things. But they are also special because they do other things, like climbing and running around and talking non-stop, so much better than other children. How they will make sense of their history when they get older I cannot say. We will just have to wait and see.

Getting the right support

We have been incredibly lucky. We have managed to access effective educational resources for both our children. This has not been easy to achieve, but it will make the biggest difference for their life chances. We have also been fortunate to access a support group which has helped. Even though we do not get to the group often it gives us so much. I would definitely recommend anyone taking on children with special needs to find a support group.

Finally we have been so fortunate to access good health support. Through this and the support group we have accessed specialist resources for FASDs through Dr Mukherjee. This formal assessment has opened doors and given us that all important paper to wave at educationalists and budget holders, with a specialist name at the bottom that says these parents are not making this up, this child does need extra support.

Seeing family life through a different lens

Writing this makes me realize how much I have changed by being surrounded at all times by FASDs. I have become more tolerant in some things, less in others. I have become more accepting of the rough and tumble, of the fights, the bumps and knocks. It is not just *having children* that has brought about this change. It is the *children I have*.

I think of the things we have achieved. I think of the joy of seeing our daughter come home after her first day at Brownies, how excited and animated she was, how proud of herself when she made her Brownie promise, and of when the tennis teacher told her she had the best backhand. I think of the first kiss she was able to give John and me. I think of her determination to ride her bike; and watching her play in the sea, her fascination with water and waves.

I also think of our son playing Joseph in the nursery play – always a tearjerker! – and the way he cannot sleep without his special teddy. I think of him tickling John – just because he can!; his love of reading books – anywhere; his constant questioning; and his ability to make us all laugh.

We have friends who have children with special needs; they share a lot of challenges we face. They do understand our frustration with trying to get resources, and the obstacles that are in the way. A difference is that FASDs are so unknown that they are either dismissed, not taken seriously, or not fully understood by many. The stigma attached to the condition is different from others too. This should not be underestimated for the parents or the children.

I once read that we have the children we are supposed to have. I do miss the peace and quiet and predictability of my life as it used to be, but I would not have missed any of this. It has made us the family we are. I love the children for that; I love what they have given to John and me; and what I have learnt about myself and the lessons yet to be learnt. I could not say to anyone that they should adopt a child with an FASD, but I would not say do not.

8

FETAL ALCOHOL SPECTRUM DISORDERS AND CHILDREN IN CARE

Good care makes a difference

Kevin Williams

Ollie's story

Ollie is 18 years old and looking forward to starting university. That of itself is not unusual. After all, nearly 40 per cent of UK citizens will graduate from tertiary education (DfE 2010, 2011a). However, for Ollie, getting to university represents a significant achievement. Ollie was in the care system and as such has managed to overcome the shocking adversity faced by Looked After Children. It is a national scandal that only 6 per cent of children in care in the UK will go into higher education (DfE 2010, 2011b).

Ollie, the eldest of three siblings, has been in care since the age of eight. He entered the care system as a result of physical abuse and neglect from both parents. He was separated from his siblings following the breakdown of his first foster placement, where his siblings remain. His early experiences in care were difficult as he was initially disruptive and was moved through a number of different foster placements. He was easily distracted and hyperactive, and many of those who worked with him in education and social care believed him to be wilfully disobedient. He seemed not to learn from his experiences and had little concept of the consequences of his impulsive behaviour. Although he had few friends, he believed himself popular and consequently exhibited inappropriate over-friendly behaviour and a limited understanding of other people's feelings. He was easily led, and was often enticed into bad behaviour. This was compounded by an apparent lack of fear which put him in danger on a number of occasions. Ollie found school hard and generally under-achieved although he excelled in areas that he was interested in. He showed a particular aptitude for art, while finding concentration in academic subjects more difficult. We will return to Ollie later in this chapter.

The nature and cause of fetal alcohol spectrum disorders (FASDs) means it has a particular prevalence among children in the care system. This is because of the often chaotic nature of those families who have children taken into care. While no research exists to estimate how many children are affected, the numbers, particularly in foster care, are significant. In 2010, there were 64,400 children in care in England and a further 5,162 in Wales. In England 47,200 (73 per cent) were in foster care with a further 4,049 (79 per cent) in Wales. Sixty-one per cent of these children were in care as a result of abuse and neglect, while 11 per cent were looked after as a result of family dysfunction. A further 9 per cent entered the care system as the family were in acute stress (DfE 2010).

Despite the system working well for many children, outcomes for children in care are often poor in comparison to the general population. They are more likely to end up homeless, resort to drug and alcohol misuse, and have mental health issues and lower educational attainment. This is not surprising given that the early life experiences of so many children involve abuse and neglect. In 2006, 63 per cent of children in care achieved one GCSE while only 12 per cent achieved five or more GCSEs compared with 98 per cent of their peer group achieving one GCSE and 59 per cent achieving five or more. This explains the poor admission rate into tertiary education mentioned above. These poor achievements can only be partly explained by the fact that 28 per cent of children in care have a Statement of Special Educational Needs (DfE 2010).

Ultimately, these differences in education have a lifetime impact and influence career and other life chances. We know that employment is a key factor in determining access to other services and activities. Those with better-paid jobs access better housing, better leisure activities and enjoy better health including mental health and emotional well being.

The Adolescent and Children's Trust (TACT)[1] believes that going into care can, and should, be positive for any child. There are reams of statistical and anecdotal evidence that shows that a stable, well-supported foster placement can transform lives (Broad 2011; Schofield *et al.* 2012). However, the overall statistics still make depressing reading. It is estimated that one in four of the adult prison population has spent time in care, that adults who have spent time in care are more likely to suffer mental health issues, more likely to end up homeless, and more likely to abuse alcohol and drugs. They are also more likely to have their own children taken into care, and at an earlier age, having been more likely to become teenage parents than their peers.

These poor long-term outcomes are the results of early life traumas and the abuse or neglect that they suffered as children. These early life difficulties are exacerbated by a care system in which, too often, placement stability is poor, with children experiencing many placement moves often resulting in school moves and disruption to friendships and family relationships.

This all makes for depressing reading so, returning to Ollie, it is worth seeing what can happen when the system works properly, particularly for children affected by FASD. Ollie had four placements before moving to his current foster carer six years ago. His behaviour continued to be challenging at times, but he also had a loving and caring nature and formed a strong bond with his single carer. He had occasional contact with his birth mother who continued to lead a chaotic lifestyle using drugs and abusing alcohol. Over time, Ollie became more settled. His carer worked closely with his school and, despite a small number of fixed-term exclusions, Ollie's work improved and he began to excel at art. After achieving six GCSEs, he went to a local college to study art further.

In 2009, six years after his placement began, his carer attended a training course on FASD. She described the experience as 'like a light coming on', as she realized that Ollie's behaviours and social interaction were classic indicators of someone affected by FASD. She was aware of Ollie's early history and his mother's drug and alcohol use. However, previously she had no reason to connect this with FASD indicators such as his sensitivity to excess stimuli and his preference for quiet environments. She has since learnt to provide a structured routine for Ollie and is now aware of the need to repeat instructions and rehearse social scenarios to help him cope. Following the training, Ollie's carer arranged a multi-agency assessment including social work, psychiatric, psychological and paediatric inputs, and Ollie was formally diagnosed as being on the fetal alcohol spectrum.

Diagnosis is vital. It not only helps to access appropriate services, but helps allow Ollie and others to have a better understanding of their behaviours and how they can be managed. Moving forward, Ollie will continue to receive support from his foster carer, and she will help him with the transition to independence via university. However, now he is an adult, he will need to manage a whole new set of relationships. He will need to manage a range of new social situations as well as the many practicalities of living independently such as paying the bills and budgeting. For Ollie, this presents a particular challenge as he will need to curb his instinctive urge for the immediate gratification offered by large purchases such as a new computer. These are realities for lots of young adults in Ollie's position, but most will not have the added difficulties associated with his FASD diagnosis.

Kylie's story

Kylie is a 12-year-old who came into care aged three with a history of neglect, physical abuse and sexual abuse, at the hands of her single parent mother and her associates/friends. Kylie is the oldest of three siblings and her early childhood experiences led to her having very challenging behaviour. She presented as anxious and hyper-vigilant, and had a diagnosis of 'global developmental delay'. She has experienced several fixed-term and one permanent exclusion. Her mother had a history of alcohol use and, following concerns about Kylie's behaviour from her current carers and multi-agency assessment, at the age of seven she was diagnosed as being on the FASD spectrum. Social workers worked closely with Kylie and her carers to help manage her behaviours and to adopt strategies for dealing with social and other situations. One of the main issues concerned consistency between home and school routines so Kylie's teacher and other school staff were included in developing and working with strategies to be used at home. At this stage Kylie was given a Statement of Special Educational Needs, and, at the age of ten, began to attend a local special school as a day pupil.

Exclusions are a major issue for Looked After Children. In England, only 0.02 per cent of primary school children were permanently excluded in 2009–2010. However, for Looked After Children, the figure rises to 0.16 per cent, eight times the rate. For boys in care the ratio is even higher with 0.28 per cent excluded, a staggering 14 times as many as the national average. The pattern is similar, albeit lower, in secondary schools. Overall, 0.15 per cent of all children were excluded as compared with 0.58 per cent for Looked After Children. In special schools 0.11 per cent of all children were excluded rising to 0.28 per cent for Looked After Children. The gender disparity is not reflected here although slightly more girls than boys were excluded (DfE 2010, 2011a).

These figures highlight Kylie's risk of permanent school exclusion and potential foster placement disruption. This carries not only the high human cost of a placement move, but also a high economic cost of finding a new placement, likely to be significantly more expensive. The average annual cost of a foster care placement is in the region of £26,000. This rises to £130,000 for the average cost of a residential children's home placement (Boarding Schools Association 2007; Lombard 2011).

Children like Kylie need consistency and recognition of the brain damage they have suffered. She needs to be seen as a young person who sometimes 'cannot' rather than one who 'will not'. She needs awareness of the difficulties she faces remembering routine, tasks and instructions; understanding social norms; comprehending the consequences of actions; and learning appropriate behaviour and communication.

Kylie's social worker worked with her carers and teachers to develop strategies to manage some of these behaviour traits. A regular routine and consistency are of utmost importance. Kylie's carers established a regular pattern in the mornings before school. They often used visual stimuli as reminders of activities Kylie had to do such as a picture of brushing teeth on the bathroom wall. There was repetition of activities to assist with long-term memory recall. Instructions were clear and avoided ambiguity. For example, when being asked to tidy her room she would get instructions using unambiguous language and picture prompts of where items went.

The carers and school needed to adapt how they responded to and managed Kylie. An example of how communications could be misinterpreted arose when Kylie's social worker asked her 'if her carers were different'. She replied, 'No, they look the same to me.' The social worker had meant to ask whether the carers had been behaving differently but Kylie had taken her literally. An awareness of the vagaries of language is vital in ensuring effective communication.

As in all areas of social policy, fostering and adoption exist in a political context. Historically, a desire to increase adoption rates crosses political divides. In 2000, the then Prime Minister Tony Blair ordered a review of Adoption Law, giving his personal pledge to increase numbers. In 2011 Tim Loughton, Under-Secretary of State for Children and Young Families, appointed former Barnardo's CEO, Martin Narey as 'Government Special Advisor on Adoption'. His brief was also to look at increasing the numbers of adoptions and to identify potential improvements in the adoption process.

Despite this political commitment adoption numbers have been steadily declining. In 2004–2005, there were 3,800 Looked After Children adopted, but in 2008–9 this number had fallen to 3,300 despite an increase in the number of children coming into care. Almost 60 per cent of children adopted in 2010 were aged between one and four years compared with 41 per cent in 2000 (DfE 2011b). This shows a reduction in the number of older children being adopted. Arguably this is in part due to the complex needs of children over five years old in the care system. The Consortium of Voluntary Adoption Agencies has identified the highest additional need of children being adopted was due to maternal substance abuse during pregnancy.

Pete's story

Pete was adopted when he was 10 months old. His birth mother had mental health problems and was diagnosed with schizophrenia. She had been homeless and a sex worker. She had been in care herself, and admitted to cocaine, opiate and other substance abuse since her early teens. She also abused alcohol, drinking over a litre of vodka a day. During pregnancy she did not attend antenatal appointments regularly, and Pete was born at 36 weeks gestation. He was delivered by emergency caesarean after fetal distress in labour. Pete was born with low birth weight (4 lbs 4 oz) with dysmorphic facial presentation. Features of fetal alcohol syndrome (FAS) were noted at birth. Despite knowing that Pete had organic brain damage, potential adopters were identified, and he moved in with them aged three months.

An issue of particular importance for adoptive families of FASD-affected children is the support available. At the age of six years, Pete required continued access to a range of services, from health, including specialist dentists and opticians, to education, while his adoptive parents required a range of supports, particularly from FASD peer support groups and social workers to help manage the range of interventions and to offer them ongoing moral support as parents of a child with very complex needs. He has been assessed on a number of occasions. At two years old and again aged five, he was specifically assessed by The Adolescent and Children's Trust Fetal Alcohol Team. In his earlier assessment the carers were much less concerned about Pete's behavioural presentation. They felt that in many ways Pete was just a typical toddler. They were hopeful that his behaviour would continue to improve with proper care and nurture. The local authority adoption social worker shared this view, and showed little real understanding of the long-term implications of FAS.

Pete's adopters were informed that a great deal of the behavioural anomalies would not really start becoming obvious until he was of school age. When coming for the second assessment a few months ago, aged nine, the family's main concerns about Pete were as follows:

- He has an extremely poor attention span, is easily distracted and cannot sit still for more than a few minutes.
- He is very impulsive and has no concept of personal boundaries; this is causing a number of issues in the school environment with lack of awareness of others' space and belongings. Pete is also distracted by noise and finds too much stimulus difficult.
- He has fierce temper tantrums and will defy those in authority, screaming and at times physically hitting out.
- He usually wets the bed and still wears nappies at night.
- He is over friendly with strangers and indiscriminate in his behaviour; this requires 24-hour supervision.
- His sleep is very poor; he is fussy with food and particularly dislikes some textures.
- He often becomes fixated on an object or a subject and will discuss this *ad nauseam*.
- He remembers things one day and forgets them the next.
- His language is very good; he uses complex grammar, but his ability to understand concepts is limited, and he does not really understand the meaning behind the language he uses. This gives the impression that he is more able than he actually is.

It is very apparent that Pete is extremely hyperactive. ADHD is frequently found as one of a spectrum of difficulties associated with exposure to alcohol. Alcohol can produce a whole spectrum of dysfunctions on the developing central nervous system. The concern is that because Pete appeared to be progressing well, aged two years, in spite of his diagnosis, his adoption support package was underplayed. His behaviour continues to be difficult, and as he gets older this is likely to become increasingly challenging to manage. His post-adoption support package was limited, and did not provide for his ongoing needs. His adoptive parents are needing to argue for ongoing support from their local authority.

At this stage it is difficult to predict Pete's likely progress and educational ability. The local authority have been informed, by health professionals, that he is at risk of continuing attention problems, receptive speech delay, learning difficulties and behaviour problems as he grows. They have responded by saying that they cannot provide an adoption support package for something that TACT is unable to quantify. This is an issue that has come up in many cases. It demonstrates the need for urgent, ongoing training for social workers and other professionals about the long-term implications of FASD. His family will continue to need to fight for resources for Pete throughout his life even though he had a diagnosis at birth!

While adoption can provide a stable, lifelong placement for a child it is vital to be aware that adopted children will continue to need access to services. TACT is concerned that the current legal arrangements to ensure that these children and their adopters have access to services and supports are inadequate. Pete's case also highlights the lack of knowledge and awareness of FAS and FASD among wider professionals including social workers. This is a real issue, as during assessments it is important that social workers are aware of the need to collect information about maternal drinking and drug use during pregnancy. This helps, not only with diagnosis, but also to help identify prevalence rates.

Candice's story

Candice is a five-year-old who came into care shortly after her second birthday. Candice had four placements prior to her current foster placement which has lasted approximately 14 months. One of these, which followed two disrupted foster placements, was with her birth father. This only lasted for a short period of time due to her very challenging behaviour. Social services knew little about the birth mother prior to the incident of physical abuse that led to Candice being taken into care, and little information had been collected by the social worker before the birth. At four years old, Candice was assessed as having global developmental delay. When she was placed with her current carers, Candice could not speak and was constantly active. Her birth mother had described her as a naughty child exhibiting temper tantrums and screaming. Candice would only sleep for a few hours each night, and when awake she would be destructive and aggressive. She would break toys and was considered a danger to herself. Behaviours included biting, scratching others and herself as well as episodes of head banging.

Candice attends a special school for children with profound, severe and complex learning difficulties. It was her teacher, who had worked with children with FASD, who first suggested the need for an assessment to consider FAS and FASD. The assessment was multidimensional and included ten validated psychometric screening tests. These were:

1. The four-digit diagnostic code which was developed by the FAS Diagnostic and Preventative Network at the University of Washington; this computer program accurately measures the key facial features associated with FAS based on digital photographs of the child's face.
2. The Wechsler Intelligence Scales for children, which measure intellectual abilities.
3. The Story Stems Assessment profile, which focuses on attachment and family history.
4. The Ruth Griffiths Scale of Mental Development, which assesses the developmental abilities from birth to eight years.
5. The Vineland Adaptive Behaviour Scales II, which is a measure of personal and social skills and functioning.
6. Parents' Evaluation of Developmental Status (PEDS), which is an indicator of the child's risk of developmental and behavioural problems.
7. The Social Communication Questionnaire, which is an autism screening instrument.

8. The Social Responsiveness Scale, which measures the severity of social impairment associated with autistic spectrum disorders.
9. The Developmental Behaviour Checklist, which assesses behavioural and emotional disturbance.
10. The ADHD Screening Questionnaire, administered by a TACT psychologist.

Due to Candice's behaviour it was not possible to undertake all of the assessments, but sufficient were undertaken, in particular the digital photographic recognition, which confirmed that Candice had moderate facial dysmorphology associated with FAS. This diagnosis not only enabled Candice's carers to access appropriate services, but it also helped them with behavioural management. Working with professionals with knowledge in this area has helped develop coping strategies that will improve Candice's behaviour and socialization. There is no cure for FAS or FASD but recognition of this as a lifelong condition allows those affected to be helped and managed.

Many children in care achieve their dreams and go on to live normal lives. Many foster carers become 'family' for the children they have cared for. Indeed, foster carers often remain supportive into the child's adulthood eventually becoming 'foster grandparents'. For other children, the care system provides a stable childhood from which they go on to lead enriched and happy lives despite their early life traumas. Research undertaken by TACT, *Aspirations: The views of foster children and their carers* (Broad 2008, 2011), showed that, for nearly 95 per cent of children in long-term TACT foster care placements, their current foster carer was 'very important'. This compared with nearly 87 per cent for siblings, 73 per cent for birth mothers and only 46 per cent for birth fathers. However, for a significant number, we see the cycle of the care system repeating itself. Eighty per cent of children in care are there because of abuse and neglect, family dysfunction or because families were in acute stress. As mentioned earlier we know that long-term outcomes for children in care are poor in terms of substance abuse, early pregnancy and having their own children taken into care. It follows that children in care are more likely than the general population to have parents who abuse alcohol and or drugs and that this abuse may have occurred during pregnancy. It is therefore likely that more children in care will be on the FASD spectrum with their condition often undiagnosed or misdiagnosed.

This knowledge should help us influence practice, and there is a need for social work assessments to include assessments of maternal drug and alcohol use during pregnancy. Without the collection of this information young people may miss out on the services that they require. Children taken into care where maternal drinking is a factor in the care application should have access to an assessment for FASD given the numbers who are probably undiagnosed.

There is a need to educate all young women about the dangers of drinking during pregnancy. This need is heightened for at-risk groups like young women in care. In addition, there is a need to educate professionals working with children in care about FAS and FASD. The policy implications for both children in care and foster care include the need to develop not only multi-agency assessments, but also to provide appropriate services to young people and support to carers. There is a particular need for these services to be consistent during periods of transition where routines and support systems may change.

I hope that Ollie does well at university. I am confident he will succeed through continued support from his foster carer although, now that Ollie is an adult and has left her home, she will receive no remuneration. She in turn will be able to rely on ongoing and unpaid support from her foster agency. These continued relationships are vital in helping those who cannot rely on familial ties to succeed.

Note

1   www.tactcare.org.uk

References

Boarding Schools' Association (2007) *Unit Cost of Health and Social Care*, Canterbury: Personal Social Services Research Unit, University of Kent.

Broad, B. (2008) *Aspirations: The views of foster children and their carers* (Full research report). London: London Southbank University/The Adolescent and Children's Trust.

Broad, B. (2011) *Aspirations Three Years On: The views of young people who are fostered and their carers (research report)*, London: The Adolescent and Children's Trust.

Department for Education (2010) *Outcomes for Children Looked After by Local Authorities in England, as at 31 March 2010 (Statistical first release)*, London: DfE.

Department for Education (2011a) *GCSE and Equivalent Results in England 2009/10 Revised (Statistical First Release 01/2011)*. London: DfE.

Department for Education (2011b) *Children looked after in England (including adoption and care leavers) year ending 31 March 2011 (SFR 21/2011)*. London: DfE.

Lombard, D. (2011) 'Can boarding schools help prevent children being taken into care?', *Community Care*, 4 September [online at: www.communitycare.co.uk/articles/04/09/2011/117386/can-boarding-schools-help-prevent-children-being-taken-into-care.htm; accessed: 11 January 2013].

Schofield, G., Ward, E., Biggart, L., Scaife, V., Dodsworth, J., Larsson, B., Haynes, A. and Stone, N. (2012) *Looked After Children and Offending: Reducing risk and promoting resilience*, Norwich: University of East Anglia.

PART III
Education

9

FETAL ALCOHOL SPECTRUM DISORDERS

Knowledge and referral pathways in early childhood settings in Western Australia

Kate Frances

Introduction

To date, much of the published research on fetal alcohol syndrome (FAS)/fetal alcohol spectrum disorder (FASD) in Australia has focused on determining the level of knowledge held about fetal alcohol-related disorders by both health professionals and the general population (Elliott and Bower 2004; O'Leary 2004; Payne *et al.* 2005). One such Western Australian study found that health professionals' knowledge of FAS was limited, with most suggesting the need for educational resources for themselves and for women about alcohol and pregnancy (Payne *et al.* 2005). Moreover, the dearth of diagnostic services in Australia, the lack of consensus regarding diagnostic criteria and the lack of knowledge about FASD management by health professionals have all been raised as concerns (Elliott *et al.* 2006; O'Leary 2004; Peadon *et al.* 2008; Telethon Institute for Child Health Research 2011).

Explorations of levels of knowledge of FAS/FASDs across other sectors coming into contact with this population (e.g. early childhood, education, criminal justice, community services) have, so far in Australia, been absent from the research agenda. International research, on the other hand, is moving beyond exploration of levels of knowledge, awareness and diagnosis to focus on identifying effective interventions and service responses for FASD-affected children, with some of this work focusing on the formal education sector (Adnams *et al.* 2007; Blackburn *et al.* 2009, 2012; Bohjanen *et al.* 2009; Edmonds and Crichton 2008; Healthy Child Manitoba 2010; Leslie and Roberts 2001; Ryan and Ferguson 2006) and, to a much lesser extent, on the early childhood sector (Blackburn 2009). While few of these interventions have been rigorously evaluated (Duquette *et al.* 2006; Premji *et al.* 2006; Ryan and Chionnaith 2006), there are increasing calls for training and support for teachers, teacher support staff and school psychologists to enable them to understand and implement the different approaches required to educate and support a child with FASDs (Blackburn 2009; Crawford 2008; Telethon Institute for Child Health Research 2011).

A preliminary qualitative study carried out in the UK in 2008, seeking to explore some existing educational practices of teachers in primary, secondary and special schools, reports a significant shortfall in guidance for teachers on how to educate children with FASDs (Carpenter

2011). These findings are similar to those found in a recent Canadian exploratory study conducted to document the experiences of classroom teachers, administrators, allied professionals and caregivers as recipients and communicators of effective learning strategies for children with FASDs; the authors report that significant challenges are experienced at the community and school levels including insufficient knowledge of FASDs (Job *et al.* 2011). In another UK study, which explored the support and education of children with FASDs in early years settings, it was found that, of the 161 early years staff who responded to a survey-based study, 78 per cent had little knowledge of FASDs and felt that this lack of knowledge would have a detrimental effect on their ability to meet the needs of an FASD-affected child (Blackburn 2009).

As a poorly recognized and largely undiagnosed population, most students with FASDs are, therefore, inevitably placed in regular classroom settings, with teachers often unaware of both this group of children and of how to meet their special educational needs (SEN) (Blackburn 2009; Carpenter 2011; Crawford 2008; Telethon Institute for Child Health Research 2011). Compounding this situation is the fact that FASDs are currently not recognized as a disability in Australia, unlike in the United States and Canada, with no funding available for special supports for either these children or their teachers (Crawford 2008; Telethon Institute for Child Health Research 2011). With this poor recognition of FASDs it is unsurprising, therefore, that there has been little advice for educators working with FASD-affected children and, adding support to the international studies mentioned above, Australian educators are also often ill prepared to meet the children's learning, behavioural and social needs (Crawford 2008; DEEWR undated). As places where developmental delays and social interaction issues are often identified for the first time, early childhood settings/formal education settings are very important sites in the pathway to recognition, identification and intervention services for these children and their families (Blackburn 2009; Carpenter 2011).

Resources, designed to provide information, increase knowledge and/or develop skills around the issues inherent in FASD-affected children and their families, have been developed for early years practitioners and educators, predominantly coming out of the United States and Canada. These resources are readily available on the internet, and include FASD training programmes as well as guides containing a variety of classroom strategies (for example, Alberta Learning 2004; Blackburn *et al.* 2012; Blackburn 2009; Healthy Child Manitoba 2010; Yukon Department of Education 2006). Resources alone, however, are insufficient to build practitioners/educators' capacities to provide optimal learning environments and experiences for these children. Training and support, not only for practitioners/educators but for all professionals involved in providing intervention services for the child, their family and the community in which they live, are vital (Ryan and Ferguson 2006). This is especially so in the context of Australia, if it aims to meets its commitment to children, their families and society more broadly to:

> extend and enrich children's learning from birth to 5 years and through the transition to school. The Council of Australian Governments has developed this [Early Years Learning] Framework to assist educators to provide young children with opportunities to maximise their potential and develop a foundation for future successes in learning. In this way, the Early Years Learning Framework ... will contribute to realising the Council of Australian Governments' vision that ... 'All children have the best start in life to create a better future for themselves and for the nation'
>
> *(DEEWR 2009: 5)*

This Early Learning Framework draws upon international evidence-informed understandings of: early childhood as a vital period in children's learning and development; how children develop and learn; and what conditions and experiences children need to do this well (DEEWR 2009: 5). Within this Framework, emphasis is placed upon the importance of early years practitioners working in partnership with children, families and other professionals to identify and assess children who may need additional support and to both choose/provide appropriate teaching strategies and to assist families to access specialist help where needed (DEEWR 2009: 17). While this Framework is still in the introductory stage, practitioners in early learning and care settings are expected to familiarize themselves with it and, in time, develop their own strategy for its implementation, taking their own unique context into consideration.

Study objectives

The objectives of the project were to explore knowledge of FASDs in early learning and care settings in Western Australia, to explore awareness of referral pathways for children with suspected FASDs in those settings, and to identify use of services and incidence of referrals for children with suspected FASDs in those settings.

Methods

The study was carried out between January 2011 and April 2012 and involved the collection of primary data through a questionnaire to early learning and care settings in Western Australia. Early learning and care settings included community and assisted playgroups, long day care and occasional care, and kindergartens and preschools (administered by the Western Australian Department of Education). In total, questionnaires were sent to 1,083 sites with an overall response rate of 22 per cent achieved (see Table 9.1).

The Fetal Alcohol Spectrum Disorders Survey

The questionnaire was adapted from the questionnaires developed for the Fetal Alcohol Syndrome Study, Telethon Institute for Child Health Research, Western Australia, and Building Bridges with Understanding: Foetal Alcohol Spectrum Disorders (FASD), Sunfield Research Institute, UK. Permission was sought and given by authors of these questionnaires for their adaption/use in this project. The survey was piloted with 15 early learning and care practitioners to assess face validity.

TABLE 9.1 Survey sample and response rates per sector

Settings	Invitations	Responses	% response rate
Community/assisted playgroups	55	21	38
Kindergartens/preschools	469	123	26
Long day care/occasional care	559	83	15

The questionnaire contained a combination of closed- and open-ended questions providing for both qualitative and quantitative data collection. Closed-ended questions included demographic data (including sex, age, qualifications, employment status, and location and type of early learning and care setting), awareness of FASDs, sources of knowledge of FASDs, and experiences of working with FASD-affected children. A Likert scale was also used in exploring participants' knowledge about the range of possible effects of FASDs and their opinion on whether they felt they were equipped with appropriate skills and knowledge to support children who have FASDs and their families. Here participants were asked to indicate their degree of agreement to a set of statements (for example, 'people with FASD have a set of birth defects' and 'people with FASD have these effects throughout their lives') by checking one of five response categories (categories included 'strongly agree', 'tend to agree', 'not sure', 'tend to disagree' and 'strongly disagree').

The scope of open-ended questions, designed to allow participants to record their own experiences and knowledge of FASDs, included: the types of formal and/or informal processes that were followed in the event they identified/suspected an FASD-affected child in their setting; the types of strategies found to be effective in supporting children with FASDs; and opinions on the types of resources that could be developed to support early years practitioners working with children with FASDs.

Data analysis

Each questionnaire was assigned a unique identifier (case number). Quantitative and qualitative (which tended to consist of single words or brief phrases) data were extracted from each of the completed questionnaires and entered into the SPSS database (Statistical (software analysis) Package for the Social Sciences). Descriptive statistics were generated to provide both percentages of the proportion of participants who answered in a certain way, and the frequency with which participants answered any given question (some participants omitted to answer some questions). The research questions provided the focus for the qualitative data analysis: the qualitative data were organized by each (relevant) question, across all participant responses, to identify consistencies and differences. The themes that emerged were then coded in order to organize the data into categories, and then sorted into categories.

From the quantitative data, the most surprising theme to emerge was the discrepancy between the majority of participants' response to a question relating to their knowledge of FASDs (the majority ticked the box corresponding with 'I know a little bit about FASD', suggesting that they did not have a high degree of knowledge) and the relatively high degree of knowledge displayed when asked opinions on the effects of FASDs (see Table 9.4 for results).

Ethics

Approval for the study was obtained from Curtin University Human Research Ethics Committee, and the Government of Western Australia, Department of Education.

Results

Response to survey

A final sample size of 236 responses was achieved. Given the challenges the early learning and care sector in Australia experiences in attracting, retaining and developing early learning and care professionals (DEEWR 2011), the achieved sample size was considered a good result, and represented adequate power from which to conduct analysis and interpret results.

Settings in which participants worked

The majority of participants both worked in the Western Australian Government's formal kindergarten/preschool sector, and were located within the Perth metropolitan region (57.2 per cent). See Table 9.2 for self-reported knowledge of FASDs by type of setting.

Knowledge of FASDs

Of the 236 participants, the majority reported that they had some knowledge of FASDs, 19 reported that they knew a lot about FASDs, 15 reported that they had heard of FASDs but did not know what they were, and two participants reported that they had never heard of FASDs. One hundred and two participants reported that they had gained their knowledge through the media, and 76 through children's services support agencies. Thirty-three participants indicated that they had gained their knowledge from their employer. For a summary, see Table 9.3.

TABLE 9.2 Self-reported knowledge of FASDs by type of setting

Setting	Frequency	%
Kindergarten/preschool	135	57.45
Long day care centre	81	34.47
Supported playgroup	6	2.55
Aboriginal-specific playgroup	5	2.13
Other	5	2.13
Community-led playgroup	3	1.28

TABLE 9.3 Self-assessment of amount of knowledge of FASDs

Knowledge	Frequency	%
Know a little about FASD	199	84.3
Know a lot about FASD	19	8.1
Heard of FASD but do not know what it is	15	6.4
Never heard of FASD	2	0.8

Knowledge of the effects of maternal alcohol consumption during pregnancy

It has been acknowledged in the literature that the severity of the effects of maternal alcohol consumption during pregnancy may differ for the individual child and factors such as the pattern and quantity of alcohol consumption, timing of intake, the stage of development of the fetus at the time of exposure, and socio-behavioural risk factors such as poverty and smoking may all act as permissive influences that increase the likelihood of FASDs (Abel and Hannigan 1994; Chudley et al. 2005).

The majority of participants indicated that they strongly agreed/tended to agree with a range of adverse effects for those affected with FASDs across the physical, behavioural and cognitive domains (see Table 9.4).

Levels of skills/knowledge to support children with FASDs

When asked to indicate whether they felt they were equipped with appropriate skills and knowledge to support children who have FASDs and their families, the majority of participants indicated that they did not believe that they did. Additionally, 89 per cent of participants also indicated that they had received no training in the past year to equip them with strategies for supporting children who have FASDs, while 83 per cent indicated that there were no alternative resources or special education strategies in their setting to support children who have FASDs. Those who did report employing strategies they found to be effective (31 participants) noted regular routines, continuity of carers, behaviour management plans, working with families, and supports from other agencies. For a summary, see Table 9.5.

TABLE 9.4 Knowledge[1] of effects of maternal alcohol consumption during pregnancy on the developing fetus

Effect	Frequency	%
Affects a person's ability to learn (n = 225)[2]	195	86.7
Affects a person's memory (n = 224)	186	83.0
Affects a person's understanding (n = 224)	177	79.0
Affects a person's ability to reason (n = 225)	172	76.4
Affects a person's motor skills (n = 225)	171	76.0
Affects a person's judgement (n = 226)	169	74.8
Affects a person's ability to plan	167	74.6
Affects a person's ability to interact socially (n = 225)	163	72.4
Complex medical needs (n = 219)	154	70.3
Intellectual disability (n = 224)	150	67.0
Will have these effects throughout their lives (n = 224)	147	65.6
Brain damage (n = 225)	142	63.1
Set of birth defects (n = 223)	139	62.3
Affected physically (n = 223)	139	62.3
Affects a child's imaginative play (n = 226)	138	61.1

Notes
1 Categories 'strongly agree' and 'tend to agree' combined.
2 n refers to the number of participants who actually responded to the statement out of the 236 completed questionnaires. Out of those who did respond, the frequency refers to how many participants indicated knowledge of the effects of FASDs.

TABLE 9.5 Working with children who have FASDs[1]

Opinion	Frequency	%
Disagree that I have received training in past year directed specifically at strategies for working with children who have FASD (n = 225)[2]	210	93.3
Disagree that I have appropriate skills/knowledge to support the families of children who have FASD (n = 227)	169	87.7
Disagree that I have appropriate skills/knowledge to support children who have FASD (n = 229)	197	86
Disagree that there are alternative resources or special education strategies in my setting to help children who have FASD (n = 226)	188	83.2

Notes
1 Categories 'strongly disagree', 'tend to disagree' and 'not sure' combined.
2 n refers to the number of participants who actually responded to the statement out of the 236 completed questionnaires.

On the other hand, almost half the participants (49 per cent) identified that they felt they had the support of their organization/co-practitioners to support those children presenting with (suspected) FASDs.

Identification of child with suspected FASDs

Of the 236 participants, 72 indicated that they had identified/suspected a child in their setting as having an FASD, with a further 80 participants noting that they had suspected FASDs but 'took it no further'. Only 38 participants indicated that they had actually cared for an FASD-affected child.

Suspicions about FASD

Issues that raised participants' suspicions in their identification of a child having a (suspected) FASD included delayed developmental milestones, behavioural difficulties, facial features (anomalies) and height/weight challenges (Astley and Clarren 2000). Other indicators were noted as learning difficulties, family history and information provided by carers and/or other agencies in touch with the child and their family. For a summary, see Table 9.6.

TABLE 9.6 Type of suspicions which alerted participants to possible FASDs

Suspicions	Frequency	%
Delayed developmental milestones	69	29.2
Behavioural difficulties	62	26.3
Facial features (anomalies)	48	20.3
Height/weight challenges	32	13.6

Use of referral pathways

Of the 72 participants who indicated that they had identified/suspected a child in their setting as having an FASD, 31 indicated that they had referred families and children to other services (including one who noted that channels were in place at the school level). Five participants noted that, as well as the professionals to whom they had referred children and families, they were also aware of other agency involvement, including: Juvenile Justice, Disability Services Commission and the Department for Communities. As well as direct referrals, other processes followed through after identification/suspicion of FASDs included observations and documentation of the child's behaviours and discussions with family/carers and/or colleagues. Five participants noted that they did not know what to do and/or that there were no formal processes in place. For a summary, see Table 9.7.

However, 74 per cent of the 236 participants indicated that they could not identify the services that were available for children with FASDs/suspected FASDs in their region.

Resources

Of the 236 participants, 75 per cent provided us with information on the types of resources that they believed could be developed/made available to support early childhood professionals in working with and supporting children with FASDs and their families. Analysis of this qualitative data showed that the majority (55 per cent) would like to see: FASD-specific training included as a formal, ongoing component of professional development activities; FASD-specific training made available through regular workshops and seminars; and/or health promotion/awareness campaigns targeted at early childhood professionals, parents/carers and the wider community.

Forty-one per cent of responses referred specifically to the development/availability of resources (to include booklets, pamphlets, brochures and audio/visual material) providing information on causes, symptoms, signs, referral processes and screening options. Human

TABLE 9.7 Frequency of referrals by participants

Referral pathway	Frequency
Allied health professional[1]	6
Pediatrician	6
GP	5
Child Development Centre	4
School psychologist	3
Department for Child Protection	3
School nurse	2
Other	2

Note
1 In Australia, Allied Health professionals work alongside doctors and nurses and include audiologists, chiropractors, dieticians, exercise physiologists, occupational therapists, orthoptists, orthotists and prosthetists, osteopaths, hospital pharmacists, podiatrists, psychologists, sonographers, social practitioners and speech pathologists (www.ahpa.com.au).

resources were also referenced by 16 participants, citing additional teacher aids in the classroom, closer collaboration between health professionals/children's services and schools, and support from a professional FASD expert. For a summary, see Table 9.8.

Discussion

The purpose of this study was to explore: knowledge of FASDs in early learning and care settings in Western Australia; awareness of referral pathways for children with suspected FASDs in those settings; and to identify use of services and incidence of referrals for children with suspected FASDs in those settings. While the majority of participants indicated a high level of knowledge on the range of effects associated with FASDs across the physical, behavioural and cognitive domains, we believe that it will come as no surprise to those working within this area in Australia that the findings of this study support others that found significant gaps in skills and knowledge in those professionals/practitioners working with FASD-affected children (and their families) (for example, Blackburn 2009; Carpenter 2011; Job et al. 2011).

It is also unsurprising, when contextualized within these studies overall, that only 26 of the 236 participants of this study had actually referred a child and their family for intervention services/supports, and that there does not appear to be a consistent approach to the strategies employed to support a child with FASDs in the various early learning and care settings in Western Australia.

To reinforce the call for training and support for all those working with children and families affected by FASDs, several participants of this study provided information additional to that asked for in our survey. One respondent in particular provided information to the author, in a confidential email, confirming that many of the early childhood educators with whom they worked did not understand (suspected) FASD-affected children's behaviours, and/or did not have the skills to manage those behaviours. Individual learning programmes to meet the child's need and include them in the service/classroom were 'never developed', more likely a 'behaviour management plan [was] implemented' with expectations that the child would comply, when in reality they could not. Consequently the (very young) children were often labelled as 'naughty' and then excluded from the service (personal correspondence, 2011). This is a very disturbing trend and one that does not bode well for those children in their transitions to formal schooling.

This study also supports the conclusion of the study carried out by Payne and colleagues (2005) into health professionals' knowledge, practice and opinions about FAS and alcohol consumption in pregnancy and the authors' assertion that, until this lack of knowledge is addressed for the health sector, opportunities for diagnosis and prevention of FAS will be

TABLE 9.8 Possible resources/resource issues suggested by participants

Resources	Frequency	%
FASD-specific training/awareness campaigns	96	54.5
Development and/or availability of resources	73	41.4
Human resources	16	9.1

limited; similarly, until this lack of knowledge is addressed for the early years sector, opportunities for intervention will be limited and FASD-affected children's opportunities to 'have the best start in life to create a better future for themselves' (DEEWR 2009: 5) will continue to be denied.

Conclusion

As the first exploratory study of its kind (that we know of) to have been carried out in Western Australia, the findings provide a baseline of knowledge upon which further research can be conducted into examples of effective interventions, appropriate professional development and support materials for staff in early learning and care settings in Australia.

References

Abel, E.L. and Hannigan, J.H. (1994) 'Maternal risk factors in fetal alcohol syndrome: provocative and permissive influences', *Neurotoxicology and Teratology*, 17(4): 445–62.

Adnams, C.M., Sorour, P., Kalberg, W.O., Kodituwakku, P.W., Perold, M.D., Kotze, A., September, S., Castle, B., Gossage, J.P. and May, P.A. (2007) 'Language and literacy outcomes from a pilot intervention study for children with FASD in South Africa', *Alcohol*, 41(6): 403–14.

Alberta Learning (2004) *Programming for Students with Special Needs Book 10. Teaching Students with Fetal Alcohol Spectrum Disorder: Building strengths, creating hope*, Edmonton, Alberta: Alberta Learning [online at: www.education.alberta.ca/admin/special/resources/FASD.aspx; accessed: 29 March 2012].

Astley, S.J and Clarren, S.K. (2000) 'Diagnosing the full spectrum of fetal alcohol-exposed individuals: introducing the 4-Digit Diagnostic Code', *Alcohol and Alcoholism*, 35(4): 400–10.

Blackburn, C. (2009) 'Foetal alcohol spectrum disorder: focus on strategies', in Blackburn, C. (2009) *Building Bridges with Understanding*, Clent, Worcestershire: Sunfield Research Institute and Worcestershire County Council [online at: www.sunfield.org.uk/pdf/FASD_Building_Bridges.pdf; accessed: 29 March 2012].

Blackburn, C., Carpenter, B. and Egerton, J. (2009) *Facing the Challenge and Shaping the Future for Primary and Secondary Aged Students with Foetal Alcohol Spectrum Disorders (FAS-eD Project): Literature review*, London: National Organisation on Fetal Alcohol Syndrome UK [online at: www.networks.nhs.uk/nhs-networks/foetal-alcohol-syndrome-an-spectrum-and-associated/documents/FAS-eD%20PROJECT%20LITERATURE%20REVIEW-1.pdf; accessed: 1 July 2012].

Blackburn, C., Carpenter, B. and Egerton, J. (2012) *Educating Children and Young People with Fetal Alcohol Spectrum Disorders: Constructing personalised pathways to learning*, Abingdon: Routledge.

Bohjanen, S., Humphrey, M. and Ryan, S.M. (2009) 'Left behind: lack of research-based interventions for children and youth with fetal alcohol spectrum disorders', *Rural Special Education Quarterly*, 28(2): 32–8.

Carpenter, B. (2011) 'Pedagogically bereft! Improving learning outcomes for children with foetal alcohol spectrum disorders', *British Journal of Special Education*, 38(1): 37–43.

Chudley, E., Conry, J., Cook, J., Loock, C., Rosales, T. and LeBlanc, N. (2005) 'Fetal alcohol spectrum disorder: Canadian guidelines for diagnosis', *Canadian Medical Association Journal*, 172(5): S1–S21.

Crawford, K. (2008) *Education of Students with Fetal Alcohol Spectrum Disorder (Churchill Fellowship report)*, Karratha, Western Australia [online at: www.churchilltrust.com.au/site_media/fellows/Crawford_Kym_2008.pdf; accessed: 1 June 2012].

DEEWR (Australian Government Department of Education, Employment and Workplace Relations) (2009) *Belonging, Being and Becoming – The Early Years Learning Framework for Australia*, Canberra: DEEWR.

DEEWR (Australian Government Department of Education, Employment and Workplace Relations) (2011) [online at: www.deewr.gov.au/policy-agenda/; accessed: 18 June 2013].

DEEWR (Australian Government Department of Education, Employment and Workplace Relations) (undated) *What Works. The Work Program: Core issues 8 – Education and student health: the big picture*, Abbotsford, Victoria: What Works, National Curriculum Services.

Duquette, C., Stodel, E., Fullarton, S. and Hagglund, K. (2006) 'Persistence in high school: experiences of adolescents and young adults with fetal alcohol spectrum disorder', *Journal of Intellectual and Developmental Disability*, 31(4): 219–31.

Edmonds, K. and Crichton, S. (2008) 'Finding ways to teach to students with FASD: a research study', *International Journal of Special Education*, 23(1): 54–73.

Elliott, E.J. and Bower, C. (2004) 'FAS in Australia: fact or fiction?', *Journal of Paediatric Child Health*, 40(1/2): 8–10.

Elliott, E.J., Payne, J., Haan, E. and Bower, C. (2006) 'Diagnosis of foetal alcohol syndrome and alcohol use in pregnancy: a survey of paediatricians' knowledge, attitudes and practice', *Journal of Paediatrics and Child Health*, 42(11): 698–703.

Healthy Child Manitoba (2010) *What Early Childhood Educators Need to Know about FASD*, Winnipeg, Manitoba: Healthy Child Manitoba [online at: www.gov.mb.ca/healthychild/fasd/fasdearly_en.pdf; accessed: 1 February 2012].

Job, J., Carter-Pasula, B., Brandell, D., Pei J., Poth, C. and Macnab, J. (2011) 'Toward better collaboration in the education of students with fetal alcohol spectrum disorders: perspectives of teachers, administrators, caregivers, and allied professionals', presentation at the Edmonton Public School Board Brown Bag Lunch, 1 February [online at: http://research.epsb.ca/datafiles/HICE_Presentation_February_2011.pdf; accessed: 1 July 2012].

Leslie, M. and Roberts, G. (2001) *Enhancing Fetal Alcohol Syndrome (FAS)-related Interventions at the Prenatal and Early Childhood Stages in Canada*, Ottawa, Ontario: Canadian Centre on Substance Abuse.

O'Leary, C. (2004) 'Fetal alcohol syndrome: diagnosis, epidemiology, and developmental outcomes', *Journal of Paediatrics and Child Health*, 40(1/2): 2–7.

Payne, J., Elliott, E., D'Antoine, H., O'Leary, C., Mahony, A., Haan, E. and Bower, C. (2005) 'Health professionals' knowledge, practice and opinions about fetal alcohol syndrome and alcohol consumption in pregnancy', *Australian and New Zealand Journal of Public Health*, 29(6): 558–64.

Peadon, E., Fremantle, E., Bower, C. and Elliott, E.J. (2008) 'International survey of diagnostic services for children with fetal alcohol spectrum disorders', *BMC Pediatrics*, 8(12): 1–8.

Premji, K., Benzies, K., Serrett, K. and Hayden, K.A. (2006) 'Research-based interventions for children and youth with a fetal alcohol spectrum disorder: revealing the gap', *Child: Care, Health and Development*, 33(4): 389–97.

Ryan, S. and Chionnaith, M.N. (2006) 'On the spectrum: similarities and differences between students with fetal alcohol spectrum disorders and autism spectrum disorders in Ireland', *Journal of International Special Needs Education*, 9: 43–52.

Ryan, S. and Ferguson, D. (2006) 'On, yet under, the radar: students with fetal alcohol spectrum disorder', *Exceptional Children*, 72(3): 363–79.

Telethon Institute of Child Health Research (2011) 'Telethon Institute for Child Health Research Submission WA Education and Health Standing Committee 2011' [online at: www.parliament.wa.gov.au/parliament/commit.nsf/(Evidence+Lookup+by+Com+ID)/75A14495940F5F29482579800018A3F7/$file/Submission+14+-+Clinical+Professor+Carol+Bower+(Telethon+Institute+for+Child+Health+Research).pdf; accessed: 2 April 2012].

Yukon Department of Education (2006) *Making a Difference: Working with students who have fetal alcohol spectrum disorders*, Whitehorse, Yukon: Yukon Department of Education [online at: www.education.gov.yk.ca/pdf/fasd_manual_2007.pdf; accessed: 29 March 2012].

10

WALKING THROUGH A MOONLESS NIGHT

Fetal alcohol spectrum disorders and early childhood intervention

Carolyn Blackburn

> When we are not protective of mothers' experiences during pregnancy, our communities may give birth to the reflection of those experiences.
>
> *(Karr-Morse and Wiley 1997: 97)*

Introduction

Early Childhood Intervention (ECI) has the potential to alter the developmental trajectory and support familial relationships for vulnerable children, optimizing individual potential and community quality. This chapter will argue that although universal ECI services offer valuable support to children with fetal alcohol spectrum disorders (FASDs) and their families, co-existing and overlapping conditions and complex family structures require that such services be enhanced to ensure they meet their unique needs. Most importantly, children's development needs to be planned for from conception, placing healthy fetal and child development at the ecological epicentre of government policy to prevent children with FASDs becoming another 'stolen generation' (Stanley 2008, in Hope 2008). This is even more important in socio-cultural populations which rely on memory and cognition to maintain cultural traditions.

There is insufficient scope in this chapter for a discussion about the use of 'labels' and the concern relating to stigma and over-use. However, reference to some of the general debates can be found (Dittrich and Tutt 2008; Laughlan and Boyle 2007) and in relation to FASDs and early diagnosis in particular (Blackburn *et al.* 2012; Blackburn and Whitehurst 2010). Also outside the scope of this chapter are issues requiring urgent debate such as paternal alcohol consumption, societal and cultural perceptions of alcohol consumption, and policy to control the way alcohol is portrayed, priced and so easily available.

FASDs and child development

Healthy early child development is influenced by factors such as early infant–caregiver relationships, cognitive and language stimulation, nutrition and safe and healthy environments

(Whitebread and Bingham 2011). The influence of maternal health and well-being is significant. In particular prenatal maternal alcohol consumption[1] is known to result in a variety of birth anomalies which can evolve and become more pronounced as children mature, limiting children's participation in a range of educational and social settings (Blackburn *et al.* 2012; Clarren 2004; Karr-Morse and Wiley 1997; Kleinfeld and Westcott 1993; Streissguth and Kanter 1997).

The significance of FASDs in this regard is thought to be higher when fetal damage is undetected and therefore not supported with intervention (Karr-Morse and Wiley 1997). This is the case for most children affected as only one-third of children with FASDs receive a correct diagnosis and only 11 per cent receive a diagnosis before the age of six years (www.nofasct.org).

The literature on neuroscience (Goswami 2008) and ECI (Guralnick 2005) notes that early identification of any child at risk of developmental delays and difficulties, when supported with subsequent intervention, results in significant gains in that child's development. ECI can improve opportunities for social inclusion, participation and the development of key life skills and independence, which benefit longer-term outcomes such as education and employment.

In the absence of inclusion and participation, as children mature they can become isolated and insular (Egerton, Chapter 12, this publication). Dorris (1989: 264) described his adult son's perspective on his disability and in particular his grasp on reality:

> My son will forever travel through a moonless night with only the roar of the wind for company. Don't talk to him of mountains, of tropical beaches. Don't ask him to swoon at sunrises or marvel at the filter of light through leaves. He's never had time for such things and he does not believe them … a drowning man is not separated from the lust for air by a bridge of thought – he is one with it – and my son, conceived and grown in an ethanol bath, lives each day in the act of drowning. For him there is no shore.

Such profound accounts of emotional and physical detachment from the natural world illustrate the difficulties faced by Adam in his adolescent and adult years, and his father's enduring empathy and humbling dedication to his son. Dorris (ibid.) narrated his life with Adam honestly and poignantly through his book, *The Broken Cord*, the reading of which left me with one burning question: *how different would this family's experience have been if Adam's condition had been recognized earlier, allowing them to benefit from ECI services?*[2]

Early intervention or early childhood intervention?

Generally ECI is understood to consist of a set of supports, services and experiences to prevent or minimize long-term difficulties as early as possible in early childhood (Dunst and Trivette 1997; Guralnick 1997). Those in receipt of such services are typically at risk for developmental, emotional, social, behavioural and school problems due to biological and/or environmental factors (Guralnick 2004). This is distinct from early intervention (EI), which refers to intervention being used to support any child and their family as early as possible during *any time* in their education (European Agency for Development in Special Needs Education 2005).

ECI focuses on children's early development (Carpenter and Egerton 2005), and acknowledges the ever-widening population of very young vulnerable children (Guralnick 2005). In the context of this chapter, ECI specifically focuses on vulnerable children from conception until the age of six years. Due to the rapid growth which takes place in children's early development the gains from ECI at this stage are unique and not evident in later stages of childhood. Infancy is a crucial developmental stage when an individual forms the core of conscience, develops the ability to trust and relate to others, and lays down the foundation for life-long learning and thinking (Karr-Morse and Wiley 1997). Allen notes the importance of early brain development: 'The early years are far and away the greatest period of growth in the human brain. The connections or synapses in a baby's brain grow 20 fold from having 10 trillion at birth to 200 trillion at age three' (Allen 2011a: 6).

In terms of prevention, the crucial period of development during which ECI could be most powerful (i.e. pregnancy) is best viewed as a 'staging period for well-being and disease in later life' (Murphy 2010: 5). In some Asian cultures, a child is considered a one-year-old at birth and the parent–child relationship to commence nine months earlier. As we understand more about the profound developmental processes occurring in the womb, conception, rather than birth, is increasingly perceived as the very beginning of child development. The womb is the first environment that a child is exposed to. Despite the notion of the protective nature of the womb, there is significant risk potential for sensory, neurodevelopmental and organ damage from toxic stimuli. A more appropriate focus for intervention services might be 'Fetal and Early Childhood Intervention' (FECI) (including the early germinal and embryonic stages). With this focus, ECI would then encompass both preventative and educational or therapeutic measures.

Intervention at any point in a child's life is recommended as worthwhile and effective. The emphasis in this chapter is on identification and support *in pregnancy and early childhood* in order to reduce or (where possible) prevent immediate risk, and improve development and outcomes in both the short and long term. Perceiving a developing fetus as a sentient being should be a fundamental principle of this objective.

Who benefits from ECI?

Intervening early in childhood has the potential to prevent, ameliorate or reverse developmental problems in children thought to be at risk. The questions of how and when to intervene to achieve optimum effect, how to measure the effect, and who benefits from the intervention, all need to be considered in the context of children's development.

Ecology of child development

Children grow and develop within the context of multiple interacting levels of influence on the dynamics of their development (Bronfenbrenner 1979; Cuthbert *et al.* 2012). These influences interact with each other and the developing child in a transactional bi-directional manner. They also change over time as children develop and mature, and family dynamics and structure change. The harmonious interaction of these multiple layers of influence is crucial. If ECI services fail to work in harmony with families or policy agendas, at the very least the consequence will be failure to achieve optimum outcomes. Theoretically, the child is at the centre of ecological models (see Figure 10.1).

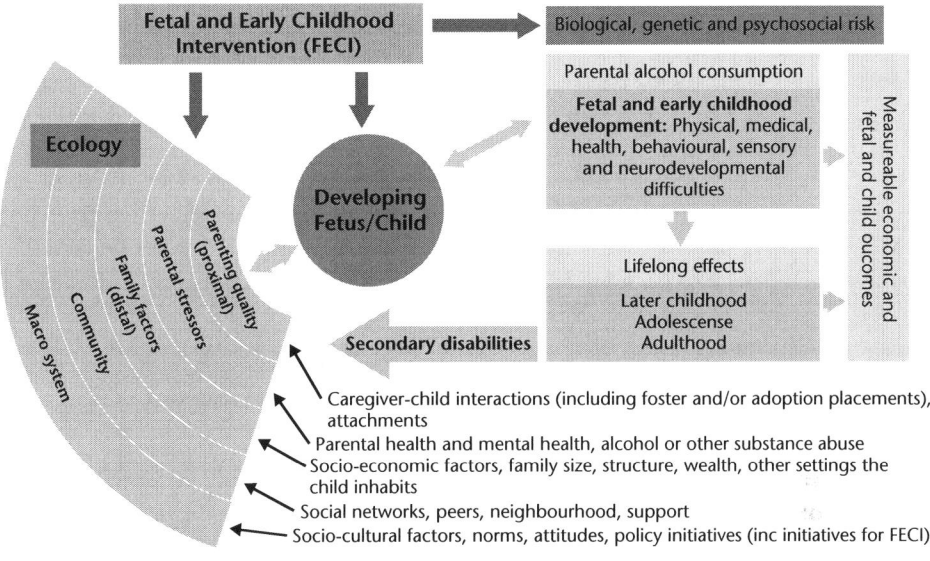

Blackburn, 2012

FIGURE 10.1 An ecological model of fetal and early childhood development and intervention for children with FASDs.

The greatest impact on children is found in the influence of family life and relationships,[3] including factors such as maternal health during pregnancy, parenting capacity, family stressors (mental health, substance use, domestic stability/violence) and other family factors (size, structure, income, assets, housing). Other settings such as early childhood education and care settings are also important. All of the above factors can provide positive or negative influences on children's development. For example, 'good enough' or warm, sensitive, attuned parenting is a positive influence, whereas parental neglect and abuse place development at risk. Some factors present simultaneous protection and risk. The removal of an abusing husband protects mother and child, but risks plunging them into poverty.

Not enough is known about maternal risk in relation to FASDs. However, risk has been described as 'multidimensional' (May and Gossage 2011) and as including factors related to: quantity, frequency and timing of alcohol exposure; maternal age; number of pregnancies; number of times the mother has given birth; the mother's body size; nutrition; socioeconomic status; metabolism; religion; spirituality; depression; other drug use; and social relationships. In particular low socio-economic status (SES), under-nutrition, advanced maternal age, high parity, and overall weathering (the cumulative effect of poor living conditions, inadequate nutrition and high levels of stress on childbearing) are reported to increase the risk for FASD trait expression (Abel and Hannigan 1995).

More research is needed to define more clearly what type of individual behavioural, physical and genetic factors are most likely to lead to having children with FASDs (May and Gossage 2011). However, animal research has shown that the genetic profiles of both the mother and fetus are important for determining the potential for risk of prenatal mortality, alcohol-related physical birth defects, and learning and other neurobehavioural problems in the offspring (Warren et al. 2011). Further risks from prenatal alcohol exposure include prematurity of birth, low birth weight and birth complications.

For some children, maternal alcohol consumption represents a risk in addition to pre-existing biological, genetic and/or psychosocial influences, such as psychological trauma and impoverished environment, rendering them vulnerable to a toxic cocktail of risk factors. Such children have a biological or genetic predisposition to experience learning, social and/or behavioural difficulties which are not ameliorated by a supportive, nurturing environment conducive to the development of healthy attachments and relationships with others. Parent–child attachments are dependent on reciprocal inter-subjective interactions between caregiver and child and are crucial for the healthy development of children's social relationships, emotional well-being, cognition and language. This is sometimes difficult to achieve when infants are irritable, cry persistently, are difficult to feed and have poor sleep patterns, which are common difficulties for children with FASDs. It is exacerbated when caregivers experience mental ill-health, inadequate coping strategies, insensitive parenting skills or substance addition or dependency; for example:

> When I was pregnant I couldn't get up in the morning without throwing up and having a drink and I knew that I shouldn't, but I couldn't function without a drink … mentally I was unfit, I had suicidal thoughts, I had thoughts about harming my son, was seeing things, I was a mess. Having a baby and trying to deal with my head was difficult.
>
> *(Anonymous birth mother, pers. comm.)*

Lack of healthy attachments may add to parental stress factors adding further risk to development. Consequently, these children may lack the resilience which would help them to overcome life challenges. Societies and communities which fail to understand the complex transactional interplay between the impact of the cumulative effects of this toxic mix on the development of individual children and the quality of the human environment and communities that these children inhabit are failing in their responsibility to these children. They are also participating in their own destruction. Such children are vulnerable to exhibiting violent, aggressive and criminal behaviour in later life (Karr-Morse and Wiley 1997).

Other more distal influences such as community activities, as well as local and national policies affect children and their families. The influence of culture, beliefs and attitudes to childhood, parenting and family functioning pervade all settings that children inhabit. In this regard, cultures that rely on the recall and verbal transmission of traditional stories (such as aboriginal cultures) are at increased risk due to the impairment of memory associated with FASDs.

How and when to intervene

If FASDs are not identified, diagnosed and supported with appropriate intervention *early in childhood*, secondary disabilities result (see Carpenter, Chapter 11, and O'Malley, Chapter 19, this publication), which encourage the development of a trans-generational process (O'Malley, ibid.). Children with FASDs become adults with FASDs and raise children of their own. Karr-Morse and Wiley (1997) note that women who themselves have FASDs have difficulty using counselling due to their inability to link cause and effect or think ahead, making treatment for alcohol or drug addiction during pregnancy problematic. As noted earlier, pregnancy is a crucial period of child development.

Intervention can include universal primary preventative measures to reduce the likelihood of women drinking during pregnancy, health visiting and midwifery services to monitor the progress of pregnancy and fetal development, and provide crucial information to expectant mothers, as well as assessing maternal mental health and well-being. Secondary preventative measures may be targeted at specific, socio-economic and socio-cultural or other vulnerable groups. Tertiary measures might include therapy with a mother after her child's birth to support reduction in alcohol or poly-substance abuse/addiction (smoking and other illicit drugs or over the counter medications are often used alongside alcohol) and to address the specific therapeutic and educational needs of individual children.

Benefits for children and families

The benefits of EI and ECI in particular to children and families are now well documented in the UK (Allen 2011a, 2011b; Allen and Duncan Smith 2008; Field 2010, Munro 2011). Allen (2011a) notes that ECI impacts on children's long-term social and emotional development, equipping them with better parenting skills in preparation for raising children of their own. As noted above, this influences the ecology of development at a trans-generational level and, for children already born with FASDs, reduces the possibility of secondary disabilities:

> If we intervene early enough, we can give children a vital social and emotional foundation which will help to keep them happy, healthy and achieving throughout their lives and, above all, equip them to raise children of their own, who will also enjoy higher levels of well-being.
>
> *(Allen 2011a: ix)*

Furthermore, families have reported improved confidence in their child's current and long term progress as a consequence of being involved in ECI programmes (Bailey *et al.* 2006, in Bruder 2010).

The particular benefits for early identification and diagnosis of FASDs are noted in the introduction to this chapter. In an unpublished survey conducted by the author with the European Birth Mothers Network (EuroBMSN) (Blackburn and Williams 2013), one mother commented on the heartache that could have been saved if professionals had listened to her and *diagnosed* her son earlier, while another was dismayed that professionals had not warned her of the 'poisonous' effects of alcohol so that her son's brain damage and birth defects could have been *prevented*. A further benefit is that identification of one affected child in the family allows the opportunity for *prevention* of subsequent children being exposed to alcohol in pregnancy through maternal and family interventions (Western Australia Department of Health 2010).

An important aspect of ECI is the focus on improvements in child development resulting from well-funded, integrated, socio-educational programmes which improve the cognitive and social functioning of children at risk (Whitebread and Bingham 2011), rather than policy initiatives designed to 'control the diversity with which children enter school' (ibid.: 1). For governments and policymakers, the importance of evidence-based ECI programmes which provide financial as well as human outcomes cannot be ignored.

Benefits for society

From a policy perspective, the reported benefits to society as a whole of providing ECI services are a reduction in the number of adults in need of life-long support, in contact with the criminal justice system and/or in long-term unemployment (Allen 2011a). These benefits can be measured in terms of return on investment. Early education programmes have noted benefit-to-cost ratios as high as 17:1 (Lynch 2005). Although some research suggests that the benefits of ECI can be measured only in the short term (Wise *et al.* 2005), long-term benefits are more likely if the quality of life-long learning and education are high, and interventions are followed up with ongoing support for vulnerable groups. Moreover, although cognitive and intellectual improvements for children are often shown to diminish in longitudinal evaluation studies, reductions in crime statistics and an increase in employment during early adolescence and adulthood are often associated with ECI (ibid.) particularly in relation to home-based visiting education programmes such as the American Head Start and Portage programmes. The simple reason for this is that they commence in early childhood and include parents and families in delivery, thereby strengthening relationships and bonds within families (Karr-Morse and Wiley 1997). It goes without saying that prevention of FASDs would provide cost as well as human benefits, though in the UK, statistics are not available to substantiate this. However Lupton and colleagues (2004) (www.fasdcenter.samhsa.gov) have estimated the lifetime cost of caring for a person with an FASD to be at least $2 million, and the overall annual cost of FASDs to the US healthcare system to be more than $6 billion.

Children, families, government and society would seem to benefit from ECI programmes. There is an inherent difficulty with FASDs in providing an evidence base of 'tested and trialled' programmes, when it is difficult to identify the children concerned due to lack of identification and consequent under-diagnosis (BMA 2007) and professional knowledge is not widespread (Blackburn *et al.* 2012; Carpenter 2011). This highlights the need to discover the extent of current professional knowledge.

Professional knowledge of FASDs

In order for ECI provision to be effectively planned, organized and delivered, knowledge about the characteristics and needs of specific service users must be established and professionals providing such services trained and skilled accordingly. The professionals involved in delivering ECI programmes are employed in the health, social care and education sectors, including – and arguably most importantly for prevention and early identification purposes – early childhood practitioners and health practitioners.

Knowledge of health professionals

In discussing the knowledge of health professionals and how they advise pregnant women, it is important to note the delicate and often difficult position health professionals are placed in. Plant (pers. comm.) notes that if someone does have a drinking problem denial is a very powerful mechanism, and we are all subject to selective deafness. In many situations where people ask intimate questions the two questions they find most uncomfortable to answer are 'How much do you earn?' and 'How much do you drink?' They are also often the questions people are most unhappy asking. A major problem for midwives is that if they ask, they have to act, and depending on their experience or training this knowledge might actually prevent them from exploring further even if they do have alarm bells ringing. Midwives are, first, human beings and, second, midwives, and sometimes it is easier not to talk about alcohol because the midwife may not want to 'upset' the woman or make her anxious. Learning how to do something in a classroom and having to do it in a busy noisy antenatal clinic are two very different things. It is important to note that the emphasis must be on how to address these issues openly, rather than on promoting a culture of blame. Nevertheless, the perspective of birth mothers is important, and sadly the attitude of these professionals towards birth mothers emerged as a theme in the Blackburn and Williams (2013) study. This study included 12 biological mothers of children and young people (CYP) with FASDs (Blackburn and Williams 2013).[4] Attitudes included perceived hostility and value judgements from midwives, and mothers feeling let down by a complete absence of professional knowledge and understanding. Some mothers commented that this limited the possibilities for them and other parents to make informed choices about their alcohol consumption during and after pregnancy as well as their ability to receive appropriate support for themselves and their children following birth.

All mothers reported that none of their health professionals mentioned FASDs. In five cases professionals knew that the mother was an alcoholic; one of these mothers was provided with an alcohol diary. In two of these cases, mothers were informed that drinking was harmful to their baby; however one mother was informed that her drinking would not present a problem, but was advised not to drink or eat particular foods (such as soft cheese or pâté). Four mothers out of the 12 were advised not to smoke and/or were informed of the detrimental effects of particular foods.

When asked directly about knowledge among professionals, mothers described professional knowledge as non-existent or flaky. One mother commented that although her child was diagnosed at birth, she was not provided with information about her child's care and development needs, while other mothers reported that the paediatrician or breast-feeding nurse were aware of FASDs indicating that there are discrete pockets of knowledge. One mother reported that professionals had to seek advice about FASDs from the internet. Parents highlighted the essential service provided by support groups in the absence of government and local authority provision and the need for professionals to be aware of the link between mental ill-health in adolescence and adulthood, and FASDs.

Despite mothers being aware that their children were developing differently from their peers between birth and the age of six, professional acknowledgement of mothers' concerns was not common. In relation to diagnosis, where professional knowledge existed and physical rather than neurological effects were evident, diagnosis occurred within a matter of hours. However this was in a minority of cases. In the absence of professional knowledge and overt signs diagnosis took between one and nine years after professional suspicion of FASD. The most common reason given for long delays or children not being diagnosed was 'no one is listening, even though I have told them I drank'. Where diagnosis had taken place, this had occurrred between birth and 20 years with the majority taking place in middle to late childhood. In two cases, diagnosis is ongoing as still 'no-one is listening' seven years and 30 years respectively after parents raised FASDs as a possibility. Two mothers commented that their children were diagnosed without their knowledge, and they were informed a number of years later, or that FASDs had been mentioned in the early stages by a health visitor or general practitioner but mothers did not understand the term and a diagnostic assessment was not forthcoming. One of the children is currently being assessed multiprofessionally.

Even so, the issues for children who are not diagnosed or not diagnosed early are complex. Two young people now aged 23 years do not want to go through the diagnostic process, believing it will achieve nothing. This is the very real issue of whether a diagnosis of FASDs is truly a diagnosis or simply a label. One mother is in consultation with the professionals in the secure mental health unit where her child is placed; the professionals believe his behaviour is attributable to his own drug addiction. Another mother is being shunted between professionals who attribute her child's behaviour to environmental issues (living in an alcoholic household). Of course this situation will add to the problems the child faces and may make the diagnosis more difficult, but it does not change the original cause of difficulties.

Mothers commented that their opinion is not valued by professionals responsible for referring their child for diagnostic assessment.

Mukherjee and colleagues (2010), in a UK study investigating public and healthcare knowledge of FASDs, found that out of 500 professionals the majority (93.8 per cent) were aware of FASDs. However, 75 per cent were not aware of the high prevalence rates. Furthermore, 72 per cent (of 417 respondents) did not feel confident that they had sufficient information to advise pregnant mothers about alcohol consumption. In conclusion, Mukherjee *et al.* suggest that although there is a reasonable knowledge at a superficial level about where to seek help for children with FASDs, a proportion of healthcare workers would not know where to turn, and clearer care pathways are needed. Moreover, there is ongoing confusion related to long-term outcomes and support needs of people with FASDs which has wider implications for training.

In a UK study investigating midwives' knowledge of FASDs and alcohol intake during pregnancy (Winstone 2012), less than 2 per cent felt very prepared to deal with this topic (n = 624 midwives working in East Anglia). Out of the remaining 98 per cent, 64 per cent did not feel prepared at all in this area of health promotion (see Fleisher, Chapter 15, this publication, for further discussion of midwives' professional development).

It is clear that there is a paucity of consistent appropriate service provision for families, and a pressing need to examine the current level of service provision.

Knowledge of education professionals

In a study conducted in the UK (2009), 78 per cent of early childhood practitioners (164 participants) reported that they knew little or nothing about FASDs and therefore would have found it difficult to plan for and support a child with an FASD attending their early childhood setting (Blackburn and Whitehurst 2010). This study included Early Childhood Leaders in Sure Start[5] Children's Centres where one practitioner admitted honestly that she felt 'ignorant to work in a Children's Centre and not know about something like this [FASD]' (Blackburn and Whitehurst 2010: 126). In a more recent study conducted in Western Australia (Frances, Chapter 9, this publication) of 236 early childhood practitioners, the majority of participants had a high level of awareness of the effects of maternal alcohol consumption during pregnancy on the developing fetus, but did not believe they had the appropriate skills and knowledge to support children with FASDs.

This paucity of knowledge transcends different disciplines for those professionals involved with individuals with FASDs across the life span. Blackburn (2010) reported families' concern that many professionals available to support their children were not knowledgeable about the condition. These included professionals within educational settings across the age range as well as those supporting short-break services, and out of and after-school services.

This suggests that the possibility or likelihood that families will receive ECI services which are planned and organized for their particular needs is limited by lack of professional knowledge. This view is reinforced by the BMA (2007: 11) who noted that 'a lack of knowledge about FASDs will limit opportunities for diagnosis, prevention and early intervention'. This influences the ecology of development at micro level impacting on early identification, assessment, diagnosis and, since these practitioners are not likely to have sufficient knowledge and skills to adequately support parents, also impacts on parenting capacity and family stressors.

This chapter will now address the current international position on ECI services in this sector highlighting any particular strengths, identifying gaps and determining which approaches would be most appropriate to meet the needs of children and families, as well as prevailing policy agendas.

Current international ECI provision

The current provision of ECI for children and families affected by prenatal alcohol exposure (as with other areas of vulnerability and disability) varies internationally. In countries such as Canada and the US, there is extensive guidance and a well-developed system of ECI provision.[6]

In Western Australia, a non-government initiative supported by a number of government departments, including the Departments of Health, Corrective Services and the Aboriginal and Torres Strait Health Department, provides support and intervention for families experiencing the effects of drug and alcohol abuse (www.palmerston.org.au). The Palmerston Association stresses the importance of acknowledging the cultural needs of a wide range of family members affected by alcohol and drug abuse in their family and parenting programmes, including grandparents, parents, step-families, uncles, aunts, cousins, close family friends and carers. These developments indicate that there are strengths in service provision in some countries.

However, in South Africa, despite having the highest prevalence of FASDs worldwide (De Beer 2008; Pienaar 2003; Viljoen *et al.* 2003), there is a shortage of early identification services as well as insufficient services dedicated to families affected by alcohol-related problems (De Beer 2008). This is surprising given that FASD is listed as one of the priority conditions targeted for prevention, early detection and the provision of appropriate intervention in the *Human Genetics Policy Document for the Management and Prevention of Genetic Disorders, Birth Defects and Disabilities* (Ntsabula 2001).

In the UK, the alcohol consumption habits of women are worryingly high (Plant, Chapter 4, this publication). The prevalence of FASDs in the UK is unconfirmed as data is not routinely collected (BMA 2007), but it is reported that the condition may account for as many as one in 100 children (Autti-Ramo 2002). Furthermore, around 79,000 babies under the age of one year in England are living with a parent who is classified as a 'problematic', 'hazardous' or 'harmful' drinker, and around 26,000 babies under the age of one year in England are living with a parent who would be classified as a 'dependent' drinker (Cuthbert *et al.* 2012). Not all parents classified as problematic or harmful drinkers experience problems with parenting skills, neither is the author suggesting that all children with FASDs are born into households where parents are hazardous, harmful or dependent drinkers, as many are not. However, it is noteworthy that a study of 268 serious child protection case reviews in England found that 22 per cent involved parental alcohol misuse (Brandon 2009, in Cuthbert *et al.* 2012). The likelihood that some children with FASDs will have experienced neglect and abuse during early childhood should be noted by those planning training for professionals and programmes for children and families.

Charities and ECI leaders in the UK have made policy calls for government to both maintain and improve ECI services for vulnerable babies (Cuthbert *et al.* 2012) and to support children with special educational needs in emerging categories 'such as those born with substance abuse or alcohol addictions' (Carpenter 2005: 176). Despite this, ECI is currently concentrated in discrete areas of professional or voluntary services, rather than being initiative-driven or goal-directed by government, and few are aimed at supporting the developing fetus.

These charities include the three, major, parent-led FASD organizations in the UK – NOFAS-UK (www.nofas-uk.org), the FASD Trust (www.fasdtrust.co.uk) and FASAware (www.fasaware.co.uk). These groups provide guidance and support for parents through local support groups, training opportunities for parents and professionals and telephone support. The European Birth Mother Support Network (www.eurobmsn.org) launched in 2010 from the UK, is a network of women who drank alcohol during pregnancy and may have children with FASDs. The network is a place where mothers can share their experiences and support each other.

The first FASD clinic in the UK being led by Dr Raja Mukherjee[7] offers specialist advice on the behaviour management and diagnosis of FASDs. The service aims to identify the disorder in childhood thus helping prevent secondary social and psychological conditions such as social exclusion and mental ill-health developing in the long term. The service is available through the National Health Service (NHS) to any family who has a referral from their general practitioner (GP) or other professional or can pay for the service independently.

The Parents Under Pressure (PUP) programme is a 20-week home-delivery programme which works with parents receiving drug or alcohol treatment and who have a child under two in their full-time care. It is underpinned by an ecological model of child development and targets multiple dimensions of family functioning. Therapists work with parents to help them develop parenting skills and safe, caring relationships with their babies. They will report any signs of child abuse or neglect to children's services. The programme is currently being provided on a trial and evaluation basis to families in selected locations in the UK to determine its efficacy (Cuthbert *et al.* 2012).

The 'Alcohol in Pregnancy – Training for Midwives Project' is an initiative of NOFAS-UK (NOFAS-UK 2010) designed to provide useful positive health information about the consumption of alcohol in pregnancy to midwives who play an important role in ECI. This must surely represent the most positive aspect of ECI as 'maternity care is the earliest intervention of them all' (Lewis 2007: 4).

Recognition of the importance of understanding the needs of children with FASDs and their families is changing in the UK (Blackburn *et al.* 2012). Recent educational research projects (Blackburn 2009, 2010; Carpenter *et al.* 2011; Egerton 2009) have left in place resources for educators to support and engage children with FASDs (including those with the most complex needs) and their families in educational settings from birth to six years (Blackburn 2009; Egerton 2009).

Primary intervention universal services in the UK such as midwifery and health visiting, those nested in children's centres such as speech and language therapy, together with targeted secondary intervention home-based services such as the Family Nurse Partnership (aimed at vulnerable children in the prenatal, pregnancy and postnatal period up to two years of age) have positive effects on many children and families (Cuthbert *et al.* 2012).

However, at the macro level, there remains a shortage of government-directed and -funded initiatives to plan for the specific needs of children and families affected by FASDs. This is despite the responsibility of governments to respect the rights of children to crucial services in line with the Convention on the Rights of the Child (United Nations 1989) and the Convention on the Rights of Persons with Disabilities (United Nations 2006). These conventions seek to ensure that all children and their families with special needs and disabilities have access to appropriate support services and also that each child's culture, language, ethnicity and family structure are valued. The imperative for interventions is stressed in some UK policy reports (Allen 2011a, 2011b; Munro 2011), but many are directed at parents who abuse or misuse alcohol and other substances, rather than children already born with the sometimes devastating effects of maternal alcohol consumption, or ensuring healthy pregnancies. As already noted, not all children with FASDs are born to mothers who are harmful or problematic drinkers. Moreover, emphasis is often placed on economic and fiscal benefits of intervention, or on ensuring children's school or life readiness, with less attention paid to children's enjoyment of childhood or enhancing their social participation by ensuring that life (or society) and school (or any educational/social setting) are ready for the children. Economics are at the ecological epicentre (see Figure 10.1) of these policies, placing healthy fetal and child development in a subordinate position on the sidelines. The introduction of the UK Foundation Years website resulting from the government's acknowledgement that pregnancy is a crucial stage of children's development might be perceived as a beacon of hope for future policy direction (www.foundationyears.org.uk).

Clearly, in some countries, there are gaps in service provision, while in others there are strengths. This suggests the possibility for professional networking and collaboration across countries to share effective practice and evidence-based approaches, and highlights the need for debate to identify elements of successful programmes that can be modified or adapted for particular socio-cultural and socio-economic contexts.

Approaches to ECI: current and emerging trends

In its fairly brief history, the field of ECI has undergone rapid change in response to social and policy agendas. During this evolutionary process, a number of emerging trends have been documented (Moore 2008). Of particular relevance to this chapter, significant trends are noted in Table 10.1 (Bruder 2010; Guralnick 2005; Moore 2008).

These trends illuminate possible policy and practice implications for the planning and delivery of services for children and families with FASDs. Evidence can be found in UK policy documents of the value of these approaches. For example, the outcomes-based approach mentioned above is recommended by Allen (2011b: 50), and one suggested (hypothetical) outcome in the EI strategy of preparing children to be 'life ready' is a 'reduction in expenditure on child abuse, fetal alcohol syndrome (FAS) and drug-dependent babies' measured by 'cashable savings in years one to five' of implementation and 'reductions in SEN

TABLE 10.1 Emerging FASD approaches and implications for practice

Previous approach	Emerging approach and implications for practice
Clinical approach	**Natural learning environments approach:** the clinical service model, where children are assessed and treated in clinical surroundings, is replaced with a natural learning environments approach in which specialists identify and utilize natural learning opportunities that occur in the course of children's everyday home and community routines, enabling children with disabilities and their families to live life very differently.
Fragmented services	**Seamless service integration:** for families with complex needs ECI services need to become part of a collaborative network of services that work in harmony to provide holistic integrated services to families.
Interdisciplinary approaches	**Trans-disciplinary approaches** with a key worker coordinator: involves several professionals providing an integrated service to the child and family, with one professional taking on the role of the key worker. This is considered to be more cost effective and families report benefits of the key worker approach.
Service-based approach	**Outcomes-based approach:** enables services to plan their work according to agreed outcomes (such as child and family improvements) and select the form of delivery accordingly.
Tradition-based approach	**Evidence-based approach:** ECI services are planned and delivered based on methodical evaluation of what has been most effective from research evidence data.
Professional skill-based approach	**Relationship-based approach:** includes consideration of the relationship between professionals and families, as well as the importance of caregiver–child interaction, and there is awareness on the part of professionals of their own role in working with infants and families where relationships are at risk.
Deficit-based approach	**Assessment for eligibility to a response-to-intervention approach:** children are assessed on their responses to increasingly intensive evidence-based intervention programmes and are not considered to have a learning difficulty or disability until it is proven that they do not respond appropriately by demonstrating progress. This ensures that those with limited early stimulation are not labelled inappropriately at an early age.
Authoritative expert stance	**Reflective practice:** practitioners reflect on their own previous and current practice to ensure that they are working optimally to achieve agreed outcomes. This also requires reflective supervision.

statements and numbers entering fostering and care' in years 6 to 11. There is also mention of relationship-based approaches (Field 2010; Munro 2011) and the need for evidence-based approaches (Allen 2011a, 2011b).

These emerging approaches to ECI provide a framework for some suggested elements of ECI programmes for children and families with FASDs, which are provided here as platform for debate among stakeholders in the FASD community.

Finding the shore: where do we want to be?

The need for ECI services to be available to children with FASDs and their families has been argued for in this chapter. Blackburn and Williams (2013) found that the need for professional knowledge about FASDs, and information and education for women about alcohol consumption during and after pregnancy are the most important dimensions of ECI stressed by the majority of mothers. When asked to rank the most important factors in the provision of early support, following the need for professional knowledge of FASDs, mothers valued early diagnosis, access to child care and education appropriate for the needs of a child with FASDs, professional knowledge of child development, maternal alcohol use and misuse, and understanding of birth mother perspective and feelings of guilt. Slightly less important but still significant were professional respect for birth mothers and other family members, access to home-based intervention programmes such Portage and therapies such as play therapy, music therapy and occupational therapy. The proximity to the family home of therapy and health services and professional appreciation of cultural diversity were rated as least important.

The question of the content, structure and most effective delivery model of such services will now be considered in light of evidence presented, intervention models already suggested and successful programmes recorded by researchers and therapists. Dimensions of provision such as workforce development, information and advice provided to families, particular programmes offered to families and location of services will be suggested.

Suggested ECI approaches for children and families with FASDs

1 PROFESSIONAL KNOWLEDGE AND CONTINUING PROFESSIONAL DEVELOPMENT

Professionals involved in ECI programmes should have:

- understanding of the relationship between women's alcohol consumption and complex psycho-social issues including aspects of women's history and culture. Knowledge of the needs of the whole population, as well as specific groups: school-age children and adolescents, women of child-bearing age, pregnant women and high-risk women (those with alcohol and poly-substance abuse histories) (Western Australia Department of Health 2010);
- training, knowledge and continuing professional development related to assessing and supporting children with FASDs and children exposed to maternal alcohol and poly-substance use who are not diagnosed with FASDs;
- the ability to suggest and implement a number of intervention programmes based on children's and families' strengths in order to determine which children are developmentally delayed because of lack of appropriate experience and those who will benefit from comprehensive health screening and diagnostic assessment;
- knowledge of appropriate and available referral pathways (Frances, Chapter 9, this publication) and relevant 'touchpoints' (Brazelton and Sparrow 2003) for children and families to ensure early detection, assessment, diagnosis and support and that

particular attention is provided at sensitive and vulnerable periods (such as times of transition or expected changes in children's pattern of development);
- knowledge of child neglect and child abuse, and the needs of children who are fostered or adopted. Knowledge of child protection and safeguarding, child development and developmental differences (from conception to age six years), and educational and therapeutic approaches suitable for children with a range of medical, physical, neurodevelopmental, communication, mental health and sensory needs;
- the ability to view children and families as a diverse group with individual cultural, spiritual and communication needs (Frances and Staggers 2011) rather than as a homogenous group of service users.
- interest in and the skills required to work in trans-disciplinary teams to achieve optimal outcomes for children and families from a diverse range of socio-economic and socio-cultural backgrounds;
- knowledge and skills to work with young children and their families in their natural environments and to provide counselling and coaching to families and colleagues;
- the ability to reflect on their own practice to assess whether outcomes and goals are being achieved. In particular, the skills and interest to seek new approaches to early detection such as those suggested by Hepper (Chapter 5, this publication) and De Beer (2008) of observing fetal startle responses *in utero* and observing young children's communication profiles to determine early differences;
- an interest in investigating and implementing new and emerging screening and diagnostic tools (Western Australia Department of Health 2010) to ensure windows of opportunity for early detection are not missed. Additional support should be provided for families who already have a child with an FASD as this a risk indicator that further children may be vulnerable (Viljoen, Chapter 22, this publication);
- the skills to ensure that terminology used for families is accessible and meaningful to them, for example the terms 'support' and 'advice' are less hostile terms for many families than 'counselling' (Frances and Staggers 2011);
- the knowledge and skills to develop professional relationships with foster and adoption agencies and understand the needs of birth and adoptive families;
- the ability to promote healthy relationships with families and within families for the benefit of all family members (Moore 2008);
- the ability to plan transitions from ECI service to mainstream services/other services in a way which minimizes disruption and maximizes support, clarity and confidence for families (Bruder 2010).

2 INFORMATION/EDUCATION PROGRAMMES

Information/education programmes should:

- be promoted to all interest groups and stakeholders involved in the FASD community (Frances and Staggers 2011);
- place families at the heart of provision and include and consult with them on all aspects of ECI services offered to them in ways which demonstrate dignity and respect as well as inclusion and participation (a key aspect of this is observing children's rights to have their voices heard in line with the United Nations Convention on the Rights of the Child);
- inform families about healthy pregnancies and maternal health issues in the pregnancy and postnatal periods, including healthy breast-feeding (Allen 2011a; NOFAS-UK 2010);
- inform families and the professionals who support them about the effects of prenatal alcohol exposure and fetal exposure to other substances (Blackburn *et al.* 2012);
- provide information for families about child development, the developmental implications of FASDs for their child/children including the importance of early attachment and caregiver–child interactions (Cuthbert *et al.* 2012).

3 ASSESSMENT, INTERVENTION, EDUCATION, THERAPY AND RELATED SERVICES

Therapies and other services should:

- provide a range of therapeutic care and educational services to address the holistic learning and developmental needs of children with FASDs across developmental domains. This would ideally be delivered through an interdisciplinary approach and be based on the child's strengths and successes as well as needs. There should be a focus on children's rights and potential to develop their identity and personality within their diverse communities. Improvements in children's attention span, sensitivity to touch and capacity to play in productive and educational ways (Kleinfeld 1993) have been noted as a result of particular therapeutic interventions in children's early years;
- commence as soon as possible either during pregnancy or after birth (Murphy 1993) in order to address children's sensory needs. The objective should be to identify and promote activities which prevent the child from becoming over- or under-stimulated both mentally and physically, by increasing tolerance to touch as well as the tolerance for noise in the environment through a staged introduction to noises when children are relaxed;
- value families' contribution to interventions and programmes delivered by play therapists and teachers working together which will improve the sustainability of interventions that can be embedded within a family context and used to help generalize learning from school/ECI setting to home (Hinde 1993);

- provide comprehensive health screening services for pregnant women and infants as well as early diagnostic services (BMA 2007; Kleinfeld and Westcott 1993);
- provide opportunities for parents and carers (and children) to socialize with and seek advice from and support each other in a safe, supportive environment (Frances and Staggers 2011);
- provide advocacy services for children and families (Frances and Staggers 2011);
- sensitively support all families and be aware of the particular needs of those who abuse alcohol (and other substances) (Cuthbert et al. 2012);
- provide counselling services for families in relation to family issues. This would include birth families, foster carers and adoptive families and address any feelings of guilt which may be evident in birth families;
- provide mental health services (Cuthbert *et al.* 2012);
- provide early childhood care and education services for children which identify their strengths, successes and needs, provide developmentally and contextually appropriate opportunities to enable children to enjoy positive early years experiences (Whitebread and Bingham 2011);
- provide community-based educational services in order for the neighbourhood systems which children inhabit to understand the needs of children and families affected by FASDs.

The provision of these services in locations convenient for family access delivered by professionals who can empathize with and respect a range of family needs and structures might serve to minimize the loneliness and isolation for individuals with FASDs described by Dorris (1989) in the introduction to this chapter.

Conclusion

ECI for children and families affected by FASDs can help to 'create a firm foundation' (Kleinfeld 1993: 319) for children's learning and development. Early identification in particular is pivotal as it results in a perceptual shift in societal views about children with FASDs, enabling people to understand their challenging behaviour and find ways to maximize their potential (Malbin 1993: 269).

Kleinfeld (1993: 219) warns that ECI should not be viewed as an 'inoculation that protects the child forever more', as it cannot overcome the damage of alcohol, although it can 'dramatically improve the child's life skills and lay the foundations for later development' (Hinde 1993: 147). However, this assertion assumes that child development commences postnatally and ECI excludes professional care for the developing fetus. It has been argued in this chapter that a perceptual shift is required towards including the prenatal period in the developmental time-line. Complacency and misunderstanding about the risks associated with prenatal alcohol consumption appear to pervade society at all levels, including professionals responsible for the care of fetal development. The term 'Fetal and Early Childhood Intervention' (FECI) might serve to highlight the importance of the critical development occurring in pregnancy and reduce the number of children vulnerable to prenatal toxic assault.

Children with FASDs are talented, skilled and have many valuable attributes. These skills and attributes must provide a mechanism to enable parents to look positively towards the future and see a way for their child to find the shore that eluded Adam (Dorris 1989).

Among families of children with FASDs, some parents have found strength and direction in becoming advocates for their children, refusing to give up the fight for their rights to crucial ECI and educational services. Such parents know 'that they cannot undo the biological damage that prenatal alcohol abuse has done'. But they can 'observe and invent and help their children achieve everything possible' (Kleinfeld 1993: 321). Birth mothers are calling for all women to be educated about the effects of drinking while pregnant and about FASDs in particular (Blackburn and Williams 2013), though it is acknowledged that some women are not aware of their pregnancy in the early stages (see Plant, Chapter 4, this publication). However, women naturally expect that their reporting of persistent or problematic drinking and concerns over their children's development to professionals, in whom they place their trust, will result in appropriate action and advice. This is not currently the experience of some mothers (Blackburn and Williams 2013).

Governments and policymakers must ensure that ECI initiatives and programmes are evidence-based and the professionals employed in them are knowledgeable about FASDs and the implications for families and are equipped to support them. The approach must be based on providing informed choice and partnerships of equity and equality with families. ECI services should respect the battles both biological or adoptive families affected by FASDs face and provide the support and resources for them to realize that the situation 'is not hopeless' and the parent and child are 'not helpless' (ibid.).

Reducing the number of children born prenatally exposed to alcohol must surely be a primary intervention goal for all governments, followed by positive education and therapeutic programmes for those already affected. This should yield long-term benefits for children, families, communities and society.

Notes

1 Although there is some evidence to suggest that paternal alcohol consumption has negative effects on a developing fetus (Karr-Morse and Wiley 1997) research in this area remains insubstantial in comparison to studies relating to maternal alcohol consumption. However animal studies indicate that there may be a link between paternal alcohol consumption and the likelihood of alcoholism in offspring as well as some indication of fetal damage (ibid.: 228).
2 Dorris (1989) notes that he had assumed that Adam's learning and behavioural difficulties were associated with his medication for seizures and the neglect he experienced in early childhood. Not until Adam was five years old did he realize that his 'real adversary was the lingering ghost of Adam's biological mother, already dead of acute alcohol poisoning' (1989: 45).
3 High numbers of children with FASD enter the social care system, resulting in children being placed in long-term foster care, multiple family placements or being adopted. Children with FASD, therefore, sometimes have two families, the family they are placed with and their birth family. The implications of this for children and families are discussed in Blackburn et al. (2012).
4 It should be noted that this study involved a survey of the European Birth Mothers Network. It is a limitation of the study that it is small scale (there are only 12 members) and the participants are self-selected. It is not suggested that this is a representative sample.
5 Sure Start is a UK government programme which provides services for preschool children and their families. It works to bring together early education, childcare, health and family support. Services provided include advice on healthcare and child development, play schemes, parenting classes, family outreach support and adult education and advice.

6 To highlight a few: the Florida Center for Early Childhood Fetal Alcohol Diagnostic and Intervention Clinic at: www.thefloridacenter.org/fetalalcohol.htm; The Government of Alberta Government and Youth Services initiatives at: www.fasd-cmc.alberta.ca/home/; the Canada Northwest FASD Partnership at: www.cnfasdpartnership.ca/index.php. See also Grant and Clarren, Chapter 20, this publication.
7 See: www.sabp.nhs.uk/services/specialist/fetal-alcohol-spectrum-disorder-fasd-clinic.

References

Abel, E.L and Hannigan, J.H. (1995) 'Maternal risk factors in fetal alcohol syndrome: provocative and permissive influences', *Neurotoxicology and Teratology*, 17(6): 445–62.

Allen, G. (2011a) *Early Intervention: The next steps (an independent report to Her Majesty's Government)*, London: HM Government.

Allen, G. (2011b) *Early Intervention: Smart investment, massive steps*, London: HM Government.

Allen, G. and Duncan Smith, I. (2008) *Early Intervention: Good parents, great kids, better citizens*, London: Centre for Social Justice and the Smith Institute.

Autti-Ramo, I. (2002) 'Foetal alcohol syndrome: a multifaceted condition', *Developmental Medicine and Child Neurology*, 44(2): 141–4.

Blackburn, C. (2009) *Building Bridges with Understanding – Foetal Alcohol Spectrum Disorders (FASD): Focus on strategies*, Worcester: Sunfield Research Institute/Worcestershire County Council [online at: www.worcestershire.gov.uk/cms/PDF/49598%20FASD%20Strategy%20web1.pdf; accessed: 9 August 2012].

Blackburn, C. (2010) *Facing the Challenge and Shaping the Future for Primary and Secondary Aged Students with Foetal Alcohol Spectrum Disorders (FAS-eD Project)*, London: National Organisation on Fetal Alcohol Syndrome (UK) [online at: www.nofas-uk.org; accessed: 27 July 2011].

Blackburn, C. and Whitehurst, T. (2010) 'Foetal alcohol spectrum disorders (FASD): raising awareness in early years settings', *British Journal of Special Education*, 27(3): 122–9.

Blackburn, C. and Williams, P. (2013) 'Survey of European Birth Mothers Network: FASD and early childhood intervention' (unpublished).

Blackburn, C., Carpenter, B. and Egerton, J. (2012) *Educating Children and Young People with Fetal Alcohol Spectrum Disorders (FASD)*, Abingdon: Routledge.

BMA (British Medical Association) (2007) *Fetal Alcohol Spectrum Disorders: A guide for healthcare professionals*, London: BMA.

Brazelton, T.B. and Sparrow, J. (2003) *Touchpoints Model of Development*, Boston, MA: Brazleton Touchpoints Center.

Bronfenbrenner, U. (1979) *The Ecology of Human Development*, Cambridge, MA: Harvard University Press.

Bruder, M.B. (2010) 'Early childhood intervention: a promise to children and families for their future', *Exceptional Children*, 76(3): 339–55.

Carpenter, B. (2005) 'Early childhood intervention: possibilities and prospects for professionals, families and children', *British Journal of Special Education*, 32(4): 176–83.

Carpenter, B. (2011) 'Pedagogically bereft! Improving learning outcomes for children with foetal alcohol spectrum disorders', *British Journal of Special Education*, 38(1): 37–43.

Carpenter, B. and Egerton, J. (2005) 'Introduction', in B. Carpenter and J. Egerton (eds) *Early Childhood Intervention: International perspectives, national initiatives and regional practice*. Coventry: West Midlands SEN Regional Partnership.

Carpenter, B., Egerton, J., Brooks, T., Cockbill, B., Fotheringham, J. and Rawson, H. (2011) *The Complex Learning Difficulties and Disabilities Research Project: Developing meaningful pathways to personalised learning (Final Report)*, London: Specialist Schools and Academies Trust (SSAT).

Clarren, S.G.B. (2004) *Teaching Students with Fetal Alcohol Spectrum Disorder: Building strengths, creating hope*, Edmonton, Canada: Alberta Learning.

Cuthbert, C., Raynes, G. and Stanley, K. (2012) *All Babies Count: Prevention and protection for vulnerable babies*, London: National Society for the Prevention of Cruelty to Children (NSPCC).

De Beer, M.M. (2008) *Communication Profiles of a Group of Young Children (0–5) with Foetal Alcohol Spectrum Disorders* (masters dissertation), Pretoria, SA: University of Pretoria [online at: http://upetd.up.ac.za/thesis/available/etd-02212011-175152/unrestricted/dissertation.pdf; accessed: 11 September 2011].

Dittrich, W.H. and Tutt, R. (2008) *Educating Children with Complex Conditions*, London: Sage.
Dorris, M. (1989) *The Broken Cord*, New York: Harper and Row.
Dunst, C.J. and Trivette, C.M. (1997) 'Early intervention with young at-risk children and their families', in R. Ammerman and M. Hersen (eds) *Handbook of Prevention and Treatment with Children and Adolescents: Intervention in the real world*, New York, NY: Wiley.
Egerton, J. (2009) *Building Bridges with Understanding – Foetal Alcohol Spectrum Disorders (FASD): Information Sheets*, Worcester: Sunfield Research Institute/Worcestershire County Council [online at: www.worcestershire.gov.uk/cms/early-years-and-childcare/information-for-providers/inclusion-equality-and-diversity/sen-information-and-resources.aspx; accessed 5th June 2013].
European Agency for Development in Special Needs Education (2005) *Early Childhood Intervention – Analysis of Situations in Europe: Key aspects and recommendations* (summary report) [online at: www.european-agency.org/publications/ereports/early-childhood-intervention/eci_en.pdf; accessed: 4 June 2013].
Field, F. (2010) *The Foundation Years: Preventing poor children becoming poor adults*, London: HM Government.
Frances, K. and Staggers, S. (2011) *Evaluation of Palmerston Association Yarning And Parenting Program for Parents and Children Experiencing Drug and Alcohol Problems*, Perth, WA: National Drug Research Institute, Curtin University.
Goswami, U. (2008) *Learning Difficulties: Future challenges (Mental Capital and Wellbeing Project)*, London: HMSO/Government Office for Science.
Guralnick, M. (1997) 'Second generation research in the field of early intervention', in M.J. Guralnick (ed.) *The Effectiveness of Early Intervention*, Baltimore, MD: Paul H. Brookes.
Guralnick, M. (2004) 'Introduction: what is early intervention?' in M. Feldman (ed.) *Early Intervention: The essential readings*, Oxford: Blackwell Publishing.
Guralnick, M. (2005) *The Developmental Systems Approach to Early Intervention*, Baltimore, MD: Paul H. Brookes.
Hinde, J. (1993) 'Early intervention for alcohol-affected children birth to age three', in J. Kleinfeld and S. Wescott (eds) *Fantastic Antone Succeeds! Experiences in Educating Children with Fetal Alcohol Syndrome*, Fairbanks, AK: University of Alaska Press.
Hope, A. (2008) *Coronial Inquest into 22 Deaths in the Kimberley (ref no: 37/07)*, Perth, WA: Coroner's Court of Western Australia.
Karr-Morse, R. and Wiley, M.S. (1997) *Ghosts from the Nursery: Tracing the roots of violence*, New York, NY: Atlantic Monthly Press.
Kleinfeld, J. (1993) 'Conclusion', in J. Kleinfeld and S. Wescott (1993) (eds) *Fantastic Antone Succeeds! Experiences in Educating Children with Fetal Alcohol Syndrome*, Fairbanks, AK: University of Alaska Press.
Kleinfeld, J. and Wescott, S. (eds) (1993) *Fantastic Antone Succeeds! Experiences in Educating Children with Fetal Alcohol Syndrome*, Fairbanks, AK: University of Alaska Press.
Laughlan, F. and Boyle, C. (2007) 'Is the use of labels in special education helpful?' *Support for Learning*, 22(1): 36–42.
Lewis, I. (2007) 'Foreword', in Department of Health, *Maternity Matters: Choice, access and continuity of care in a safe service*, London: DH.
Lynch, R. (2005) *Early Childhood Investment Yields Big Payoff*, San Francisco, CA: WestEd.
Malbin, D. (1993) 'Stereotypes and realities – positives outcomes with intervention', in J. Kleinfeld and S. Wescott (eds) *Fantastic Antone Succeeds! Experiences in Educating Children with Fetal Alcohol Syndrome*, Fairbanks, AK: University of Alaska Press.
May, P. and Gossage, J.P. (2011) 'Maternal risk factors for fetal alcohol spectrum disorders: not as simple as it might seem', *Alcohol Research and Health*, 34 (1): 15.
Moore, T.G. (2008) *Early Childhood Intervention: Core knowledge and skills (CCCH Working Paper 3)*, Parkville, Victoria: Centre for Community Child Health.
Mukherjee, R. et al. (2010) 'Knowledge of FASD in UK general public and healthcare practitioners', presentation at the first European Conference on 'FASD: Growing Awareness in Europe', 3–5 November 2010, Netherlands.
Munro, E. (2011) *The Munro Review of Child Protection: Final Report – A child-centred system*, London: Department for Education [online at: https://www.education.gov.uk/publications/eOrderingDownload/Munro-Review.pdf; accessed 4 June 2013].

Murphy P.A. (2010) *Origins: How the nine months before birth shape the rest of our lives*, London: Hay House.
Murphy, M. (1993) 'Shut up and talk to me', in J. Kleinfeld and S. Wescott (eds) *Fantastic Antone Succeeds! Experiences in Educating Children with Fetal Alcohol Syndrome*, Fairbanks, AK: University of Alaska Press.
NOFAS-UK (2010) *Alcohol in Pregnancy: Information for midwives*, London: NOFAS-UK.
Ntsabula, A. (2001) *Human Genetics Policy Document for the Management and Prevention of Genetic Disorders, Birth Defects and Disabilities*, Pretoria, SA: Department of Health.
Pienaar, A. (2003) 'n Dop wat kind Skop', *BEELD*, 22 October: 9 [online at: http://152.111.1.88/argief/berigte/beeld/2003/10/22/B1/09/01.html].
Streissguth, A. and Kanter, J. (eds) (1997) *The Challenge of Fetal Alcohol Syndrome: Overcoming secondary disabilities*, Seattle, WA: University of Washington Press.
United Nations (1989) *Convention on the Rights of the Child*, New York, NY: United Nations [online at: http://treaties.un.org/Pages/ViewDetails.aspx?src=TREATY&mtdsg_no=IV-11&chapter=4&lang=en; accessed: 22 October2012].
United Nations (2006) *Convention on the Rights of Persons with Disabilities*, New York, NY: United Nations [online at: http://treaties.un.org/Pages/ViewDetails.aspx?src=TREATY&mtdsg_no=IV-15&chapter=4&lang=en; accessed: 22 October 2012].
Viljoen, M.D., Craig, P., Hymbaugh, M.P.H, Boyle, C. and Blount, S. (2003) 'Fetal alcohol syndrome – South Africa 2001', *Morbidity and Mortality Weekly Report (MMWR)*, 52(28): 660–2.
Warren, K.R., Hewitt, B.G. and Thomas, J.D. (2011) 'Fetal alcohol spectrum disorders: research challenges and opportunities', *Alcohol Research and Health*, 34(1): 4–14.
Western Australia Department of Health (2010) *Fetal Alcohol Spectrum Disorder Model of Care*, Perth, WA: Health Networks Branch, Department of Health.
Whitebread, D. and Bingham, S. (2011) *School Readiness: A critical review of perspectives and evidence (occasional paper no. 2)*, Canterbury: TACTYC – Association for the Professional Development of Early Years Practitioners.
Winstone, A. (2012) 'FASD: are we getting the message across?', presentation at the 'Missing a Trick: Stepping up to the Challenge of FASD' Conference, Coventry, September.
Wise, S., da Silva, L., Webster, E. and Sanson, A. (2005) *The Efficacy of Early Childhood Interventions (AIFS research report no. 14)*, Melbourne, Victoria: Australian Institute of Family Studies [online at: www.aifs.gov.au/institute/pubs/resreport14/aifsreport14.pdf; accessed 5 August 2012].

11
EVOLVING PEDAGOGY FOR CHILDREN AND YOUNG PEOPLE WITH FETAL ALCOHOL SPECTRUM DISORDERS

Barry Carpenter

Many educators are unaware that they have taught children and young people with fetal alcohol spectrum disorders (FASDs). However, with the widely accepted prevalence of FASD as 1 in 100 children (British Medical Association 2007), it is likely that they will have done so without realizing it. Kieran O'Malley (2007) has described young people with FASDs as clinical masqueraders, meaning that they are often misdiagnosed with other conditions based upon their symptoms alone. Misdiagnoses may include: attention deficit/hyperactivity disorder (ADHD), autistic spectrum disorders (ASD), conduct disorder, social emotional behavioural disorder (SEBD) or oppositional defiant disorder (ODD), among others (Coles 2011; Dubovsky 2009; O'Malley 2007).

Although some professionals are concerned about the stigma of a fetal alcohol syndrome (FAS) diagnosis, Alberta Education (2009: 7) describes a true diagnosis as a protective factor which 'can increase understanding of the individual's needs and strengths, and be a catalyst for the individual receiving the supports he or she needs'. Most children and young people with FASDs are diagnosed around nine years old (Paley and O'Connor 2009), and while appropriate intervention at any age can produce life improvements (Grant *et al.* 2004; Grant and Clarren, Chapter 20, this publication), Streissguth *et al.* (1996) found that diagnosis, preferably before the age of six years, reduced the risk of poor outcomes. Without diagnosis, a lack of awareness by professionals and families of young people's difficulties can lead to consistently unrealistic expectations of them (Streissguth and O'Malley 2000) resulting in serious behavioural, cognitive, and psychological secondary disabilities, which may include mental health problems, disrupted school experience and trouble with the law (Dossetor *et al.* 2011). As SAMHSA (2010: slide 24) points out:

> inaccurate diagnosis can be harmful. Persons with an undiagnosed FASD may be mislabeled as noncompliant, uncooperative, or unmotivated. In addition, treatments are selected on the basis of the diagnosis. If the diagnosis is not correct, the treatment will not be correct. For example, medications for ADHD may not help a person whose attention deficits stem from prenatal alcohol exposure.

The challenge

Whatever the background, the challenge remains: how do we optimize learning for these children and young people? Even more so, we have to ask, how do we teach them? Despite the attention given to diagnosing FAS and describing these young people's characteristics, there has been no systematic investigation of their educational needs of or of best educational strategies for effective teaching and learning (Ryan and Ferguson 2006). Often teachers, being unaware of this group of young people, do not identify them or plan specifically to meet their learning needs (Blackburn 2012).

Until recently, there was no direct guidance from any government agency in the UK to teachers on how to educate children and young people with FASDs. However, in October 2010, NOFAS-UK (www.nofas-uk.org) published a significant report offering guidance to educators in all age phases (Blackburn 2010), and in 2012, Blackburn, Carpenter and Egerton published *Educating Children and Young People with Fetal Alcohol Spectrum Disorders* largely based upon that work, and also with reference to the Complex Learning Difficulties and Disabilities Research Project (Carpenter *et al.* 2011).

The impact of FASDs upon learning

Brain damage is the most serious aspect of FASDs (see Figure 11.1). This damage is permanent. It can be accommodated, but not reversed. FASDs affect cognition, behaviour and social skills. It is a pervasive developmental disorder with lifelong implications for schooling and beyond. Whereas the facial features of the child or young person with FAS make it easier to

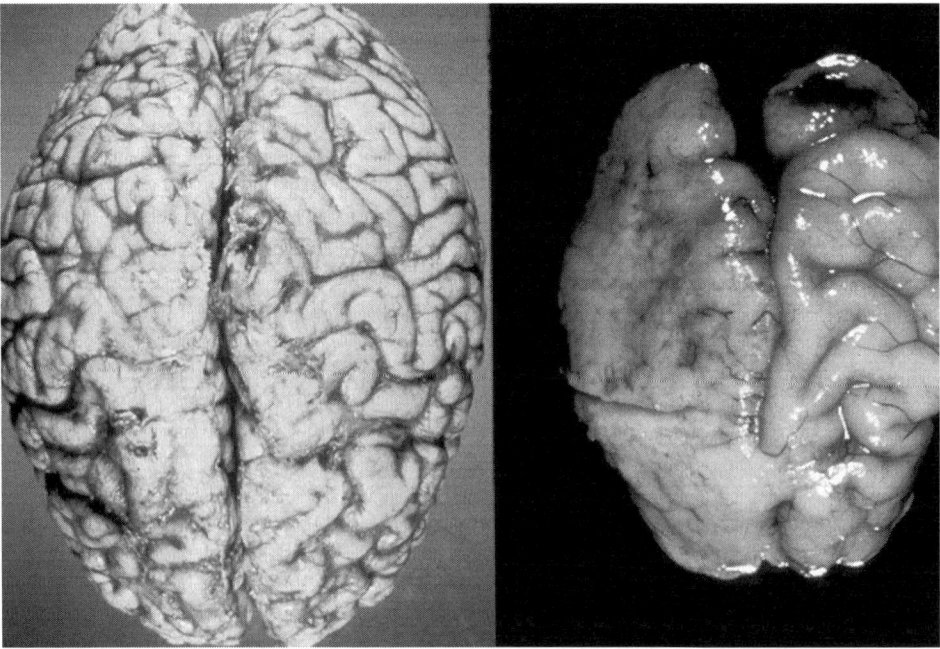

FIGURE 11.1 Comparison between the brain of a typically developing baby and that of a baby with FAS (courtesy of Dr Sterling Clarren).

identify, for those elsewhere on the spectrum, who may not have these facial features, it is usually the intensity of the school learning situation which highlights their particular needs.

It is also important that educators are aware of the true extent of the hidden impairments of FASDs, so they can recognize, understand and accommodate children and young people's learning needs. The developmental profile of young people with FASDs is uneven. This means that they are difficult to accommodate within any Key Stage of the English National Curriculum. They may score within normal limits on measures of IQ, and give the appearance of functioning at a level consistent with their chronological age. However, their academic abilities are often well below that suggested by their IQ, and their living skills, communication skills and adaptive behaviour levels are even further below (Streissguth *et al.* 1996) (see Figure 11.2). They appear physically mature, their expressive language may be in advance of their actual age, and their reading skills may be chronologically appropriate. However, while they are apparently articulate, their verbal communication typically lacks complex meaningful content and their actual comprehension is often significantly compromised (Gibbard *et al.* 2003). Mathematical and numerical concepts are particularly challenging for this group of young people in that, for some, the parietal lobe, which controls numeracy and computational activity in the brain, may have significantly reduced functioning (Kopera-Frye *et al.* 1996). In areas such as social skills and emotional maturity, they may be performing at half of their developmental age.

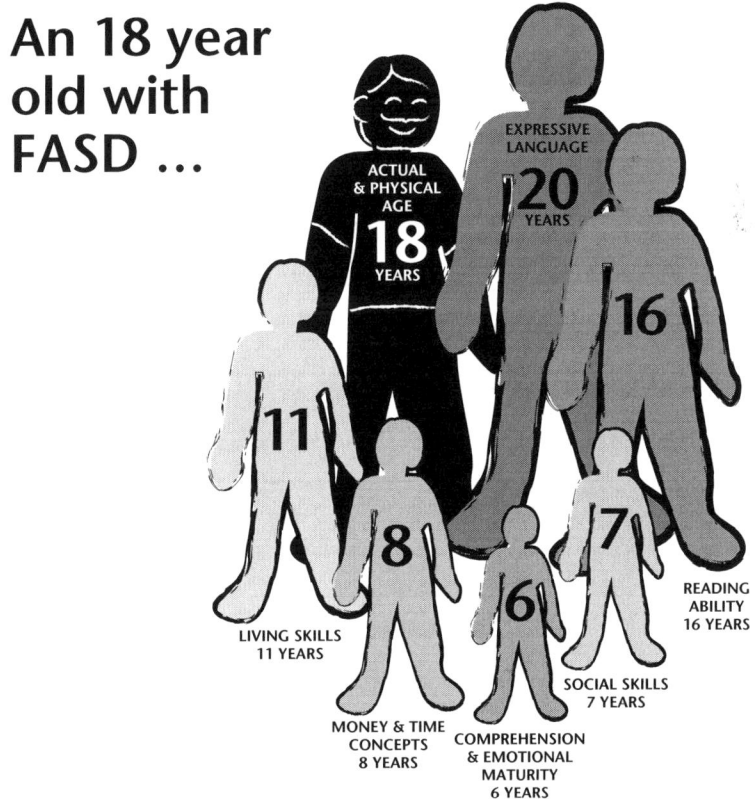

FIGURE 11.2 Developmental profile of an 18-year-old with an FASD (*Source*: Jodee Kulp, www.betterendings.org).

In their articles, Gibbard *et al.* (2003) and Kodituwakku *et al.* (2006) summarize the findings of a wide range of neuropsychological research in relation to the impairments experienced by children and young people with FASDs, and these are presented in Table 11.1.

TABLE 11.1 Possible impairments experienced by children and young people with FASDs

Possible cognitive impairments	• Impaired auditory learning
	• Impaired nonverbal intellectual ability
	• Impaired IQ
	
	• Memory function impairment – including visual, short-term, working memory, explicit memory functioning, conscious memory recall
	• Impaired strategic manipulation of information to improve recall
	• Impaired initial encoding of information
	• Visual-motor integration and visual-perceptual deficits, including reading disorders, impaired visual-spatial perception
	
	• Slow information processing
	• Impairment of higher level receptive and expressive language
	• Impaired comprehension
	• Impaired arithmetical reasoning, and mathematical skills (e.g. money management and telling time)
	
	• Cognitive inflexibility
	• Poor executive function ('dysexecutive syndrome'):
	  — Impaired concept formation
	  — Poor abstract reasoning/metacognition
	  — Impaired ability to plan

Possible behavioural/ emotional difficulties	• Difficulty in focusing attention and maintaining attention in the presence of distractors • Poor impulse control/response inhibition • Disorganization • Impaired persistence • Perseverative behaviour • Attention Deficit Hyperactivity Disorder (usually earlier-onset, inattention subtype; often unresponsive to medication) • Developmental, psychiatric, and medical conditions Attachment Disorder, Post-Traumatic Stress Disorder • Anxiety disorders

Possible social difficulties	• Emotional immaturity (e.g. age inappropriate emotional interactions and responses)
	• Lack of effective reciprocal social behaviour (leading to alienation from others)
	• Difficulty in understanding the social consequences of behaviour
	
	• Lack of social perception including difficulties with:
	  — Detecting and understanding nonverbal communication/subtle social cues
	  — Understanding another's perspective
	  — Self-reflection and
	  — insight into own actions

Other possible difficulties	• Gross and fine motor function difficulties • Sensory processing difficulties

Developing education support strategies for children and young people with FASDs

Each child or young person with FASDs has a unique profile with their own strengths and challenges, developmental levels and family context (Gibbard 2009). They tend to be very erratic and unpredictable learners, and it is necessary to reframe our traditional expectations. The symptoms of FASDs can be wide-ranging and highly variable between individuals. Prenatal damage through alcohol can occur anytime within the nine-month gestation period with different impacts depending on the developmental stage of the fetus and the dose of alcohol. As a result, one of the difficulties with devising educational approaches for young people with FASDs is that the condition currently has no identified core deficits, although Kodituwakku (2009) proposes a global deficit in the processing and integration of information. Current educational strategies therefore have to be symptomatically based (Hannigan and Berman 2000), and a personalized approach to assessment and intervention is needed (Carpenter *et al.* 2011). Paley and O'Connor (2009: 259) emphasize the importance of 'thorough assessments that are designed to evaluate functioning across multiple domains'.

Strategies adopted must take into consideration neurological differences. Due to their sensory processing difficulties, we need to consider how children and young people with FASDs make sense of, and use of, information from the sensory world (Jirikowic 2007). Young people with FASDs often overreact, even to simple things like a fly landing near them. They may startle if someone approaches them from behind. They may be driven to seek or avoid certain sensations. There is also significant emotional dysregulation in children with FASDs, and they are prone to significant mood swings. Their capacity for self-regulation is impaired; they find it difficult to self-calm, and seem not to respond well to parental calming techniques such as hugging. Classrooms have to be carefully designed to accommodate their learning and behavioural needs. Some teachers have developed 'safe areas' in their classrooms to provide a personal space for the young person with an FASD, containing cushions and favourite activities known to have a calming effect (Carpenter 2011).

The following broad educational strategies have been suggested when working with children and young people with FASDs (Blackburn *et al.* 2012; Clarren *et al.* 2000; Evensen and Lutke 1997; Paley and O'Connor 2009):

- keep teaching and instruction simple and specific;
- break down stories or lessons into smaller parts;
- employ adaptive teaching techniques which focus upon the child's interests, strengths and developmental stage;
- use consistent and predictable language to support understanding;
- use visual cues and aids to accompany verbal instructions;
- provide concrete learning resources and opportunities to support learning;
- use pre-learning, rehearsing and practising of desirable skills and behaviours;
- engineer repetition;
- note strategies used by the student and teach more effective alternatives;
- give instructions to the individual in small steps to support understanding and executive function;
- give warning and instructions well ahead of transitions, and give support;
- provide a structured learning environment (e.g. classroom spaces, time, work, etc.);

- have consistent and predictable routines (e.g. providing visual schedules of activities);
- make cause and effect explicit (e.g. outcomes of decisions);
- supervise;
- reward effort rather than achievement.

In *Educating Children and Young People with Fetal Alcohol Spectrum Disorders* (Blackburn et al. 2012), mentioned above, there are detailed primary and secondary education intervention frameworks based upon research with teachers of young people with FASDs in nine UK schools.

WORKING WITH A CHILD WITH COMMUNICATION DIFFICULTIES: THINGS TO REMEMBER

Before you speak
- make sure you have the child's attention before you speak to them;
- make sure you are facing the child and are at their level so that they can see facial expressions and gestures;
- have all necessary visual aids available either on the work surface or ideally attached to a wrist strap or belt

When you speak
- say the child's name at the beginning of an instruction or sentence;
- only give one instruction at a time;
- keep instructions short, use the minimum number of words;
- say exactly what you want the child to do (e.g. instead of saying 'tidy up', say 'put the wooden bricks in the blue box') and back this up with pictures if necessary;
- give the child time to think about what you have asked of them;
- use positive communication, instead of saying 'don't run', say 'walk';
- use exaggerated facial expressions and gestures to give the child clues as to your meaning;
- use visual prompts such as puppets for story telling;
- if you are interrupted while giving an instruction go back to the beginning of your sentence;
- the child's ability to repeat an instruction back to you does not signify understanding.

(Blackburn 2009)

Important considerations

Any educational programme for children and young people with FASDs should not overlook the additional factors which make them such complex learners. In addition to their learning difficulties, their family context, their impaired social understanding and FASD-related health issues may also impact on their ability to learn. Health complications may result in time away from school. Mental health difficulties might arise from attachment disorders associated with, for example, initial infant–maternal bonding difficulties, a disrupted home environment, multiple foster placements, etc. (Blackburn *et al.* 2012). The cognitive impairments of young people with FASDs also give rise to social difficulties; social strategies need to be supported through rehearsal and coaching at school and at home (O'Connor *et al.* 2006) to promote positive life outcomes.

There have been few formal evaluations of skills programmes for children and young people with FASDs, but Table 11.2 shows some recent trials and their outcomes.

TABLE 11.2 Trials of educational and social programmes with positive outcomes

Programmes with positive outcomes	Related areas of difficulty for children with FASDs	Outcomes	Reference
Cognitive Control Therapy (CCT)	Ability to acquire and organize information more effectively	Improvements in function but no significant difference	Paley and O'Connor 2011
Language and literacy intervention	Language and literacy skills	Improved phonic awareness and early literacy test scores	Adnams *et al.* 2007
Alert Programme (adapted)	Self-regulation skills and executive functioning	Significant effect on executive functioning (parent report measure)	Williams and Shellenberger 1996
Sociocognitive mathematics programme	School-based mathematics intervention	Significant mathematics knowledge gain	Original study: Kable *et al.* 2007; follow-up: Coles *et al.* 2009
Working memory through rehearsal strategies	Working memory	Significantly increased digit span test outcomes	Loomes *et al.* 2008
Children's Friendship Training (adapted)	Social understanding (e.g. social cues, processing social information and communicating in social contexts)	Significantly improved knowledge and skills	O'Connor *et al.* 2006
Safety skills	Impulsivity, lack of behavioural inhibition, poor judgement, and difficulty generalizing skills across contexts	Improved knowledge of fire and street safety; only fire safety knowledge retained after one week	Coles *et al.* 2007
Safety skills	As above	Showed knowledge gain in response to a virtual fire simulation	Padget *et al.* 2006
Social communication intervention	Social communication: strategies for social situations; use of mental state verbs	More strategies and increased number of verbs used	Timler *et al.* 2005
Attention Process Training	Sustained attention, nonverbal reasoning	Significant improvement	Vernescu 2007

Source: compiled from Paley and O'Connor 2011 and Peadon *et al.* 2009.

Identifying learning needs

In 2008, the author carried out a preliminary piece of qualitative research, seeking to explore some existing educational practice concerning FASDs in the West Midlands – what teachers had identified as the key learning issues for these children and young people in their classrooms, and what their effective teaching strategies were. The purposive sample comprised 20 teachers in primary, secondary and special schools, all of whom were currently working with a young person with a diagnosis of FASDs or had done so within the previous two years. Information was gathered through semi-structured interviews with teachers and, where possible, the young people themselves, and through direct, periodic, nonparticipant observations of teachers and young people in classroom environments (Carpenter 2011).

In the semi-structured interviews, teachers were asked to identify the challenges to the classroom learning environment presented by the children and young people. The following is a list of the top ten challenges reported by these teachers:

1. hyperactivity;
2. short attention span;
3. erratic mood swings;
4. poor memory;
5. lack of social skills;
6. auditory/vocal processing;
7. visual sequencing;
8. sensory integration difficulties (particularly lack of coordination);
9. poor retention of task instruction;
10. numeracy/mathematical difficulties.

It was very obvious that retention and overlearning were not key features of the learning pattern of the young person with FASDs. As one teacher said, 'It's very much "here today, gone tomorrow"!'

Regardless of the difficulties identified, how we optimize the learning of these children and young people remains the challenge. The observations in class, alongside an extensive international literature survey which reported teaching young people with FASDs, led to the identification of ten major teaching responses to the ten learning needs profiled above. These were:

1. a calm learning environment, free from clutter;
2. focused tasks presented in small steps;
3. personal space for the young person with plenty of support and praise;
4. visual structuring (e.g. visual timetables; highlighting key aspects of the task/activity);
5. scripting/role play;
6. short, key information-carrying word instructions;
7. visual clarity and graphic simplicity;
8. frequent, short exercise programmes during the day;
9. a breakdown of tasks with visual and tactile clues, and time given for the young person to complete the task;
10. multisensory learning – giving messages through a variety of sensory pathways.

As one young person with an FASD said:

> When a teacher uses visual clues, I can understand the topic. I learn better when things are presented in a visual way. My brain does not always cope with the words the teacher says. I would say to teachers, 'Please show me, don't tell me…'

Managing the child with an FASD in the classroom environment

Observations indicated that the structure of the classroom was absolutely key to how children with FASDs functioned in their learning environment. As Kalberg and Buckley state: 'It is helpful to think of the environment as an external nervous system of the child, a place where external (environmental) supports can be implemented to bolster the deficit areas of the child' (Kalberg and Buckley, in Paley and O'Connor 2011: 67–8).

Where teachers had carefully considered physical structure, deployment of staffing, visually based resources, groupings of young people and their teaching styles, then the levels of engagement of young people with FASDs were considerably higher than in classrooms where this did not happen.

Discussions with teachers showed that when considering these five points, in relation to physical structure, they had thought through the lighting of the classroom, creating distraction-free environments, and any sensitivity to colour that the child or young person may show. For example, when deploying staff they knew that mathematics was a particularly challenging curriculum area for the young person and therefore ensured that a teaching assistant was available to support during these sessions. As manual dexterity may not be a strength of young people with FASDs, pencil holders were provided. In order to strengthen visual learning, visual clutter on tables was kept to an absolute minimum.

Peer groupings were inevitably the major problem area. The child or young person with an FASD is often irrational, yet longs for friendships. Ten teachers reported that they had tried 'buddy systems', but, in several instances, this had led to the buddy actually being physically or verbally abused by the young person with an FASD. Most teachers adopted a rotational system, where the young person joined different groups for different curriculum areas. This was easier to achieve in the secondary school context than in the primary school context.

An overriding message in relation to teaching staff is that the child or young person with an FASD is a visually dominant learner – not in the same pronounced way as the young person with ASD, but their visual processing was certainly more efficient than their auditory/vocal processing. These teacher interventions to mediate the learning environment mirror the advice offered by Kleinfeld and Wescott (1993) for managing the young person with an FASD in the classroom. They suggest:

- seating the child at the front of the classroom, always in the same seat;
- minimizing distractions (e.g. visual, auditory, etc.);
- providing a calm space;
- ensuring visually clear display;
- using tape on the floor to define spatial boundaries;
- keeping the classroom door closed;
- closing blinds partially (in bright light);
- avoiding bells.

An inquiry approach

Schools need to capitalize on their status as places of enquiry, innovation and development. We need to structure our approach to teaching children and young people with FASDs so that it begins to build a bedrock of evidence from which every learner with FASDs can move forward. Our adoption of strategies to support these young people should not be impulsive and haphazard but informed and consistent. While there are many suggested strategies for working with young people with FASDs available, there is relatively little hard evidence of their success in the classroom. As educators we need to systematically investigate, record, reflect and share what benefits the young people we teach, so they can avoid pitfalls and fast-track to successes.

As reflective practitioners, our daily practice is based on inquiry. We identify an issue in our classroom, and think about how to improve it. We read about and reflect on it, identify possible adaptations or solutions, collect evidence based on assessment and evaluations, and consider its implications, and then reflect on these outcomes and whether it can be improved. These are the principles of the Accessible Research Cycle (ARC) (Jones et al. 2012; see Figure 11.3). However, often our inquiry is informal, low priority and takes place in the background. We do not record the process of discovery that we have been through, and we do not have the evidence to share with others showing the journey from implementation to outcome.

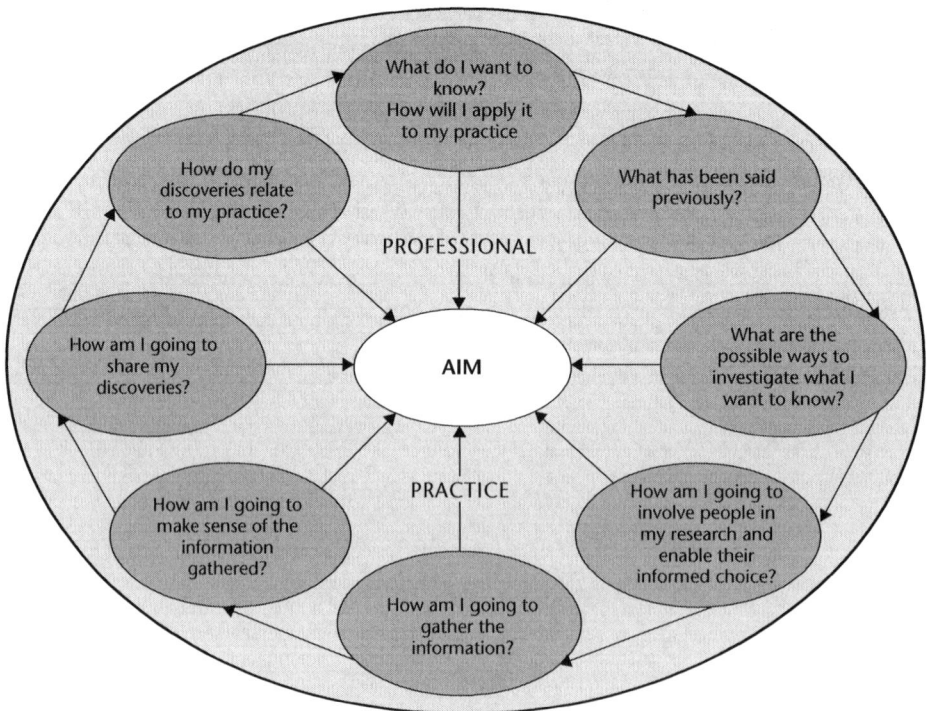

FIGURE 11.3 Accessible Research Cycle (source: Jones et al. 2012).

Michael Guralnick, Professor in Early Childhood Education at the University of Washington has said (2004): 'We now know so much about childhood disability that we must move to second generation research. This must be practitioner led and evidence based.'

While this is may be a daunting prospect, it recognizes the expertise of practitioners and the needs of young people in the real world of the classroom. For our most complex learners, there are no off-the-peg, proven-to-work approaches.

As places of learning, twenty-first century special schools should be about evolving a framework for teaching and learning for these children and young people which is relevant and realistic. Special schools need to become pedagogical think-tanks – nurturing, shaping and framing approaches that are dynamic and innovative, and that transform these young people into active participants in the process of learning (Carpenter 2013). As Hargreaves (2006) suggests, schools need to transform their response to the learner from the largely standardized to the profoundly personalized. Children's engagement in learning will be the benchmark for assessing whether we have achieved this goal. As a gold standard, our approaches must be:

- research informed
- inquiry focused
- evidence based
- practice led.

The following case study illustrates the benefits of some of these approaches, which allowed 15-year-old Naseem (not his real name), to achieve learning success. It describes an intervention devised by his class team, and structured and monitored using the Engagement Profile and Scale (Carpenter *et al.* 2011, 2014; http://complexld.ssatrust.org.uk). The intervention resulted in his increased engagement and independence in learning, and was able to be generalized to other lessons.

Introduction

Naseem, a young man of 15 years, was diagnosed with an FASD and moderate learning difficulties, made more complex by attachment disorder and behavioural emotional and social difficulties (BESD) as well as health issues. The teacher and teaching assistant reviewed Naseem's learning, and concluded that one of his most significant barriers to learning was his apparent inability to complete tasks and activities. Therefore completing an activity became Naseem's priority learning need, and the focus for the intervention.

Using the Engagement Profile and Scale

The Engagement Profile and Scale works on the principle of enabling a child or young person's engagement in an activity or learning task through personalization, which enables the young person to attain their learning targets. It offers a way of recording the pathways and monitoring outcomes of personalizing learning through an engagement score.

Completing the Engagement Profile

An Engagement Profile was drawn up for Naseem that described his behaviour when engaged in a favourite activity, and allowed all educators to recognize the level of engagement that Naseem was capable of and the kind of behaviours they were aiming for in other activities. It helped them to develop high expectations for Naseem.

Establishing a priority learning need

His teacher and teaching assistants identified his individual strengths, difficulties and motivators so that another activity, in which Naseem engaged in with difficulty, could be personalized to increase his engagement with it. This was done by transferring some of the characteristics of activities in which he was able to engage highly to the low engagement activity. His difficulties, in common with many students with FASDs, were a high level of distractibility, and the need for continual reminders and prompts from the staff working with him to keep him on task.

Naseem's first target was to complete his class job of setting the table for break time. Keeping in mind Naseem's barriers, the teacher used the following strategies – introduced one by one over a number of sessions – to allow Naseem to achieve success:

1. She developed a series of visual photographic prompts for each part of Naseem's task to aid his memory retention. The photographs were initially sequenced in the right order as he found sequencing difficult, but in later sessions, to extend Naseem's independence, he was given the responsibility for sequencing the photos.
2. The teacher physically modelled and rehearsed with Naseem how to use them to build on his kinaesthetic learning strengths, rather than relying on auditory instruction which Naseem struggled to process and retain.
3. Students with FASDs need repetition of facts or requests many times, as they have difficulties with retaining learning. Use of the visual prompts allowed a continuing permanent reminder to Naseem of the task he was doing and the steps he needed to make to complete it. It is important to 'script' the task or activity so that the young person can link fragments of knowledge and make a 'whole' response.
4. The teacher praised Naseem, increasing his self-esteem and self-confidence. It is also important to share a young person's achievement with their family, so that they can further reinforce the successes.

In this way, the teacher supported Naseem to keep active as a learner and to experience success.

Monitoring outcomes using the Engagement Scale

Naseem's baseline engagement was documented using the Engagement Scale prior to the intervention taking place. This allowed the teacher to show Naseem's progress from his original level of engagement with the activity before the intervention to his post-intervention level once the intervention was in place.

Figure 11.4 shows the intervention engagement outcomes for Naseem over a two-month period. The pre-intervention marker ('Pre'), shows Naseem's level of engagement before his teacher put the interventions in place.

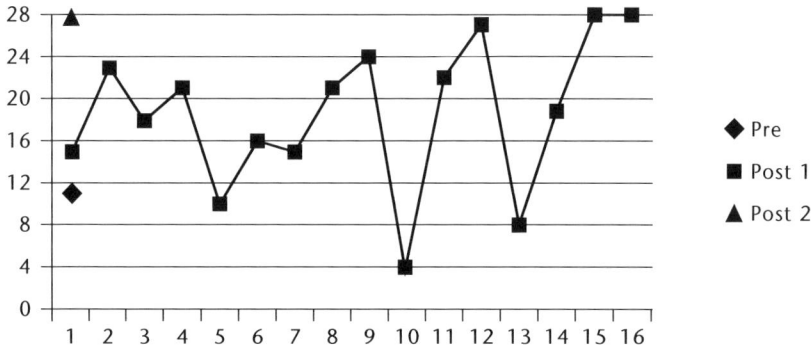

FIGURE 11.4 Graph showing Naseem's Engagement for Learning outcomes monitored using the Engagement Profile and Scale.

The post-intervention line ('Post 1') shows Naseem's progress in completing his classroom job. As Naseem increased in his ability to engage with the activity, the teacher added new elements to extend and expand his learning. These extensions broadly correspond to dips in his engagement as each unfamiliar element was included within his photographic task instructions, and then increasing engagement as his confidence grew. The extensions to the task were introduced as follows:

TARGET 1: TO COMPLETE ALLOCATED CLASS JOB (see Figure 11.4, 'Post 1')

Strategy 1: Visual schedule – eight photographs in correct order to support completion of activity (Session 1)
Strategy 2: Eight photographs in incorrect order to support independence in completion of activity (Sessions 2–6)
Strategy 3: Peers instructed not to interact with Naseem (Session 6)
Strategy 4: Additional job: to make drinks to give more responsibility (Session 7)
Strategy 5: Fewer photos (five) (Session 8)
Strategy 6: Additional job: putting cups out (Session 9)
Strategy 7: One additional photo introduced for additional element of task (Sessions 10–11)
Strategy 8: Additional job: to pour drinks (Sessions 12–16).

Following Naseem's success using the sequenced photo cues for completing his class task, the teacher decided to generalize this strategy to his science lessons. Previously, Naseem had never been able to set up the equipment for his science experiments, so it was hoped that the photo cues strategy would be effective in this situation. His teacher created a set of photos showing each piece of science equipment needed for a practical and where in the classroom they were to be found, with a final photo of how the equipment should look when it was set up.

Naseem entered the science room, set out his photos and collected the equipment. He got only one piece wrong, bringing a glass rod rather than a thermometer, but he was able to correct this when questioned what the photo was. He then set up the equipment perfectly apart from putting the thermometer in upside down.

The second post-intervention marker ('Post 2') in Figure 11.4 shows the success of this intervention. His teacher noted in the Engagement Scale comment boxes: 'Naseem went straight to where his photos kept, put them out in correct order and looked at them… He started task without being needed to be told… It was a massive improvement; he completed the whole task without the teacher needing to intervene and keep him on task.'

The teacher concluded of the intervention: 'It was an amazing success. I will now start to photograph all practicals to have a set of photo packages for all CYP [children and young people] to use.' This case study overview shows the benefits for both a young person and his educators of personalizing learning using appropriate strategies (concrete visual cues; modelling; praise) to meet the acknowledged learning strengths (visual/kinaesthetic learning style) and needs (distractibility; difficulties with memory), based on the concept of Engagement in Learning.

A research approach brings intensity to evidence-based practice. It allows educators to prioritize a key aspect of a student's learning. The investigation takes place within a specific time frame with an agreed practice commitment (e.g. an agreed frequency and conditions of intervention, consistency and rigour of recording, high priority in relation to other activities, additional resources if needed). It allows educators to innovate and trial alternative approaches, under the approval of the senior leadership team, without a long-term commitment to an intervention that may prove unhelpful. If successful, the interventions can be generalized to other areas of the student's curriculum.

By taking a formal inquiry approach, we can not only tell people – parents, colleagues, the wider educational and multidisciplinary communities – but also evidence and demonstrate what practices have been effective for that child or young person as a learner. It forms a basis for professional dialogue, and the possibilities of other young people benefiting from the intervention. A successful intervention can no longer be brushed aside or forgotten as one educator's 'pet theory', but can become part of a school's core evidence-based offer to support a young person throughout their school career and into adulthood.

Practitioner research is a dynamic process owned by all staff working with young people and families (Carpenter 2007). From their different perspectives comes a greater appreciation of specific contextual detail and its implications for the young people. All have a contribution to make to transdisciplinary research along a continuum of involvement. Including practitioners who have traditionally been excluded from research – for example, school dinner ladies (Smith 2002) – within a research context brings insight from alternative perspectives which can address problematic issues and add value to the evidence base. As educators experience the difference that alternative approaches can make to young people's lives, their openness to thinking about and trialling new approaches increases.

The lens of understanding

Without looking at behaviours through the lens of FASDs, it is easy for teachers to assume they are dealing with a child or young person who 'could do better', 'could try harder' or is acting out. Young people's behaviours are often misinterpreted as disrespectful and subversive. However it is essential to be highly aware of the impact of FASD impairments, and to reinterpret behaviours from this perspective (Paley and O'Connor 2009). For example, in a classroom situation, a young person may be able to repeat back instructions to you but seems unwilling – but is really unable – to carry them out. Repeating and doing are different brain tasks (SAMHSA 2007). The appropriate response for a young person with an FASD would not be to assume they are defiant, but to:

- make the instructions concrete and literal;
- break down the work into specific steps;
- discuss with the student how to approach each step.

(SAMHSA 2007)

SAMHSA (2007) provide an excellent chart, available online, which compares appropriate expectations for a child with typical development with those for a child with an FASD between the ages of 5 and 18 years.

It is important to personalize teaching approaches to recognize an individual's needs and abilities to allow success. Morgan Fawcett, a 19-year-old with an FASD, describes the impact of supportive approaches on his ability to learn:

> Even with my disabilities, because I have support, because we're doing things differently, I've become profoundly successful. Right now, at this point, I am a 4.0 student – first time in my life; in college – because we were able to adapt my learning style to my course work. While we know and realize that it takes me longer to do something. That's okay. I can work steady for a few days, but after that I need rest. Because there comes a point when my brain no longer functions.
> *(National Organisation on Fetal Alcohol Syndrome 2012)*

Children and young people with FASDs have many, many positive qualities, and through intensive and collaborative support from family, friends, education, social and health professionals, can enter adulthood with dignity, self-respect and self-esteem, in full knowledge of their strengths and skills, and the part they can play in the adult world. Through well-planned, engaging activities, we can personalize the pathways to learning for young people with FASDs, leading to success, achievement and a sense of self-worth. However difficult the journey with the student is, we must never lose sight of the fact that every child achieves, and it should be celebrated.

Acknowledgements

Some of this material has previously appeared in Blackburn *et al.* (2012) and Carpenter (2011). My thanks to Carolyn Blackburn and Jo Egerton for agreeing to the inclusion of some of their material from our shared publication.

Bibliography

Adnams, C.M., Sorour, P., Kalberg, W.O., Kodituwakku, P., Perold, M.D., Kotze, A., September, S., Castle, B., Gossage, J. and May, P.A. (2007) 'Language and literacy outcomes from a pilot intervention study for children with fetal alcohol spectrum disorders in South Africa', *Alcohol*, 41(6): 403–14.

Alberta Education (2009) *Re: Defining Success: A team approach to supporting students with FASD*, Edmonton, Alberta: Alberta Education. Learning and Teaching Resources Branch.

Benz, J., Rasmussen, C. and Andrew, K. (2009) 'Diagnosing fetal alcohol spectrum disorder: history, challenges and future directions', *Paediatric Child Health*, 14(4): 231–7.

Blackburn, C. (2009) *Building Bridges with Understanding – Foetal Alcohol Spectrum Disorders (FASD): Focus on strategies*, Worcester: Sunfield Research Institute/Worcestershire County Council [online at: www.worcestershire.gov.uk/cms/PDF/49598%20FASD%20Strategy%20web1.pdf; accessed: 9 August 2012].

Blackburn, C. (2010) *Facing the Challenge and Shaping the Future for Primary and Secondary Aged Students with Foetal Alcohol Spectrum Disorders* (FAS-eD Project), London: NOFAS-UK [online at: http://nofasaa1.miniserver.com/~martin/documents/FAS-eD%20PRIMARY%20FRAMEWORK.pdf; accessed: 11 June 2013].

Blackburn, C. (2012) 'Drinking it in', *SEN Magazine*, 60(September): 80–83.

Blackburn, C., Carpenter, B. and Egerton, J. (2012) *Educating Children and Young People with FASD*, Abingdon: Routledge.

British Medical Association (2007) *Fetal Alcohol Spectrum Disorders: A guide for healthcare professionals*, London: BMA.

Carpenter, B. (2007) 'Developing the role of schools as research organisations: the Sunfield experience', in B. Carpenter and J. Egerton (eds) (2007) *New Horizons in Special Education: Evidence-based practice in action*, Clent: Sunfield Publications.

Carpenter, B. (2011) 'Pedagogically bereft! Improving learning outcomes for children with foetal alcohol spectrum disorders', *British Journal of Special Education*, 38(1), 37–43.

Carpenter, B. (2013, in press) 'Inquiry-based leadership', *School Matters*.

Carpenter, B., Egerton, J., Brooks, T., Cockbill, B., Fotheringham, J. and Rawson, H. (2011) *The Complex Learning Difficulties and Disabilities Research Project: Developing meaningful pathways to personalised learning (Project report)*. London: Specialist Schools and Academies Trust (now The Schools Network) [online at: http://complexld.ssatrust.org.uk/project-information.html; accessed: 21 March 2012].

Carpenter, B., Egerton, J., Brooks, T., Cockbill, B., Fotheringham, J. and Rawson, H. (2014) *Children and Young People with Complex Learning Difficulties and Disabilities: A resource book for teachers and teaching assistants*, Abingdon: Routledge.Clarren, S.K., Carmichael, H., Olson, S., Clarren, G.B. and Astley, S.J. (2000) 'A child with fetal alcohol syndrome', in M.J. Guralnick (ed.) *Interdisciplinary Clinical Assessment of Young Children with Developmental Disabilities*, Baltimore, MA: Paul H. Brookes.

Coles, C.D. (2011) 'Discriminating the effects of prenatal alcohol exposure from other behavioral and learning disorders', *Alcohol Research and Health*, 34(1): 42–50 [online at: http://pubs.niaaa.nih.gov/publications/arh341/42-50.htm; accessed: 26 September 2011].

Coles, C.D., Kable, J.A. and Taddeo, E. (2009) 'Math performance and behavior problems in children affected by prenatal alcohol exposure: intervention and follow-up', *Journal of Developmental and Behavioral Pediatrics*, 30(1): 7–15.

Coles, C.D., Strickland, D.C., Padgett, L. and Bellmoffv L. (2007) 'Games that "work": using computer games to teach alcohol-affected children about fire and street safety', *Research in Developmental Disabilities*, 28(5): 518–30.

Dossetor, D., White D. and Whatson, L. (eds) (2011) *Mental Health of Children and Adolescents with Intellectual and Developmental Disabilities: A framework for professional practice*. Melbourne: IP Communications.

Dubovsky, D. (2009) 'Co-morbidities with mental health for an individual with FASD', in E. Jonsson, L. Dennett and G. Littlejohn (eds) *Fetal Alcohol Spectrum Disorder (FASD): Across the lifespan (Proceedings from an IHE Consensus Development Conference 2009)*, Alberta, Canada: Institute of Health Economics [online at: www.ihe.ca/documents/FASDproceedings.pdf; accessed 17 September 2011].

Egerton, J. (2009) *Foetal Alcohol Spectrum Disorder Information Sheets*. Worcester: Sunfield Research Institute/Worcestershire County Council.

Evensen, D. and Lutke, J. (1997) *Eight Magic Keys: Developing successful interventions for students with FAS*. Homer, AK: Fasalaska Project FACTS (Fetal Alcohol Consultation and Training Services) [online at: www.fasdcenter.samhsa.gov/documents/EightMagicKeys.pdf; accessed: 16 September 2012].

Gibbard, W.B. (2009) 'FASD: Extent and impact on child development', presentation to the IHE Consensus Development Conference, 'Fetal Alcohol Spectrum Disorder (FASD) – across the lifespan', Edmonton, Alberta (7–9 October).

Gibbard, W.B., Wass, P. and Clarke, M.E. (2003) 'The neuropsychological implications of prenatal alcohol exposure', *Canadian Child and Adolescent Psychiatry Review*, 12(3): 72–6.Grant, T., Huggins, J., Connor, P., Pedersen, J.Y., Whitney, N. and Streissguth, A. (2004) 'A pilot community intervention for young women with fetal alcohol spectrum disorders', *Journal of Community Mental Health*, 40(6): 499–511.

Guralnick, M. (2004) 'Early intervention for children with intellectual disabilities: current knowledge and future prospects', address to the 12th IASSID World Congress, Montpellier, France, 15 June.

Hannigan, J.H. and Berman, R.F. (2000) 'Amelioration of fetal alcohol-related neurodevelopmental disorders in rats: exploring pharmacological and environmental treatments', *Neurotoxicology and Teratology*, 22(1): 103–11.

Hargreaves, D (2006) *A New Shape for Schooling?* London: SSAT.

Jirikowic, T. (2007) 'Sensory integration and sensory processing disorders', in K.D. O'Malley (ed.) *ADHD and Fetal Alcohol Spectrum Disorders*, New York, NY: Nova Science Publishers.

Jones, P., Whitehurst, T. and Egerton, J. (eds) (2012) *Creating Meaningful Inquiry in Inclusive Classrooms: Practitioners' stories of research*, Abingdon: Routledge.

Kable, J.A., Coles, C.D. and Taddeo, E. (2007) 'Socio-cognitive habilitation using the math interactive learning experience program for alcohol affected children', *Alcoholism: Clinical and Experimental Research*, 31(8): 1425–34.

Kleinfeld, J. and Wescott, S. (eds) (1993) *Fantastic Antone Succeeds! Experiences in educating children with fetal alcohol syndrome*, Fairbanks, AK: University of Alaska Press.

Kodituwakku, P., Coriale, G., Fiorentino, D., Aragon, A.S., Kalberg, W.O., Buckley, D., Gossage, J.P., Ceccanti, M. and May, P.A. (2006) 'Neurobehavioral characteristics of children with Fetal Alcohol Spectrum Disorders in communities from Italy: preliminary results', *Alcoholism: Clinical experimental research*, 30(9): 1551–61.

Kodituwakku, P.W. (2009) 'Neurocognitive profile in children with fetal alcohol spectrum disorders', *Developmental Disabilities Research Review*, 15(3): 218–24.

Kopera-Frye, K., Dehaene, S. and Streissguth, A.P. (1996) 'Impairments in number-processing induced by prenatal alcohol exposure', *Neuropsychologia*, 34(12): 1187–96.

Loomes, C., Rasmussen, C., Pei, J., Manji, S. and Andrew, G. (2008) 'The effects of rehearsal training on working memory span of children with fetal alcohol spectrum disorder', *Research in Developmental Disabilities*, 29(2): 113–24.

National Organisation on Fetal Alcohol Syndrome (2012) 'Morgan Fawcett on living with FASD'. National Washington, DC: Organization on Fetal Alcohol Syndrome [online at: www.youtube.com/watch?v=K0VrkLQfkFg&feature=player_embedded; accessed: 16 September 2012].

O'Connor, M.J., Frankel, F., Paley, B., Schonfeld, A.M., Carpenter, E., Laugeson, E.A. and Marquardt, R. (2006) 'A controlled social skills training for children with fetal alcohol spectrum disorders', *Journal of Consulting and Clinical Psychology*, 74(4): 639–48.

O'Malley, K. (2007) *ADHD and Fetal Alcohol Spectrum Disorders*. Hauppauge, NY: Nova Science Publishers.

Padgett, L.S., Strickland, D. and Coles, C.D. (2006) 'Case study: using a virtual reality computer game to teach fire safety skills to children diagnosed with fetal alcohol syndrome', *Journal of Pediatric Psychology*, 31(1): 65–70.

Paley, B. and O'Connor, M.J. (2009) 'Intervention for individuals with fetal alcohol spectrum disorders: treatment approaches and case management', *Developmental Disabilities Research Reviews*,15(3): 258–67.

Paley, B. and O'Connor, M.J. (2011) 'Behavioral interventions for children and adolescents with fetal alcohol spectrum disorders', *Alcohol Research and Health*, 34(1): 64–75.

Peadon, E., Rhys-Jones, B., Bower, C. and Elliott, E.J. (2009) 'Systematic review of interventions for children with Fetal Alcohol Spectrum Disorders', *BMC Pediatrics*, 9,35 [online at: www.biomedcentral.com/content/pdf/1471-2431-9-35.pdf; accessed: 17 September 2012].

Ryan, S. and Ferguson, D.L. (2006) 'On, yet under, the radar: students with fetal alcohol syndrome disorder', *Exceptional Children*, 72(3): 363–5.

SAMHSA (Substance Abuse and Mental Health Services Administration) (2007) *Reach to Teach: Educating Elementary and Middle School Children with Fetal Alcohol Spectrum Disorders*. Rockville, MD:

Center for Substance Abuse Prevention, Substance Abuse and Mental Health Services Administration [online at: www.fasdcenter.samhsa.gov/documents/Reach_To_Teach_Final_011107.pdf; accessed: 15 September 2012].

SAMHSA (Substance Abuse and Mental Health Services Administration) (2010) 'Fetal Alcohol Spectrum Disorders (FASD): The basics' (PowerPoint presentation) [online at: http://fasdcenter.samhsa.gov/educationTraining/fasdBasics.aspx; accessed: 11 September 2011].

Smith, N. (2002) 'Transition to the school playground: an intervention programme for nursery children', *Early Years: an international journal of research and development*, 22(2): 129–46.

Streissguth, A.P. and O'Malley, K. (2000) 'Neuropsychiatric implications and long-term consequences of fetal alcohol spectrum disorders', *Seminars in Clinical Neuropsychiatry*, 5(3): 177–90.

Streissguth, A.P., Barr, H.M., Kogan, J. and Bookstein, F.L. (1996) *Understanding the Occurrence of Secondary Disabilities in Clients with Fetal Alcohol Syndrome (FAS) and Fetal Alcohol Effects (FAE) (Final Report to the Centers for Disease Control and Prevention (CDC))*, Seattle, WA: University of Washington, Fetal Alcohol and Drug Unit.

Timler, G.R., Olswang, L.B. and Coggins, T.E. (2005) '"Do I know what I need to do?": a social communication intervention for children with complex clinical profiles', *Language, Speech, and Hearing Services in Schools*, 36(1): 73–85.

Vernescu, R. (2007) 'Attention process training in young children with fetal alcohol spectrum disorders', presentation to the 2nd Annual Conference on Fetal Alcohol Spectrum Disorders, Victoria, British Columbia, 10 March.

Williams, M.S. and Shellenberger, S. (1996) *How Does Your Engine Run?: A leader's guide to the Alert Program© for self-regulation*, Albuquerque, NM: TherapyWorks.

12

A STEP IN TIME

Fetal alcohol spectrum disorders and transition to adulthood

Jo Egerton

Fetal alcohol spectrum disorders (FASDs) are a lifelong disability. As young people grow towards adulthood, most begin to assume more responsibility for managing their own lives and determining their life course. However, for young people with FASDs, the difficulties that set them apart from their peers and challenged them during their primary and secondary education continue to challenge them in adolescence (Lutke and Antrobus 2004). As they approach adulthood the impact can be much more serious and long-lasting, affecting their long-term success and quality of life in the community. Difficulties with memory, planning and causal understanding mean that they can find it hard to devise and execute plans to fulfil their aspirations, and learn to avoid detrimental situations (Morley 2006). Difficulties with impulsiveness, poor judgement and poor self-esteem, combined with a desire for excitement, novelty and friends can draw them into law-breaking behaviour. Community Living British Columbia (2011: 4) state:

> The life experiences of individuals with FASD vary greatly. Many are successful, happy, contributing members of families and communities – electricians, teachers, counsellors, parents, skilled workers and others. However, without identification and appropriate supports, there is often a sad trajectory of failure, loss, and confusion. This often results in multiple placements and in secondary defensive behaviours that lead to involvement with the justice system and multiple mental health diagnoses.

In her longitudinal research with 415 individuals with FASDs, Streissguth and colleagues (2004) identified a range of secondary disabilities which increase in severity for many young people with FASDs in adolescence and adulthood. Kellerman (2002) lists the categories as: mental health problems, disrupted school experience, trouble with the law, incarceration, inappropriate sexual behaviour and substance misuse.

Researchers have noted that stories of stability in adult life among young people with FASDs are comparatively few, and many who enjoy positive adult life outcomes experience a rollercoaster life pattern (Kleinfeld 2000). Barriers, depression, law-breaking, etc. can be overcome only through courage and commitment from the young person, and intensive support from family and services. The danger is that, as young people overcome difficulties and experience success in the context of service and community support structures, service providers wrongly perceive the young person has learned how to cope. The subsequent removal of services is commonly followed by a devastating breakdown in the young person's coping capacity. What professionals often fail to recognize is that, with FASDs, these supports will *always* be critical to the young person's ability to function, and need to be lifelong, just as physical aids are lifelong for people who have physical disabilities.

Preparation for adult life

In common with their peers, young people with FASDs long for meaningful relationships, freedom in making life choices, independence from parents, and a job which supports their desired lifestyle (Fuchs *et al.* 2010). However, without planned support in achieving adult skills from an early age, they struggle to achieve this. Even young people with high IQ are likely to have very low levels of adaptive ability (Fast and Conry 2009; Lutke and Antrobus 2004; Streissguth *et al.* 2004) to the extent that: 'they are unable to manage the mechanics of daily life or access services or supports on their own; the process is too difficult for them' (Lutke and Antrobus 2004: 16).

Clark and colleagues (2004) discovered that while only 34 per cent of the clients in their research had an IQ below 70, 81 per cent required a moderate to high level of supported care. Spohr and Steinhausen (2008) found that 86.5 per cent (32 of 37) of their patients with FASDs had no long-term employment or were unemployed despite protective factors (e.g. diagnosis of an FASD before age six, a stable and nurturing home, caregivers who understand FASDs and seek help, etc.; Streissguth *et al.* 2004) and, in some cases, preparatory job training.

To acquire competencies which will carry them into adulthood, children and young people with FASDs need much longer and more painstaking life-skill preparation and lifelong support. This chapter focuses on four strands in supporting young people with FASDs into adulthood:

- building on young people's aspirations, interests and strengths;
- modifying and extending the 'external brain';
- developing adult skills step by step from a young age;
- involving key others, outside the family, in supporting the young person with an FASD.

Supporting aspirations

Young people with FASDs have many strengths and skills. For example, Malbin (quoted in Shepard and Hudson Breen 2012: 466) identifies 'good visual memory and verbal skills, persistence, commitment, success in low-stress, structured situations, a strong sense of fairness, and success in learning with hands-on tasks'. Blackburn (2010: 8) additionally mentions 'rote learning and long-term memory ... literacy and practical subjects, such as art, performing arts, sport, and technologies'. When the strengths of young people with FASDs are combined with their individual interests – be that beauty therapy, animal husbandry, sport, etc. – it enhances their incentive to learn, their ability to achieve, and their self-esteem (Blackburn 2010, Blackburn *et al.* 2012). As they grow up, interests can also provide a much needed oasis of respite for the young person from their academic and social struggles, and a basis for encouragement when life gets tough (Groupe Groves 2000).

During adolescence, extending their expertise in areas of interest can increase the young person's likelihood of being accepted for employment or further education. Interests can also provide the vehicle for positive peer interactions, the chance for their skills to be fully appreciated and valued by others, and a context for essential supervision and support in a form which is acceptable to the young person. In 'Matthew's story', Matthew described his joining of the Air Training Cadets (ATC), age 13, as 'the best thing I have ever done' and continued:

> The ATC provide positive structure, boundaries and support that I need to enable me to gel with my peer group. For the first time in my life I fitted in. I have been in the ATC since I was 13 and I am now 18. I am a corporal… We can do it, it just takes a little longer!
>
> *(FASAware n.d.: 12)*

Adapting and extending the 'external brain'

Dr Stirling Clarren coined the expression 'external brain' (Kellerman 2003) to describe the structure, supports and strategies that enable young people with FASDs to function and contribute successfully within their community, and gain a good quality of life. In adulthood, the external brain must expand to include key areas such as those identified below (Badry and Wight Felske 2011; Community Living British Columbia 2011; Kleinfeld 2000; Lutke and Antrobus 2004; Morley 2006). The accompanying figures (Kellerman 2002; US DHHS n.d.) show research-based indications of the percentages of people with FASDs who need support in some of these areas:

- daily living skills (e.g. shopping, 52 per cent; cooking meals, 49 per cent; leisure, 47 per cent; personal care, 36 per cent);
- dependent living (80 per cent);
- further education/vocational training/employment (80 per cent);
- social relationships (56 per cent) and sexual relationships (45 per cent);
- community participation;
- physical health (e.g. medical care, 66 per cent);
- mental health (94 per cent), addiction services (30 per cent);
- use of public services (e.g. transport, 24 per cent);
- involvement with the justice system (42–47 per cent);
- financial management;
- accessing disability services and benefits (70 per cent).

Families often find that the 'external brain' that was so successful when their child was young, can come to be seen as restrictive and unwelcome by their now-adolescent son or daughter. However, it can still be successful providing it changes (e.g. becomes more subtle) to reflect the young person's status as an adolescent/young adult and increasing awareness of peer attitudes. For Anne Ruggles Gere, and her daughter Cindy (2000), core to the success of the external brain is:

> a belief, not a strategy. I remained convinced that Cindy was a person of considerable potential, and she, in turn, believed in herself [and] a creative tension between honest

acknowledgement of the limitations imposed by FAS/E and never underestimating potential ... about what individual people can accomplish.

(Ruggles Gere and Gere 2000: 78)

Asking for help

In order to ask for assistance, the young person needs to know why they need help, who and how to ask for it, and what to do if they do not get it. As Doctor (2000) states, the ability to ask for help is critical to success or failure for young people with FASDs, but they need to be taught these skills, and to recognize that everyone exists interdependently. This allows everyone to achieve personal goals that make the best use of available resources.

Marceil Ten Eyck (2000), with and for her daughter, Sydney, developed a stepped approach to asking for assistance independently which could be taught and adapted for all situations from junior school through to employment in adulthood. It involved:

1. recognizing the need for help;
2. independently asking the person in charge (e.g. the teacher) for help in a positive but assertive way;
3. if the person in charge did not help, identifying a more senior person and asking them for help;
4. finally, if this was unsuccessful, asking her mother so they could both find someone to help.

Guiding and mentoring young people with FASDs

Despite years of practising routines and strategies, individuals with FASDs are always likely to need the support and prompting of a mentor to be able to use their strategies and structures. In the early lives of children with FASDs, support is provided largely by their immediate family and by their school. However, as they grow older and want greater autonomy, Kleinfeld (2000) advises parents to begin widening their son or daughter's support network. Community Living British Columbia (2011: 14) suggests this should include 'carefully selected, informed, understanding and accepting mentors who are in relationships with the person, not custodial roles'. A support network could include paid assistance (e.g. housekeeping), peers, mentors, family and/or friends. It is important that these people are responsive, tolerant of idiosyncrasy, affirming of abilities and willing to modify requirements in recognition of FASD-associated difficulties (Ruggles Gere and Gere 2000). Young people will often act more readily on advice from a peer or someone they admire, than from immediate family members. Moving the locus of advice from the family can also reduce teenage conflict.

One young adult with an FASD learned to recognize that when she attended professional appointments alone she easily became intimidated and confused (Doctor 2000). She therefore involved her advocate, who created the space for her to explain her needs, and ensured the professional communicated in a way that the young woman could understand. Following the meeting, the advocate would then review the meeting with her, and plan further action with her.

As young people with FASDs grow up, and the gap between their intellectual ability and adaptive abilities widen, their disability may remain largely invisible to others. People's expectations increase. Young people with FASDs may be overfaced by what is asked of them – at school and at home – leading to poor self-esteem, lack of motivation, resentment and frustration. When this is prolonged, it can lead to secondary disabilities, mentioned above. If parents and professionals observe young people closely they can pick up early signs, and discuss and resolve difficulties between the young person and others involved.

Parents may need to adjust their hopes for their son and daughter to fit in with life goals the young person has chosen (Kleinfeld 2000). It may be that learning adjustments, creative curriculum adaptations or a change of school may rekindle the young person's self-belief and interest in learning, and allow them to achieve on their terms. However, to get their son or daughter's needs met often requires strong advocacy from parents.

In adulthood, some young people with FASDs have found that they can hold down a job, but need part-time employment, because the demands of a full-time job are too emotionally demanding. One mother wrote of her daughter: 'When she works longer hours, migraine headaches appear. She needs enormous energy to pay attention, think, process, and remember on a level required to maintain employment' (Kleinfeld 2000: 25).

Research and anecdotes show that adolescents with FASDs may also have unrealistic expectations – a trait associated with much younger children. Blackburn (2010) quotes one young boy's ambition to be a superhero at age 11. A careers advisor (Tucker 2011) suggests that young people with FASDs are likely to express confidence in carrying out a skill based on minimal experience and without proven competence. They understand the desirable end result, but may not appreciate, remember or realize the existence of steps which must be taken to get there. For example, a young person may express an intention to get a flat without perceiving that there is a process to go through to achieve their goal or that there are associated expectations (e.g. paying rent). Similarly a young person may express an intention to go to college, without appreciating that the type of college and course will be a prelude to their future career. Rather than accepting what a young person with an FASD states they can do, professionals need to inquire more closely and specifically, and help the young person establish specific goal pathways (Tucker 2011).

Pre-teen strategies bridging into adulthood

Children and young people with FASDs find learning hard and often rely on strict routine and rote learning to reduce memory overload; Carpenter (2011: 39) emphasizes the effectiveness of 'scripting'. The importance of forming habits in early life which can continue into the teenage and adult years of young people with FASDs is highlighted by parents of successful adults with FASDs. They emphasize the necessity of long-term, pre-emptive, repeated real-life practice, and when possible learning sets of behaviours in childhood which do not have to be modified to make them age appropriate when older. Behaviours which are acceptable or endearing in childhood can become undesirable, unsafe, challenging or even threatening in a pre-teen or adolescent (Slinn 2000). Rather than further burdening young people with FASD with learning altered routines at a time when they are already struggling with adolescence, it can be better to introduce these rules of behaviour from a young age. For example, some parents have successfully used the following strategies with pre-teen children:

- personal care routines – e.g. introducing adolescent-appropriate bathing schedules, shaving, deodorant and sanitary wear years before they are needed (Groupe Groves 2000);
- dressing/undressing – developing rules for appropriate behaviour around dressing/undressing (e.g. always checking they are fully dressed before coming out of the bathroom) (Groupe Groves 2000);
- personal space – with their craving for physical closeness yet lack of understanding around personal space and social cues, learning specific rules from a young age about who/when/where they can hug and sit close to others can protect them from harm and from harming others (Lipow/Southern California FASD Information and Support Network 2012; Slinn 2000);
- ownership of property – discussing and teaching the importance of ownership, learning how to borrow, and always returning loaned objects without exception, can help prevent issues with 'stealing'.

Table 12.1 illustrates possible small step sequences to attaining some adult further skills from a young age.

Preparing for employment

Getting a job and remaining in employment can be difficult for young people with FASDs, and, according to Lutke and Antrobus (2004: 22) 'is not a current reality for most adults with FASD because of the lack of services and supports necessary to make it happen.' Streissguth and colleagues (1996, in Lutke and Antrobus 2004) reported the following percentage employment difficulties:

- easily frustrated (65 per cent);
- poor task comprehension (57 per cent);
- poor judgement (55 per cent);
- social problems (54 per cent);
- fired (50 per cent);
- unreliable (42 per cent);
- anger management (42 per cent);
- problems with supervisor (40 per cent);
- lying (33 per cent);
- lose jobs without understanding why (30 per cent).

Lutke and Antrobus (2004: 56) go on to say that:

> Many individuals with FASD are fired from jobs not because of their ability to do the job itself, but because of the lack of life and social skills support required to keep the job (ie: appropriate dress, unspoken rules of the workplace, lateness, fleeing when things get difficult, not asking for help, bad debts, eviction, addiction, etc.).

TABLE 12.1 Examples of possible small steps towards adult skills

Employment	Finance	Friendship and dating	Using public transport
From a young age, teach the young person how to complete chores to specific, agreed standards	Pay pocket money for chores	From a young age, talk about and develop appropriate rules for behaviour with family, friends etc. around personal space	Habitual use of public transport with the young person from a young age
Pay pocket money for chores completed to an agreed standard	Discuss financial good practice and support cheque book skills and budgeting through the teenage years	From a young age, practice social life-associated skills step by step (e.g. talking on the telephone; making arrangements; using public transport)	Discuss key elements of using public transport (e.g. waiting at the right stop; identifying the right bus; flagging the bus down; etc.)
Discuss career aspirations with the young person; establish realistic steps to realizing or accommodating aspirations (e.g. veterinary nursing rather than veterinary surgery)	Open a bank account with a double signature for the young person	Empathize with romantic interests, and attempt to steer sensitively in a realistic direction; discuss indicators of romantic interest from another person	Involve the young person in supported travel decisions appropriate for their age (e.g. buying tickets; when to get off)
With the young person, take part in community volunteer work and use opportunities to teach employment skills and promote social understanding	Increase money for chores and give young person increasing responsibility over time for buying own essentials; teach associated skills (e.g. transport; shopping for and preparing food)	Role play and practise dating behaviour/skills; practise 'going out on dates' within the family	With the young person, develop and understand concrete rules for riding on the bus
Share a Saturday job with the young person to support employment skills and promote social understanding	Increase the young person's independence in budgeting so that they can learn from mistakes in a safe environment	Initially invite a date out on a family outing	Provide visual cues/reminders/systems
Arrange a holiday job for the young person at your work place – to teach employment skills and promote social understanding	Create rules (e.g. to pay bills first; time bill payments and standing orders to coincide with salary/benefits payments)	Discuss and plan activities the young person could do to get to know their date better: initially with a high level of family involvement, and then fading this	Get to know the bus drivers on the route
			Gradually hand over responsibility for the journey to the young person
			Discuss and role play what could go wrong (e.g. missed bus; threatening or dangerous situations) and practise specific behaviours in case it does (e.g. phrases to use; people to call; etc.)

TABLE 12.1 continued

Employment	Finance	Friendship and dating	Using public transport
Arrange for extended career training within the young person's school curriculum; discuss the job regularly with the young person, and maintain supportive advocacy relationship with the employer	Teach sustainable buying habits and strategies (e.g. bulk buying to save money); teach about financial traps (e.g. gambling)	Double date with a responsible peer	First shadowing, then gradually fading your presence so the young person becomes more independent and confident, and if possible completely independent or with minimal peer support
	Set up bank balance alerts and daily/weekly withdrawal limits on the account; teach young person the importance of checking their balance regularly; avoid credit	Ongoing discussions with the young person, helping to plan appropriate activities, finding out how they feel, what they think, troubleshooting, responding to questions, advising, etc.	
Discuss how to share FASD issues and needs with the employer; parent can attend interview with the young person		Support the young person to share their FASD difficulties with their boy/girlfriend and their family in a sensitive and positive way if the relationship develops	Providing safeguards (e.g. a mobile phone with a prepaid emergency number; informing someone of the journey)
Independent evening/weekend job; discuss the job regularly with the young person, and maintain supportive advocacy and troubleshooting relationship with the employer	Employ trusted and independent financial trustees who will support the young person in adulthood		
Search for permanent part-time job/training reflecting the young person's interests	Prepare strategies in case of financial difficulties (e.g. a prepaid telephone number to call in emergencies; spending restrictions on mobile accounts)	Work with the boy/girlfriend's parents to ensure the time the couple spend with each other and their activities are appropriate to the age and stage of their relationship	
Help the young person and employer prepare strategies for successful employment	Teach strategies for getting advice on big purchases		
Continue to discuss and monitor the situation with the young person and employer; troubleshoot with the employer as necessary	Ask friends to give resources as presents (e.g. bus pass, prepaid phone card, gift certificates, food, etc.) instead of money which may be misspent		

It is important to involve key, trusted people in the workplace in supporting the young person's difficulties so that they can help them to succeed, and collaborate with an advocate or mentor who can provide essential supports, such as:

- informing and training key colleagues about FASDs
- collaboration with the young person
- defending
- planning
- monitoring from the young person's and others' (e.g. employer, college) perspectives
- prompting
- pre-empting
- intervening
- standing back
- role play/role modelling.

They need to realize that the young person succeeds *only* with the structures and strategies in place, and these supports must be maintained through staff changes. Table 12.2 describes some of the difficulties and possible solutions of employment for young people with FASD.

If the young person opts to go to college, encourage them initially to take up a college place nearby and live at home for a while, so that new routines can be supported by the family, and they still have the familiarity of home routines and expectations. At a later date, they may be ready to move out of home but remain close enough for easy support. Finally they may be ready to move further away, but it is important to help the young person build an empathetic, proactive and supportive community network wherever they live, and for parents to continue to monitor from both their son/daughter and the college's perspective. Ruggles Gere and Gere (2000) describe in very useful detail the steps they took to make college a successful experience.

Leisure and social opportunities

Leisure time may be problematic for young adults with FASDs without a mentor to help them plan and organize it. Good strategies for structuring free time from an early age – inside and outside the home – can give the young person the opportunity to combat boredom, build positive social relationships and practice social skills (e.g. talking to friends and making arrangements over the telephone). Supporting young people to identify options for structured time alone at home is important. Some young adults with FASDs who were asked about undirected leisure time (Minnesota Organization on Fetal Alcohol Syndrome 2011) variously replied variously that they practised skills related to their hobby (e.g. football), did puzzles or wandered the streets. The latter is a risky and possibly dangerous option for many young people with FASDs and could draw them into a lifestyle centred around drinking, drugs and delinquency. If your teen is liable to storm out of the house after a disagreement, agree with them 'safe houses' where they are welcome while they calm down (Toolbox Parenting 2010).

Young people with FASDs may find it difficult to form stable and safe friendships. Their difficulty in understanding subtleties of emotion, social situations and language often distance them from positive peer groups and, unless care is taken to encourage such associations,

TABLE 12.2 FASD-associated difficulties within the workplace: outcomes and solutions

Possible difficulties	Possible outcomes	Collaborative response (advocate/young person/employer)
Lack of understanding of FASDs by community contacts (e.g. employer, social services, justice system, peers/co-workers, etc.)	Unrealistic expectations; lack of supervision, environmental adaptation and support; misinterpretation of behaviours; risk of firing	*Apply to all situations below*: young person and/or their advocate to explain the difficulties and impacts of FASDs; develop and agree adaptations with employer; emphasize young person's strengths and abilities, and how to build on them; identify empathetic workplace mentors/buddies to be trained in FASD support
Impulsive responses to social situations and difficulties (e.g. aggressive outbursts)	Unacceptable/inappropriate workplace behaviours; heightened emotional responses; deteriorating relationships with colleagues	Recognize and act on early indicators of difficulty; put situation response strategies in place (e.g. opportunities for time out; rules to prevent impulsive resignation); recognize emotional strain for the young person of working – reduce hours if necessary
Young person does not work proactively or take initiative; does not follow through on work sequences	Interpreted as lack of interest/lack of motivation	Explain difficulties with planning and learning from experience; explain mismatch between apparent IQ and adaptive ability; explain need for specific rules and simple instructions; devise aids and prompts (e.g. photo sequences; written lists/schedules etc.)
Continually ignores instructions	Employee appears not to follow explicit instructions/directions about workplace behaviour; breaks workplace rules (e.g. timekeeping)	Explain young person may not understand that: general instructions or rules apply to them although they can repeat them; rules/instructions apply in all situations; the context for the instruction. They may think that they are complying. Check the young person's understanding of the instruction; personalize instructions by using their name each time; ask the young person how they plan to fulfil the instruction; provide concrete personalized examples/demonstrations/role play
Shows poor judgement	Exploited by colleagues; engages in misguided behaviour	Monitor work situation with young person and employer; inform employer about FASD-associated difficulties; intervene if difficulties arise; involve work buddy; provide support for the young person in any situations requiring a difficult judgement call

Possible difficulties	Possible outcomes	Collaborative response (advocate/young person/employer)
Difficulties with memory, understanding, thinking and decision-making related to work	Young person cannot carry out a task which he could do the previous day	Develop stable routines, strategies and systems to remind and reduce memory overload; simplify language; keep instructions short; develop interim steps to task completion; provide visual cues (e.g. text messages; written lists; photo sequences etc.); provide repeated hands-on instruction and coaching
Antisocial behaviours (e.g. 'lying', 'stealing' etc.)	Breakdown of trust between employer and employee; risk of firing	Check the young person's understanding of expectations/interpretation of instructions/situation (e.g. 'borrowing'); involve advocate; explain reasons (e.g. 'confabulation'; desire to please leading to lies; difficulties with recognizing ownership; perseveration; impulsiveness etc.); advise simple concrete teaching and leniency
Lack of causal understanding, impulsiveness	Does not change behaviour in response to sanctions and incentives (e.g. bonus systems; loss of privileges, threats)	Explain the impact of causal understanding and memory difficulties and alternative FASD logic; develop alternative solutions collaboratively with employer; establish rote rules, routines, prompts and supports.
Perseveration and difficulties with transitioning	Young person 'ignores' workplace instructions	Explain FASD-associated difficulties with perseveration; provide concrete reminders, prompts and countdowns to changes in activity
Distractibility, impulsivity	Young person does not complete required work; distracts others etc.	Involve work mentor; provide visual cues to keep on task (see examples above); develop habit-forming routines; explain FASD difficulties (e.g. distractibility; exhaustion); modify work environment to eliminate distractions as far as possible and address exhaustion.
Sensory hypersensitivity	Young person becomes distracted and cannot concentrate	Talk to employer about difficulties with sensory stimuli (e.g. light, noise, touch); make appropriate adjustments (e.g. modifying light source, wearing ear defenders, explanations to colleagues, moving work station)

Source: Kleinfeld 2000; Lally and Dubovsky 2005.

can lead them to socialize with disruptive and antisocial peers, who become negative role models. Taking part in social activities they are good at and enjoy will boost their sense of self-efficacy and self-esteem. As the young person becomes older, peers or family friends may be willing to take over the social mentoring role with training and guidance from immediate family.

Both ordinary friendships and intimate relationships may become problematic for young people with FASDs unless behaviours are discussed and taught from a young age. Apply the principles of: developing and practising unwavering concrete rules (e.g. no romantic relationships with girls more than two years younger; rules around personal space); breaking learning down into small steps; long-term, repeated role play and practice in real-life situations; ensuring subtle supervision; providing safety nets (see Table 12.1 for examples). While rules may seem restrictive, they can keep the young person safe from alienating others, help them to avoid those who would victimize or exploit them (e.g. drug dealing, criminal gangs) and protect them from unwittingly committing offences (e.g. sexual harassment, sex with minors) which could end in imprisonment (Boulding n.d.).

Help young people to know themselves and gain a sense of self-identity (Fuchs *et al.* 2010). From a young age, talk with them about what kind of a person they are and would like to be, role models they admire, what values are important to them, and the importance of finding friends who have compatible values. This can give a young person with FASDs some basis for evaluating potential friends. Socializing with trusted peers or family members close to their own age can provide positive role models and help with meeting potential friends. With the young person, work out a few questions they can ask new acquaintances to find out their values. Discuss how friends behave and what to expect of true friends (Lipow/Southern California FASD Information and Support Network 2012), and help the young person to put together a 'ladder' of activities to do as they gradually get to know friends better.

Other parents of adolescents with FASDs advise that parents stay 'support active' as long as possible in scaffolding a son or daughter's friendships (Toolbox Parenting 2010); for example: creating opportunities to meet the young person's friends early in the friendship; providing rides; becoming a volunteer for organized activities; planning appealing group activities; sensitively supporting the young person through any issues; and developing strategies in case something goes wrong. As one parent says (Kleinfeld 2000: 27), although they were not entirely comfortable with the attitudes and lifestyle of their son's friends:

> They meant he had someone to talk to and hang out with. He listened to their advice, and since they were not into illegal activity or drugs and alcohol, that had to be good enough. If he was with one of these kids, he wasn't with the ones I *really* didn't want him near.

A place to live

Appropriate accommodation is regarded by Lutke and Antrobus (2004: 9) as crucial to adult success for young people with FASDs:

> Safe, stable, secure, supported, structured, supervised, subsidized housing (7S model) should be considered the primary key to broad risk management for adults with FASD.

> The absence of housing is the absence of everything… Housing that provides various kinds of on-site staff support, peer mentoring, outreach workers, volunteers, 'relationship referees' and leisure buddies was seen as critical for efficacy.

Rented accommodation needs to be kept up to an acceptable standard. Teaching housekeeping skills and strategies from an early age will help the young person to live healthily and hygienically, and prepare them for keeping their own room or flat as an adult. As with other skills, use the principles of teaching and practising small steps from a young age. Doctor (2000) describes how a peer supporter, having directed the young person with an FASD where to put away each of her possessions one by one, then advised her simply that each time she used something to put it back in exactly the same place. The young woman was able to learn and keep to this very black/white rule.

Young people with FASDs are also likely to need support with tasks such as cleaning, grocery shopping and bill paying (US DHHS n.d.). However, as the US DHHS point out, support housing which provides help with daily living tasks is exceptional, and traditional group homes may provide a poor peer fit for young adults with FASDs who have poor adaptive skills yet an average or high IQ. As mentioned by Black (Chapter 21, this publication), Germany is unique in Europe in offering such opportunities. Additionally, assessment for services needs to take account of potential threats to housing stability arising from the young person's social difficulties (e.g. exploitative acquaintances who move in, steal and create an antisocial nuisance resulting in the young person's eviction) (Fast and Conry 2009).

Finance

The difficulties with money experienced by young people with FASDs mean they have little sense of value or budgeting. Once they get into difficulties with money, it can mean the loss of their accommodation, their job, their well-being and their safety. This difficulty will be lifelong, so it is important to plan rules, support and guidance with the young person. Table 12.1 suggests small steps towards financial stability.

The justice system

Many young people with FASDs become involved in the justice system in their teenage years through association with peers who are engaged in thrill-seeking, antisocial behaviour. With their social understanding difficulties, they are easily exploited. They may unwittingly engage in criminal activities to help out and please friends, without understanding the implications for themselves or the victims.

Some young people with FASDs were asked to comment on their experiences with the justice system (Minnesota Organization on Fetal Alcohol Syndrome 2011). The temptation to steal for one young man came through a characteristic tendency to perseverate. He stated: 'When I want something I get really focused on it and it's hard to stay away from it.' However once he had physically toured his local police station, and been warned by the police, he found that 'the more concrete example stuck with me'. Another young man said that, even after he had been made to apologize for a misdemeanour, it typically took him a day or longer to really process he had done something wrong. Another described how he tried to avoid upsetting the people who loved him by not getting caught; he had not understood that they wanted him to cease the activity. The young people argued that their previous criminal involvement was not indicative of a lack of conscience, but of their not understanding that they were hurting other people. Once they realized it in a concrete way, it made them more likely to stop.

David M. Boulding, a Canadian barrister who specializes in supporting people with FASDs warns of the lack of knowledge about FASDs in the justice system as a whole (see also Killingley, Chapter 16, this publication). He describes the criminal with an FASD as an often likeable rogue who rarely learns from experience, being unable to understand the association between their actions and the punishments meted out through the justice system (Boulding 2001). They are typically caught time and again for the same crime, are the gang stooge, do not understand their rights under law, use the same implausible excuses, confess to things they have not done to please their interviewers, confabulate their story, are unable to understand how the justice 'game' works and forget, over the course of their incarceration, what they have been interned for. He remarked on his clients' difficulty in understanding language, and their need for concrete and visual demonstrations. Fast and Conry (2009: 253) observe that:

> Language deficits have important implications for individuals with FASDs in the legal system in understanding the proceedings, understanding questions, and providing answers. Also, their superficial talkativeness may lead others (e.g., judges, lawyers) to overestimate their competence and level of understanding.

Jones (2000) suggests to protect young people with FASDs, they can be taught rules for behaviour if stopped by the police: be respectful; show a driver's licence; say 'I need a lawyer.' They should also carry and present a card to the police that states their disability, their rights not to talk and to make a completed call to their lawyer, together with the name and contact details of a specialist learning disability lawyer and the young person's advocate.

Conclusion

Transition into adulthood is often an uncertain and potentially stressful period for any adolescent, but especially so for young people with FASDs, who struggle with an understanding and adaptive skills far below their years, and also secondary disabilities as a result of their FASD. All young people with FASDs are individuals and their life experiences are varied. However, almost all need support to live successfully in the community and avoid bleak outcomes (Community Living British Columbia 2011; Streissguth *et al.* 2004).

At a younger age, all children are more receptive to teaching and accepting of parent direction, so it makes sense for families and schools to capitalize on this and prepare for the period of adolescence when teenagers with FASDs find it more difficult to learn, and strive for personal autonomy. Learning and practising skills for their adolescent and young adult years ahead of their peers, not only increases chances of success for young people with FASDs through extended practice, but increases self-esteem. Organizing older peer support can give adolescents with FASDs highly valued and safe friendships with older children, increase access to interesting activities, and widen their social circle beyond their immediate family and school classmates.

Care should be taken when removing the protective structures in young people's lives that these are not the young person's 'bearing walls' against the impacts of FASDs (e.g. impulsiveness, poor judgement etc.). Kleinfeld (2000) describes how a school's stopping one young man's lunchtime supervision against his parents' better judgement because he seemed to be coping better led to his gradual immersion in a thrill-seeking lifestyle and antisocial behaviours including stealing, cheating and social inappropriateness. As the young man would no longer cooperate with attempts to reinstate lunchtime supervision, the situation was irreversible.

Tragically, many young people with FASDs end up with mental health issues for which they will need professional medical intervention. Some may benefit from therapy providing the therapist takes a concrete, active and multisensory approach (e.g. role play, practice dialogues, play therapy), which can create new habit patterns for real-life situations (Kleinfeld 2000) and makes sure there are supports in place to prompt their use (Southern California FASD Information and Support Network n.d.). Baxter (2000) describes how therapy helped a young woman to trust herself and her skills, understand her responses, solve problems on her own, identify sources of help and access them, and trust her parents more than before.

Characteristic of many of stories of success for young people with FASDs in adulthood, are parents who introduced skills young people would need in their teenage years much earlier than usual, who made the young person's aspirations attainable by scaffolding a series of small steps to achievement, who adopted the mantras, 'supervise, supervise, supervise', 'practise, practise, practise'. However, it is important that young people with FASDs are not robbed of their autonomy. Ruggles Gere writes:

> I struggled… over whether I was helping Cindy too much. I wondered if I was teaching her a kind of helplessness so that she would not be able to act on her own behalf. I have continued to ask myself that question each time I am tempted to intervene, and if there is a way for Cindy to accomplish her goal without my aid, I happily back off… At the same time, I feel it is entirely appropriate to help her when she requests and needs my aid.
>
> *(Ruggles Gere and Gere 2000: 66)*

Kellerman (2004) and Kleinfeld (2000) report that parents observe that their sons or daughters with FASDs who are approaching their 30s begin to gain more control over their impulsive behaviour, achieve greater emotional stability, experience success, and have a more realistic view of their limitations. In all their achievements, young people with FASDs overcome great odds. As one young man says:

> If I was to run with a broken leg and finish it's going to be that much more of an accomplishment for me and [it's] similar with FAS. The little things I do might not be that important, but because of my disorder… it's just that bit more of an accomplishment.
>
> *(Minnesota Organization on Fetal Alcohol Syndrome 2011)*

References

Badry, D. and Wight Felske, A. (2011) 'Policy development in FASD for individuals and families across the lifespan', in E.P. Riley, S. Clarren, J. Weinberg and E. Jonsson (eds) *Fetal Alcohol Spectrum Disorder: Management of policy perspectives and FASD*, Edmonton, AB: Institute of Health Economics.

Baxter, S.L. (2000) 'Adapting talk therapy for individuals with FAS/E', in J. Kleinfeld (ed.) (2000) *Fantastic Antone Grows Up: Adolescents and adults with fetal alcohol syndrome*, Fairbanks, AK: University of Alaska Press.

Blackburn, C. (2010) *Facing the Challenge and Shaping the Future for Primary and Secondary Aged Students with Foetal Alcohol Spectrum Disorders* (FAS-eD Project), London: National Organisation on Fetal Alcohol Syndrome (UK) [online at: www.nofas-uk.org; accessed: 27 July 2011].

Blackburn, C., Carpenter, B. and Egerton, J. (2012) *Educating Children and Young People with Fetal Alcohol Spectrum Disorders*, Abingdon: Routledge.

Boulding, D.M. (2001) 'Mistakes I have made' [online at: www.davidboulding.com; accessed: 27 January 2013].

Boulding, D.M. (n.d.) 'Fetal alcohol and the rules for sex' [online at: www.davidboulding.com; accessed: 28 January 2013].

Carpenter, B. (2011) 'Pedagogically bereft! Improving learning outcomes for children with fetal alcohol spectrum disorders', *British Journal of Special Education*, 38(1): 37–43.

Clark, E., Lutke, J., Minnes, P. and Ouellette-Kuntz, H. (2004) 'Secondary disabilities among adults with fetal alcohol spectrum disorder in British Columbia', *Journal of FAS International*, 2(e13): 1–12 [online at: www.motherisk.org/JFAS_documents/Secondary_Disabilities_Adults.pdf; accessed: 27 January 2013].

Community Living British Columbia (2011) *Supporting Success for Adults with FASD*, Vancouver, BC: Community Living British Columbia [online at: www.communitylivingbc.ca/policies-publications/publications/other-publications/supporting-success-for-adults-with-fasd/; accessed: 9 December 2012].

Doctor, S. (2000) 'Creating an "external brain": supporting a mother and child with FAS', in J. Kleinfeld (ed.) (2000) *Fantastic Antone Grows Up: Adolescents and adults with fetal alcohol syndrome*, Fairbanks, AK: University of Alaska Press.

FASAware (n.d.) 'FASD and how to live with it: Matthew's story' (www.fasaware.co.uk) [online at: www.prestoncollege.net/fas/images/matthew_a5.pdf; accessed: 27 January 2013].

Fast, D.K. and Conry, J. (2009) 'Fetal alcohol spectrum disorders and the criminal justice system', *Developmental Disabilities Research Reviews*, 15(3): 250–7.

Fuchs, D., Burnside, L., Reinink, A. and Marchenski, S. (2010) *Bound by the Clock: The voices of Manitoba youth with FASD leaving care*, Winnipeg, MB: University of Manitoba [online at: www.southernauthorityfasd.org/pdf/Bound%20by%20the%20clock%20Final%20Report%20November%202010.pdf; accessed: 27 January 2013].

Groupe Groves, P. (2000) 'Growing up with FAS/E', in J. Kleinfeld (ed.) *Fantastic Antone Grows Up: Adolescents and adults with fetal alcohol syndrome*, Fairbanks, AK: University of Alaska Press.

Jones, M. (2000) 'Trouble with the law', in J. Kleinfeld (ed.) (2000) *Fantastic Antone Grows Up: Adolescents and adults with fetal alcohol syndrome*, Fairbanks, AK: University of Alaska Press.

Kellerman, T. (2002) 'Secondary disabilities in FASD' [online at: www.come-over.to/FAS/fasconf.htm; accessed: 7 January 2013].

Kellerman, T. (2003) 'External brain' [online at: www.come-over.to/FAS/externalbrain.htm; accessed: 27 January 2013].

Kellerman, T. (2004) 'Teens with FASD: What makes them tick?' [online at: www.come-over.to/FAS/TeensTick.html].

Kleinfeld, J. (ed.) (2000) *Fantastic Antone Grows Up: Adolescents and adults with fetal alcohol syndrome*, Fairbanks, AK: University of Alaska Press.

Lally, E.M. and Dubovsky, D. (2005) 'Addressing child welfare and mental health issues for individuals with an FASD and their families', presentation to the 'Building FASD state systems' meeting, San Antonio, Texas, 21–22 June.

Lipow, V./Southern California FASD Information and Support Network (2012) 'Sexuality' [online at: https://sites.google.com/site/socalfasdnetwork/fasd-and-social-issues/health-and-safety/sexuality; accessed: 28 January 2013].

Lutke, J. and Antrobus, T. (eds) (2004) *Fighting for a Future – FASD and 'the system': Adolescents, adults and their families and the state of affairs*, proceedings from a two-day forum, British Columbia, 19/20 June, Surrey, BC: Connections.

Minnesota Organization on Fetal Alcohol Syndrome (2011) 'Young adults living with FASD share their experiences' (video) 26 October [online at: www.youtube.com/watch?v=KBaAS2CNxbA&list=UUuSmw_FF-RT5i344bcJsxYA&index=14; accessed: 27 January 2013].

Morley, J. (2006) *A Bridge to Adulthood: Maximizing the independence of youth in care with fetal alcohol spectrum disorder*, Victoria, BC: Child and Youth Officer for British Columbia/Ministry of Children and Family Development's Vancouver Coastal Region.

Ruggles Gere, A. and Gere, C. (2000) 'The graduate: college for students with FAS/E', in J. Kleinfeld (ed.) *Fantastic Antone Grows Up: Adolescents and adults with fetal alcohol syndrome*, Fairbanks, AK: University of Alaska Press.

Shepard, B. and Hudson Breen, R. (2012) 'Youth with fetal alcohol spectrum disorder: suggestions for theory-based career practice', in R. Shea and R. Joy (eds) *A Multi-Sectoral Approach to Career Development: A decade of Canadian research*, Toronto, ON: Canadian Education and Research Institute for Counselling/Memorial University of Newfoundland.

Slinn, J. (2000) 'Reaching independence day: managing the behaviour of teenager', in J. Kleinfeld (ed.) *Fantastic Antone Grows Up: Adolescents and adults with fetal alcohol syndrome*, Fairbanks, AK: University of Alaska Press.

Southern California FASD Information and Support Network (n.d.) 'Anger and violence' [online at: https://sites.google.com/site/socalfasdnetwork/fasd-and-social-issues/health-and-safety/anger-and-violence; accessed: 27 January 2013].

Spohr, H.L. and Steinhausen, H.C. (2008) 'Fetal alcohol spectrum disorders and their persisting sequelae in adult life', *Deutsches Arzteblatt International*, 105(41): 693–8.

Streissguth A.P., Bookstein, F.L., Barr, H.M., Sampson, P.D., O'Malley, K. and Kogan Young, J. (2004) 'Risk factors for adverse life outcomes in fetal alcohol syndrome and fetal alcohol effects', *Journal of Developmental and Behavioral Pediatrics*, 25(4): 228–38.

Ten Eyck, M. (2000) 'Living independently: a mother's tale', in J. Kleinfeld (ed.) (2000) *Fantastic Antone Grows Up: Adolescents and adults with fetal alcohol syndrome*, Fairbanks, AK: University of Alaska Press.

Toolbox Parenting (2010) 'Make life easier for teenagers with FASD' [online at: www.toolboxparent.com/Articles/FASD/EasierOnTeenagers.aspx; accessed: 28 January 2013].

Tucker, M. (2011) 'Transition planning' (FASD learning series video), 14 December, Edmonton, AL: Government of Alberta [online at: www.fasd-cmc.alberta.ca/education-training/fasd-learning-series-2011-2012; accessed: 27 January 2013].

US DHHS (United States Department of Health and Human Services)/Substance Abuse and Mental Health Services Administration (n.d.) 'Independent living for people with fetal alcohol spectrum disorders' (information sheet), Washington, DC: DHHS/SAMHSA [online at: www.fasdcenter.samhsa.gov/documents/WYNKIndLiving_6_colorJA_new.pdf; accessed: 27January 2013].

PART IV
Interdisciplinary perspectives

13

FETAL ALCOHOL SPECTRUM DISORDERS
Diagnosis and complexities

Raja A.S. Mukherjee

Introduction

Fetal alcohol spectrum disorders (FASDs) represents a range of conditions that are caused by alcohol exposure to a developing fetus. The range of disorders vary from the most recognized part of the spectrum, fetal alcohol syndrome (FAS), to problems with behaviour and the brain with no obvious external signs (alcohol-related neurodevelopmental disorders, ARND) (British Medical Association 2007).

As described by Calhoun and Warren (2007), the modern story of FAS began with a case series published by Paul Lemoine in 1968 (Lemoine *et al.* 1968). A French obstetrician, reporting with his midwifery colleagues, presented findings on 127 children all exposed to alcohol prenatally. The paper, originally published in a French journal, highlighted some of the difficulties found in children exposed to heavy prenatal alcohol. It did not, however, set out the diagnostic features required to diagnose the condition. The article that did lead to a change in the recognition and definition of the condition in the English-speaking press was published in 1973. This series of articles, published in the *Lancet* in 1973 by Smith and Jones, reported on children living on an American Indian reserve who all presented with consistent features (Jones *et al.* 1973). Smith and Jones described these cases as having classic features, and in the second article (Jones and Smith 1973) they coined the term 'fetal alcohol syndrome'. All the cases described were the offspring of mothers who had consumed heavy levels of alcohol in pregnancy. The articles set out a series of criteria by which later diagnostic criteria would be defined.

The following years saw growing interest in FAS with increased recognition. Case studies considering the presentation of behavioural difficulties, neurological damage and physical characteristics of the disorder were published (Warren and Foudin 2001). Further, the recognition that alcohol could affect the brain without having facial features was also becoming clearer. This led to the debate as to whether the term fetal alcohol effect (FAE) was required (Clarren and Smith 1978). Insights were obtained both from human examination and through animal studies (Hannigan 1996). It was in this latter area that probably the greatest understandings about the effects of alcohol were achieved. This was both from a pathological point of view, but also clarification about the teratogenicity of alcohol (Hannigan 1996; Mattson *et al.* 2001; Olson *et al.* 1994; Riley *et al.* 2003). By using multiple animal models, allowing controlled experiments not possible in humans ethically, it became possible to begin to identify pathological processes, confirm cognitive profiles and explore possible therapeutic interventions (Hannigan 1996; Jacobson and Jacobson 2002; Mattson *et al.* 1997; Mattson and Riley 1998).

The Institute of Medicine came together in 1996 to define a set of criteria by which the disorder could be classified. The term 'fetal alcohol spectrum disorders' became popular at the turn of the millennium. Alongside the diagnostic criteria being established, the meeting led to a recognition that prenatal alcohol could present with a spectrum of difficulties that would vary between individuals (Calhoun and Warren 2007).

Diagnosis of FASDs

The diagnostic features of FAS are made up of a triad of facial features (short palperbral fissures, elongated and flattened philtrum and a thin upper lip vermillion), pre- and postnatal growth deficits below the tenth percentile, neuro-cognitive deficits and a history of alcohol exposure in pregnancy. It is only in the case of FAS that a confirmed knowledge of prenatal alcohol exposure is not required. Despite this, there remains disagreement between different groups as to the cut-off that is used for palperbral fissure length and what point the wider spectrum should be considered (Astley 2006; Burd *et al.* 2003; Hoyme *et al.* 2005).

Some core characteristics are agreed upon. The lip philtrum guide developed as part of the 4-Digit Code (see Figure 13.1) has been recognized as having made a significant contribution to the wider diagnostic process (Hoyme *et al.* 2005). This has led to consistency in approach and less reliance on gestalt (the use of observation of patterns to recognize the disorder).

Table 13.1 summarizes the similarities and differences between the four main diagnostic frameworks in current practice. The main difference between the groups remains whether or not the cut-off should be the tenth or the third percentile. In the UK, ninth and second percentiles are now more commonly used and implies the inherent need for local norms to be established.

Percentiles essentially stem from statistical normal distributions. This implies that for a population there is an 'even', upside-down U-shaped distribution (Figure 13.2). At the centre of the distribution is the mean with 50 per cent of the group falling on either side of this mean. Further it is noted from statistical analysis that 95 per cent of the group will lie within two standard deviations from the mean. This will leave 2.5 per cent of the group

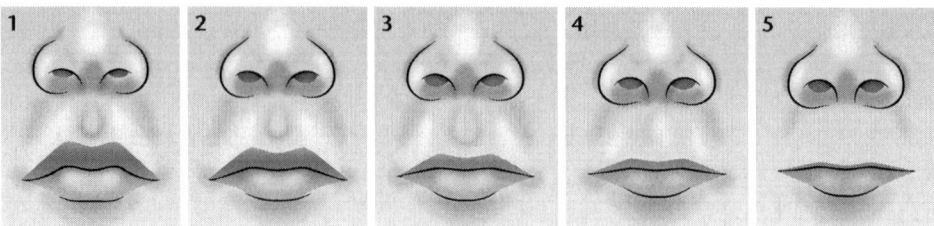

FIGURE 13.1 Lip philtrum guidance (*Source:* Wattendorf and Muenke 2005).

TABLE 13.1 Summary of the different diagnostic tools and the criterion broadly used in each

	Centers for Disease Control and Prevention (CDC)	Institute of Medicine (IoM) revised	Canadian Diagnostic Guidelines	4-Digit Diagnostic Code
Face	Tenth percentile palpebral fissure length (PFL) and rank 4/5 on lip philtrum	Tenth percentile PFL and rank 4/5 on lip philtrum	Third percentile PFL and rank 4/5 on lip philtrum	Third percentile PFL and rank 4/5 on lip philtrum
Growth	Pre/postnatal growth below tenth percentile	Pre/postnatal growth below tenth percentile	Pre/postnatal growth below tenth percentile	Pre/postnatal growth below tenth percentile
Neurological	One out of several brain parameters including orbitofrontal cortex (OFC) <10%, central nervous system (CNS) deficits	One out of several brain parameters including OFC <10%, CNS deficits or abnormal structure	More than three soft/hard neurological signs	One out of several brain parameters including OFC <3%, CNS deficits
Alcohol	Confirmed or unknown	Confirmed to be excessive or unknown	Confirmed or unknown	Confirmed or unknown

Source: Bertrand *et al.* 1994, Chudley *et al.* 2005, Hoyme *et al.* 2005, Institute of Medicine 1996.

below and 2.5 per cent above this main group. It is this level that has historically been accepted as being the cut-off for abnormality (Abidin 1995; Field 2009). For example, it is for this reason the level of 70 in terms of IQ defines the border between what is considered normal IQ range and intellectual disability, i.e. IQ has a mean of 100 with each standard deviation being 15. Thus two standard deviations from 100 equates to 30 points and a score of 70.

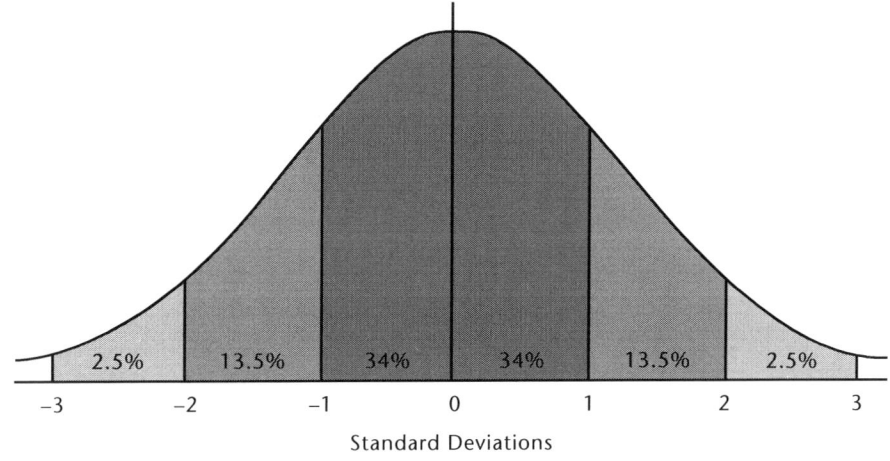

FIGURE 13.2 Normal distribution curve (*Source:* Dorland 2011).

Sensitivity and specificity

The difficulty however in this situation relates to the sensitivity and specificity of this cut-off. A sensitive test will pick up more of the true positive cases, while a specific test will rule out more of the incorrect cases (see Table 13.2). The best test is one that has both high sensitivity and high specificity (Abidin 1995; Field 2009). Unfortunately in most cases one tends to be higher than the other. Susan Astley in 2006 compared the then two main diagnostic groupings and found discrepancies according to the methods used (Astley 2006). The paper highlighted that the higher cut-off of the tenth percentile while picking up more people actually also included some false positives. The study by Astley compared 952 people using both the Hoyme and 4-digit criteria suggesting the Hoyme specificity to be 75 per cent. Of the 952 people studied four had a confirmed absence of prenatal alcohol exposure, and one (25 per cent) of those four met the Hoyme criteria for the full FAS facial phenotype (Hoyme *et al.* 2005).

What is unclear is whether this would be truly replicated by clinicians applying these criteria in a clinical setting rather than strict application in a research project. The Hoyme criteria do actually require knowledge of alcohol exposure for all conditions other than for FAS. An absence of confirmed prenatal alcohol exposure would in reality exclude a diagnosis of FAS. While this may not have been explicit in the Hoyme criterion it is an exclusion criterion for clinicians working in this field. The same issue to a degree can be claimed about the 4-digit scoring schedule in that a score of three (alcohol some risk) can be attributed to a small amount of alcohol due to the range of disorders. In reality, however, the other associated features required for a disorder are unlikely to be seen at low alcohol exposure levels and the coding score that would be achieved would not be consistent with a disorder. What these discussions do highlight is the importance of understanding the implications of these cut-offs as well as the benefits and limitations of each diagnostic framework.

Other physical characteristics

Alongside the core characteristics various physical features have been highlighted as being linked to people prenatally exposed to alcohol. The list is potentially expansive with a summary of some of the more common findings highlighted in Table 13.3 (Autti-Ramo *et al.* 2006; Kvigne *et al.* 2004; Landegard *et al.* 2010; Manning and Hoyme 2007; Spohr *et al.* 1993, 1994, 2007; Steinhaussen *et al.* 1982). Unfortunately, in many cases, these are not necessarily unique to alcohol exposure. Two features that continue to be considered as features associated with the condition are railroad ears and hockey-stick hand creases (Figures 13.3 a and b). The debate about whether or not to include them in diagnostic criteria continues.

TABLE 13.2 Sensitivity and specificity of a test to establish a characteristic being looked for

		Characteristic	
		Positive	Negative
Test	Positive	True positive (sensitivity)	False positive
	Negative	False negative	True negative (specificity)

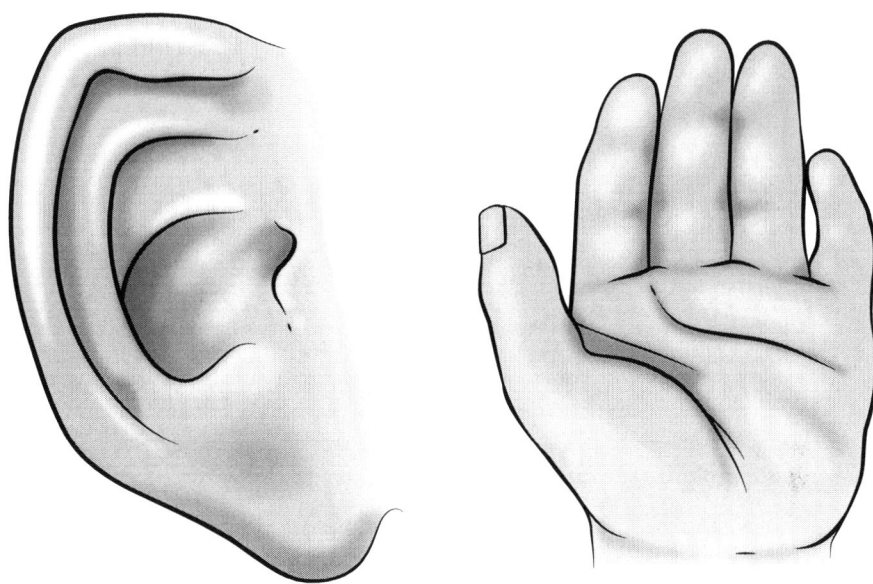

FIGURE 13.3 (a) Railroad ears and (b) Hockey-stick palmar crease (*Source:* Wattendorf and Muenke 2005).

The problem here relates to the fact that these features are not always present, thus can only be considered associated findings. The complexity of this presentation and the range of possible features highlight the need to consider alcohol exposure more when these symptoms are present, but the opposite is not necessarily true. Just because a finding is present, for example a heart defect, it cannot be said that it was necessarily caused by alcohol. For a list of common associated features see Table 13.3.

Further other disorders and genetic syndromes can present with similar symptoms, both physical and cognitive. These are summarized in Table 13.4 (Barrow and Iley 2011; Chudley *et al.* 2005).

TABLE 13.3 Summary of common physical features seen in people prenatally exposed to alcohol

Eyes	Drooping eyelids, strabismus, short-sightedness, underdeveloped optic nerve, blindness
Ears	Hearing loss, recurrent ear infections, central auditory processing disorder secondary to brain damage
Teeth	Improperly aligned and misshapen secondary teeth, faulty enamel
Musculo-skeletal	Minor problems with hands, fingers, arms and toes, foot position defects, problems with some joint movement, cervical spine abnormalities, thoracic abnormalities
Internal organs	Septal defects of heart, underdeveloped or misplaced kidneys
Genitourinary	Abnormal genital development

TABLE 13.4 List of conditions known to overlap physical characteristics with FASDs

- Aarskog syndrome
- Cornelia de Lange syndrome
- Dubowitz syndrome
- Fetal anticonvulsant syndrome
- Maternal phenylketonuria
- Noonan's syndrome
- William's syndrome
- Di George syndrome
- Opitz syndrome
- Duplication sequence of Chromosome 10q and 15q
- Trisomy 18
- Toluene embryopathy

Challenges to making the diagnosis

Despite attempts to refine diagnostic criteria several inherent difficulties related to timing of development, exposure risk and ascertainment of information continue to present challenges to the diagnosis of FASDs.

Timing of development of features

The fetus is formed from the fusion of two gametes, namely the sperm and ovum, to form the embryo which, following initial cell division, becomes the fetus (Sadler 2006). All fetuses follow a genetically programmed pathway of development that, while still showing some general individual variations in timing, tends to have periods during which specific organs are formed. For example, generally the palate has been shown to form between weeks six and eight, but some temporal variability can exist (Sadler 2006). Essentially what this means in terms of diagnosis is that there are specific periods of risk where the process of development may be interfered with. This is important because alcohol *in utero* acts as a teratogen.

A teratogen is defined as a compound that causes damage to a developing embryo or fetus (Martin 2007). Alcohol is one such compound. Numerous researchers have spent many years highlighting the effects of alcohol on the fetus if consumed *in utero*. They have shown that not only is there a direct effect of the alcohol on the development of organ systems in the fetus including the facial features required for diagnosis but that the timing of the exposure has an impact on the observed outcomes (Anthony *et al.* 2010; Cudd 2005; Gohlke *et al.* 2008; Hannigan 1996; Sulik *et al.* 2010) (see Figure 13.4). The implication here is that intermittent exposure, as seen for example with binge drinking, may not affect features such as the face which has a short exposure risk period, but may well affect the brain which has a long exposure risk period.

Information and age of presentation

A further complication that has an impact on being able to make the diagnosis is often the lack of information available. Impacting on this is the age at which the individual presents to a clinic for diagnosis. Unlike a genetic disorder, there is no specific test that can be conducted

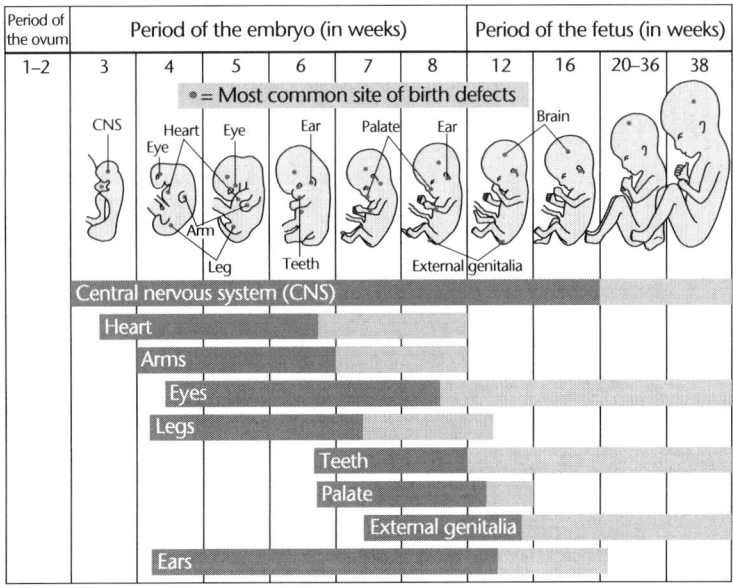

FIGURE 13.4 Diagram showing developmental periods for different organ systems during pregnancy.

to confirm FASDs. Tests such as Free Fatty Ethyl Ester (FAEE) will help to confirm alcohol exposure *in utero* in the second and third trimester to an accurate level (Hutson 2006). While this may highlight the risk it does not make the diagnosis in itself. Those types of tests have also yet to replace good clinical assessment of individuals. This leaves the clinician reliant on information gathered from records, informants and the individual themselves. The individual may not have all this required information. For example they may well not know what the level of alcohol consumption was by their mother during her pregnancy.

As things stand, at least in the UK, there is an ethical difficulty in obtaining maternal records when consent is withheld and often the required information is not recorded in paediatric notes (Morleo *et al.* 2011). For all but the diagnosis of FAS this exposure risk history is mandatory. This means that for many children, especially when taken into care, adopted or when the mother has died, this information is simply not available, making the diagnostic confirmation impossible. As will be discussed below a characteristic profile may be evident, but this cannot be considered unique unless alcohol exposure is confirmed and other factors excluded.

The argument has been made that all information that has potential developmental risks to a child should be included in perinatal discharge summaries, but this is yet to occur widely (Morleo *et al.* 2011).

A further complication was highlighted by Spohr and colleagues. They reported a 20-year follow up of individuals with FAS. Spohr followed up a cohort of 60 children. They showed that the characteristic craniofacial malformations of FAS/FAE diminish over time, namely microcephaly, a poorly developed philtrum and a thin upper lip, and, to a lesser degree, short stature. In females, adult body weight increases. Persistent mental compromise, including intellectual disability, limited occupational options and dependent living are the major sequelae that persist (Spohr *et al.* 2007). This has implications for the age of presentation and the impact on the diagnosis achieved. While the facial features were highlighted to be most obvious in the first few years of life it is not until later that there is a developmental divergence (i.e. a clear difference between those people with normal and delayed development), which again can affect the diagnosis. Complicating this is the fact that this often occurs later in life when the physical parameters have diminished.

Overlapping disorders

The use of a behavioural phenotype approach to study the effects of different aetiological disorders on clinical neurodevelopmental consequences has increased in interest and popularity recently. Several authors have highlighted the benefits of this approach in defining comparators and causal relationships between clinical 'conditions' and groups of individuals (Oliver *et al.* 2008; Turk 2007).

Phenomenological and aetiological approaches are important but need to be recognized as two different, yet complementary, ways of classifying potentially overlapping clinical presentations (see Figure 13.5). By addressing a condition from the aetiological standpoint a bottom-up approach is taken (i.e. from cause to different symptoms and signs and subsequently diagnoses). A phenomenological approach however does the opposite. A top-down approach is adopted, where the outcomes are reached from identification of clustering of symptoms, signs and phenomena without necessarily a clear understanding of cause.

The bottom-up approach has been shown to be useful in the study of behavioural phenotypes such as fragile X syndrome and velocardiofacial (22q11) syndrome (Turk 2007). Consistent with this the Royal College of Psychiatrists (UK) published a classification system in 2001 for adults with Learning Disability – the *Diagnostic Criteria for Learning Disability (DCLD)* – which takes into account the different approaches using a multi-axial format coding which includes both aetiology and outcome (Royal College of Psychiatrists 2001).

The relationship between diagnoses and the outcomes such as autism and attention deficit hyperactivity disorder (ADHD) are thus complex. It has been suggested that in the study of the similarities, as well as differences, between disorders, we can begin to identify and understand the unique nature of each condition (see Figure 13.6) (Mukherjee *et al.* 2011).

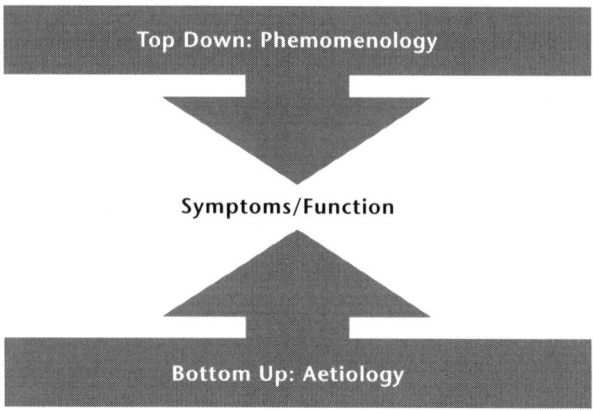

FIGURE 13.5 Relationship between symptoms, phenomenology and aetiology.

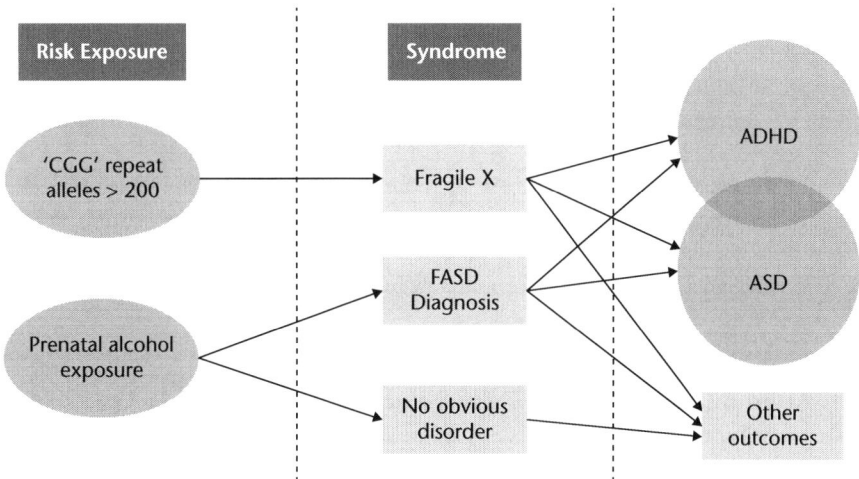

FIGURE 13.6 Diagrammatic comparison between a genetic risk and syndrome (fragile X) and prenatal alcohol to highlight relationship between risk, syndrome and outcome.

We used this approach in a clinical series of the first 21 cases seen in a UK FASD behavioural clinic run. This looked at the relationship between these disorders. The paper published highlighted that in that group 76 per cent met diagnostic criteria for ICD-10 childhood autism as well as having confirmed FASD diagnoses. The group did not, however, present with a classic social interaction style commonly seen in autism, meaning many may well be unrecognized as having an autism diagnosis. Instead they fitted into a more expansive concept of autistic spectrum disorders (ASD). While firm conclusions could not be drawn regarding aetiology the association was reported to be strong enough to warrant further exploration (Mukherjee *et al.* 2011).

Attachment

Attachment theory was first proposed by Bowlby (1969, 1973, 1980). It was further developed by Ainsworth *et al.* (1978) and further still by the addition of a fourth attachment classification from Main and Solomon (1986). Attachment theory concludes that an individual's psychosocial and emotional development can be greatly hindered if they fail to establish a strong, secure attachment with those who care for them in their childhood.

Alcohol, as well as other drugs, is a significant reason for children being taken into the care system, and high rates of FASDs may be found within children in foster care and awaiting adoption (Astley *et al.* 2002; Williams, Chapter 8, this publication). The behaviours attributed to these disorders can often be seen in people with FASDs. Despite this there is very little research with people with FASDs or those exposed to prenatal alcohol.

In the absence of robust research with FASDs, evidence from other conditions offer some insight. A study by Rutgers *et al.* (2007) reported that attachment security was lower in autistic children than other clinical samples; a finding which was unaffected by parenting style. Furthermore, Rutgers and colleagues also looked at the confounding variable of intellectual functioning and discovered that individuals diagnosed with ASD and who were also intellectually disabled were rated as less secure in their attachment than both a non-clinical sample and those who were mentally retarded but without ASD (Rutgers et al. 2007). Such a finding further stresses the importance of distinguishing between the intellectual function of individuals when exploring attachment styles in children within clinical populations including FASD.

In a population, such as those who are taken into care, where there is also prenatal alcohol exposure, leading to an increased vulnerability to postnatal environmental neglect, only increases their vulnerability to insecure attachment. This is an area of work still requiring more investigation but one which impacts on the clinician's ability to differentiate and develop appropriate intervention strategies.

Complexity and the need to understand the relationship between brain and behaviour

Ultimately the complexity of these conditions relates to the fact that prenatal alcohol causes damage to the underlying brain and body. It is the nature and degree of this damage that leads to the presentation seen clinically. Because alcohol expresses its effects in multiple ways, it is also the case that the outcomes and level of damage can vary. In this situation, when phenomenology (descriptive psychopathology) is insufficient to allow a diagnosis to be made, it is necessary to base clinical management on the underlying measurable deficits that can be found. For example the use of psychological tests or even brain imaging allows a more neurological approach to behaviour to be taken. By understanding what is going on inside the brain and how it is processing information, practitioners can understand the behaviour that individuals present within this context. Here similarities between syndromes can be useful in directing management strategies as lessons can be learnt and applied between them.

This approach is not one that is used by all. For this reason, the attempt to pigeon-hole people into diagnostic boxes leads to many simply falling through the gaps. Until society is able to adapt to this alternative way of measuring and understanding behaviour, this situation is likely to continue. The appendix suggests an alternative process for diagnosis for consideration.

Appendix

A suggested process for diagnosis and information that will help with diagnosis in the UK

PRIOR TO ASSESSMENT

1. Gather data from previous reports and assessments including:
   a   psychological testing
   b   educational reports
   c   developmental reports
   d   paediatric reviews
   e   maternal obstetric reports (subject to consent).
2. Rule out other possible causes of behavioural and cognitive presentation
   a   genetic array
   b   karyotpye
   c   fragile X.

AT ASSESSMENT

1. Complete thorough history including alcohol in pregnancy, developmental history
2. Assess wider neurodevelopmental disorders such as autism and ADHD
3. Complete physical measurements:
   a   facial features
   b   growth parameters
   c   general physical assessment.
4. Consider necessary wider investigations:
   a   general cognitive assessment including working memory and processing speed: Wechsler Adult Intelligence Scale (WAIS)/Wechsler Intelligence Scale for Children (WISC);
   b   executive function testing: continuous performance test, card sort test, trail making test, go no go test;
   c   communication: Test for Reception of Grammar (TROG), Clinical Evaluation of Language Fundamentals (CELF);
   d   scanning including MRI (if clinical indication found).

References

Abidin R. (1995) *Parental Stress Index* (3rd edition), Vero Beach, FL: PAR Publishing.
Ainsworth, M.D.S., Blehar, M., Waters, E. and Wall, S. (1978) *Patterns of Attachment*, Hillsdale, NJ: Lawrence Erlbaum Associates.
Anthony, B., Vinci-Booher, S., Wetherill, L., Ward, R., Goodlett, C.R. and Zhou, F. (2010) 'Alcohol induced facial dysmorphology in C57BL/6 mouse models of FASD', *Alcohol*, 44(7/8): 659–71.
Astley, S.J. (2006) 'Comparison of the 4-digit code and the Hoyme diagnostic guidelines for fetal alcohol spectrum disorders', *Paediatrics*, 118(4): 1532–45.

Astley, S.J.P., Stachowiak, J.R., Clarren, S.K.M. and Clausen, C.R. (2002) 'Application of the fetal alcohol syndrome facial photographic screening tool in a foster care population', *Journal of Pediatrics*, 141(5): 712–17.

Autti-Ramo, I., Fagerlaud, A., Ervalhatri, N., Loimu, L., Korkman, M. and Hoyme, H.E. (2006) 'Fetal alcohol spectrum disorders in Finland: clinical delineation of 77 older children and adolescents', *American Journal of Clinical Genetics*, 140(2): 137–43.

Barrow, M. and Iley, E.P. (2011) 'Diagnosis of fetal alcohol syndrome: emphaisis on early detection', in P.Preece and E.P. Riley (eds) *Alcohol, Drugs and Medication in Pregnancy*, London: MacKeith Press.

Bertrand, J., Floyd, R.L., Weber, M.K., O'Connor, M.J., Riley, E.P., Johnson, K.A. et al. (1994) *Fetal Alcohol Syndrome: Guidelines for referral and diagnosis*, Atlanta, FL: Centers for Disease Control.

British Medical Association (2007) *Fetal Alcohol Spectrum Disorders: A guide for healthcare practitioners*, London: BMA Publishing.

Bowlby, J. (1969) *Attachment and Loss: Attachment (vol. 1)*, New York, NY: Basic Books.

Bowlby, J. (1973) *Attachment and Loss: Separation (vol. 2)*, New York, NY: Basic Books.

Bowlby, J. (1980) *Attachment and Loss: Loss, sadness and depression (vol. 3)*, New York, NY: Basic Books.

Burd, L., Martsolf, J.T., Klug, M.G. and Kerbeshian, J. (2003) 'Diagnosis of FAS: a comparison of the Fetal Alcohol Syndrome Diagnostic Checklist and the Institute of Medicine Criteria for Fetal Alcohol Syndrome', *Neurotoxicology and Teratology*, 25(6): 719–24.

Calhoun, F. and Warren, K.R. (2007) 'Fetal alcohol syndrome: historical perspectives', *Neuroscience and Biobehavioral Reviews*, 31(2): 168–71.

Chudley, A.E., Conry, J., Cook, J.L., Loock, C., Rosales, T. and LeBlanc, N. (2005) 'Fetal alcohol spectrum disorder: Canadian guidelines for diagnosis', *Canadian Medical Association Journal*, 172(5) Supp: S1–S21.

Clarren, S.K. and Smith, D.W. (1978) 'The fetal alcohol syndrome', *New England Journal of Medicine*, 298(19): 1063–7.

Cudd, T.A. (2005) 'Animal model systems for the study of alcohol teratology', *Experimental and Biological Medicine*, 230(6): 389–93.

Dorland, W.A.N. (2011) *Dorland's Illustrated Medical Dictionary* (32nd edition), Philadelphia, PA: Elsevier Saunders.

Field, A. (2009) *Discovering Statistics Using SPSS* (3rd edition), London: Sage Publishing.

Gohlke, J.M., Hiller-Strumhofel, S. and Faustman, E.M. (2008) 'A systems based computaitonal model of alcohols toxic effects on brain development', *Alcohol Research and Health*, 31(1): 76–83.

Hannigan, J.H. (1996) 'What research with animals is telling us about alcohol-related neurodevelopmental disorder', *Pharmacology, Biochemistry and Behavior*, 55(4): 489–99.

Hoyme, H.E., May, P.A., Kalberg, W.O., Kodituwakku, P.W., Gossage, J.P., Trujillo, P.M., Buckley, D.G., Miller, J.H., Aragon, A.S., Khaole, N., Viljoen, D.L., Jones, K.L. and Robinson, L.K. (2005) 'A practical clinical approach to diagnosis of fetal alcohol spectrum disorders; clarification of the 1996 Institute of Medicine Criteria', *Pediatrics*, 115(1): 39–47.

Hutson, J. (2006) 'Meconium fatty acid ethyl esters and prediction of fetal alcohol effects', *Journal of FAS International*, 4(e15): 1–3.

Institute of Medicine (1996) *Fetal Alcohol Syndrome: Diagnosis, epidemiology, prevention, and treatment*, Washington, DC: Nation Academy Press.

Jacobson, J.L. and Jacobson, S.W. (2002) 'Effects of prenatal alcohol exposure on child development', *Alcohol Research and Health*, 26(4): 282–6.

Jones, K.L. and Smith, D.W. (1973) 'Recognition of the fetal alcohol syndrome', *Lancet*, 302(7836): 999–1001.

Jones, K.L., Smith, D.W., Ulleland, C. and Streissguth, A.P. (1973) 'Patterns of malformations in offspring of chronic alcoholic mothers', *Lancet*, 1(7815): 1267–71.

Kvigne, V.L., Leonardson, G.R., Neff-Smith, M., Brock, E., Borzelleca, J. and Wetley, T.K. (2004) 'Characteristics of children who have full or incomplete fetal alcohol syndrome', *Journal of Paediatrics*, 145(5): 635–40.

Landegard, M., Svennson, L., Stromland, K. and Andersson-Gronlund, M. (2010) 'Prenatal alcohol exposure and neurodevelopmental disorders in children adopted from eastern Europe', *Paediatrics*, 125(5): e1178–85.

Lemoine, P., Harousseau, H., Borteryu, J.P. and Menuet, J.C. (1968) 'Les enfants des parents alcoholiques: anomoloies observees a propos de 127 cas', *Ouest Medical*, 25: 477–82.

Main, M. and Solomon, J. (1986) 'Discovery of an insecure disorganised/disorientated attachment pattern: procedures, finding and implications for classification in behaviour', in M. Yogman and T.B. Brazelton (eds) *Affective Development in Infancy*, Norwood, NJ: Ablex.

Manning, M. and Hoyme, H.E. (2007) 'Fetal alcohol spectrum disorder: a practical guide to diagnosis', *Neuroscience Biobehavioural Reviews*, 31(2): 230–8.

Martin, E.A. (ed.) (2007) *Concise Medical Dictionary*, Oxford: Oxford University Press.

Mattson, S.N. and Riley, E.P. (1998) 'A review of the neurobehavioral deficits in children with fetal alcohol syndrome or prenatal exposure to alcohol', *Alcoholism: Clinical and Experimental Research*, 22(2): 279–94.

Mattson, S.N., Riley, E.P., Gramling, L., Delis, D.C. and Jones, K.L. (1997) 'Heavy prenatal alcohol exposure with or without physical features of fetal alcohol syndrome leads to IQ deficits', *Journal of Pediatrics*, 131(5): 718–21.

Mattson, S.N., Schoenfeld, A.M. and Riley, E.P. (2001) 'Teratogenic effects of alcohol on brain and behaviour', *Alcohol Research and Health*, 25(3): 185–91.

Morleo, M., Woolfall, K., Dedman, D., Mukherjee, R.A.S., Bellis, M.A. and Cook, P.A. (2011) 'Under-reporting of fetal alcohol spectrum disorders: an analysis of hospital episode statistics', *BMC Paediatrics*, 11(14) [online at: www.biomedcentral.com/1471-2431/11/14; accessed 11 June 2013].

Mukherjee R.A.S., Layton, M., Yacoub, E. and Turk, J.T. (2011) 'Autism and autistic traits in people exposed to heavy prenatal alcohol: data from a clinical series of 21 individuals and a nested case control study', *Advances in Mental Health and Learning Disability*, 5(1): 43–9.

Oliver, C., Arron, K., Sloneem, J. and Hall, S. (2008) 'Behavioural phenotype of Cornelia de Lange syndrome: case-control study', *British Journal of Psychiatry*, 193(6): 466–70.

Olson, H.C., Streissguth, A.P., Bookstein, F.L., Barr, H.M. and Sampson, P.D. (1994) 'Developmental research in behavioral teratology: effects of prenatal alcohol exposure on child development', in S.L. Friedman and H.C. Haywood (eds) *Developmental Follow-up: Concepts, genres, domains, and methods*, Orlando, FL: Academic Press.

Riley, E.P., Mattson, S.N., Li, T.K., Jacobson, S.W., Coles, C.D., Kodituwakku, P.W., Adnams, C.M. and Korkman, M.I. (2003) 'Neurobehavioral consequences of prenatal alcohol exposure: an international perspective', *Alcoholism: Clinical and Experimental Research*, 27(2): 362–73.

Royal College of Psychiatrists (2001) *Diagnostic Criteria for Psychaitric disorders in Adults with Learning Disability (DCLD)*, London: Gaskell.

Rutgers, A.H., van Ijzendoorn, M.H. and Bakermans-Kranenburg, M.J. (2007) 'Autism, attachment and parenting: a comparison of children with austistic spectrum disorder, mental retardation, language disorder and non-clinical children', *Journal of Abnormal Child Psychology*, 35(5): 859–870.

Sadler, T.W. (2006) *Langman's Medical Embryology* (10th edition), Baltimore, MD: Lippincott, Williams and Wilkins.

Spohr, H.L., Willms, J. and Steinhaussen, H.C. (1993) 'Prental alcohol exposure and long term developmental consequences', *Lancet*, 341(8850): 907–10.

Spohr, H.L., Willms, J. and Steinhaussen, H.C. (1994) 'The fetal alcohol syndrome in adolescence', *Acta Paediatrics*, 404: 19–26.

Spohr, H.L., Willms, J. and Steinhaussen, H.C. (2007) 'Fetal alcohol spectrum diorders in young adults', *Journal of Paediatrics*, 150(2): 175–9.

Steinhaussen, H.C., Nestler, V. and Spohr, H.L. (1982) 'Development and psychopathology of children with the fetal alcohol syndrome', *Development and Behavioural Paediatrics*, 3(2): 49–54.

Sulik, K.K., O'Moore-Learey, S.K., Godin, E. and Parnell, S. (2010) 'Normal and abnormal embryogenesis of the mammalian brain', in P.Preece and E.P. Riley (eds) *Drugs in Pregnancy: The price for the child*, London: MacKeith Press.

Turk, J. (2007) 'Behavioural phenotypes: their applicability to children and young people who have intellectual disability', *Advances in Mental Health and Learning Disability*, 1: 4–13.

Warren, K.R. and Foudin, L.L. (2001) 'Alcohol-related birth defects – the past, present, and future', *Alcohol Research and Health*, 25(3): 153–8.

Wattendorf, D.J. and Muenke, M. (2005) 'Fetal alcohol spectrum disorders', *American Family Physician*, 72(2): 279–85.

14

BUILDING A COMMUNITY OF CARE THROUGH DIAGNOSIS OF FETAL ALCOHOL SPECTRUM DISORDERS IN AOTEAROA NEW ZEALAND

Christine Rogan and Andi Crawford

This chapter illustrates how diverse community and professional sectors have come together and collaboratively built a multidisciplinary diagnosis capacity for fetal alcohol spectrum disorders (FASDs) in Aotearoa New Zealand. It describes the dynamic process that led up to and formed this collaboration, and presents the experience of a clinical service that integrated what they had learned into their practice. The hoped-for outcome is a more supportive environment for FASD-affected children and families, and prevention and harm reduction within the wider community.

The challenge

The detrimental effects of prenatal alcohol exposure were recognized and documented as far back as 1874 with these immortal words:

> our babies are not born healthy because the parents drink to excess and the child suffers.
>
> *(Petition of Haimonate te Aotearangito and 167 Others to the House of Representatives 1874)*

These early signs and their link to parental alcohol abuse would today be recognized as FASDs.

Drinking in twenty-first century Aotearoa New Zealand has created an overall burden of harm in health and social cost that is estimated to be $5.3 billion per annum (Law Commission 2010). However, this figure does not take account of the likely burden that is the result of prenatal exposure, which according to overseas studies is substantial and lifelong (Centre for Addiction and Mental Health 2012). The paucity of research into the prevalence and impact of FASDs appears part of a wider problem of a society failing to account adequately for the 'second-hand effects' that children suffer from the drinking of those around them (Connor 2012).

Tackling such issues is Alcohol Healthwatch, a small charitable trust based in Auckland, Aotearoa New Zealand's largest city. The Agency is contracted to the Ministry of Health to provide a range of regional and national health promotion services to reduce alcohol-related harm. The Ottawa Charter for Health Promotion (World Health Organization 1986) provides a multilayered framework for the practice of health promotion within the public health domain. This framework allows factors underpinning health inequalities to be approached ecologically. The Charter has provided the Agency with a framework for the reduction of harm from drinking during pregnancy for more than two decades.

Despite Ministry of Health advice and some generalized public awareness that alcohol is harmful to the fetus, the prevalence of drinking during pregnancy in Aotearoa New Zealand remains high. Aotearoa New Zealand research suggests that up to 60 per cent of women may 'binge' drink (4+ standard drinks per occasion) prior to pregnancy recognition, 28 per cent continue to drink some alcohol during their pregnancy, and 10 per cent continue to binge drink (Ho and Jacquemard 2009). This has been consistently shown across various surveys (Alcohol Healthwatch 2007). A recent Aotearoa New Zealand and USA cross-cultural Infant Development, Environment and Lifestyle (IDEAL) longitudinal study, which compared the outcome of methamphetamine and non-methamphetamine exposed infants, showed the rate of alcohol use by the Aotearoa New Zealand control group to be four times that of the matched USA cohorts (Wouldes 2012).

While fetal alcohol syndrome (FAS) has been discussed in Aotearoa New Zealand since its initial identification in the 1970s, the first Aotearoa New Zealand-born case was not documented in published literature until 1996 (Leversha and Marks 1995). At that time, the Pediatric Surveillance Survey identified 63 cases of FAS in pediatric care – equivalent to 0.11 cases of FAS per 1,000. However, this study used a 'passive' approach to establishing prevalence, which has been shown to estimate lower population rates of FAS than clinic-based and active case ascertainment approaches and to report only the most severe cases (May and Gossage 2001; May et al. 2011). Since no other study has been undertaken to ascertain the prevalence for the general population, this extreme underestimation still stands.

Around the same time, on the other side of the world, the Fetal Alcohol Drug Unit at the University of Washington released their findings of a longitudinal study of secondary disabilities related to FASDs in 415 individuals with FAS and fetal alcohol effects (FAE) (Streissguth et al. 1996). This lent considerable weight to the anecdotal evidence from affected Aotearoa New Zealand families and had the potential to strengthen the case for early intervention (Alcohol Healthwatch 2007). It highlighted issues that impacted areas other than health, which led Alcohol Healthwatch to engage more meaningfully with other sectors such as the Government's Justice and Education Departments. However, little changed.

The inability to identify an affected population is a barrier to strategic action, taking the form of a 'Catch 22': no prevalence = no action = no capacity to identify = no prevalence = no action, and so on. For Alcohol Healthwatch, the impact of this continuing 'no can do' situation was three-fold: the difficulty of preventing what was systematically rendered invisible; the ethical dilemma of raising awareness knowing there was inadequate follow-up; and the lack of capacity to support affected individuals and families.

Efforts to raise awareness of FASDs up to the mid-1990s were directed toward health sector education with the expectation that knowledge would be integrated into practice. Knowledge within the sector certainly increased, but barriers continued and pathways for diagnosis remained elusive. From a health promotion perspective, it was clear that diagnosis was the key to unlocking what had become a paralysing stalemate.

Trying differently

Dialogue ensued with Aotearoa New Zealand's Youth Court judges to bring to their attention the hidden nature of FASDs, the likely over-representation of FASDs among the youth offending population, and the importance of considering this in offending behaviour and rehabilitation (Fast *et al.* 1999).

Retired judge Anthony Wartnik and Kathryn Kelly, experts in FASDs and justice matters, were invited to Wellington, Aotearoa New Zealand, from the USA to present a workshop at the 2007 youth offenders conference, 'Working Together'. The workshop (Wartnik 2007) was well received. Subsequently a meeting with government ministers was called for by the Principal Youth Court Judge, seeking a mandate to conduct a prevalence study among the Aotearoa New Zealand youth offending population. This met with a familiar and disappointing response: 'a research project involving medical assessment of Youth Court Offenders for FASD may be ineffective due to the lack of diagnostic capacity at this time' (Ministry of Health 2008).

Continuing to build connections, further FASD and justice workshops brought forward clinicians with a different level of interest: those whose job was to assess young offenders for the courts. Their reports needed to stand up to cross-examination, and therefore the imperative to improve clinical knowledge and accuracy was great. Alcohol Healthwatch set about making that possible.

A successful bid secured a special grant enabling FASD diagnostic capacity to be explored by a multidisciplinary group. The aim of this initial investigative project was to ascertain the clinical elements required to establish an adequate yet robust multidisciplinary approach to FASD diagnosis in Aotearoa New Zealand, and to ensure clinicians and policy-makers were better informed as a result. Clinicians were able to learn from FASD experts in Canada and the USA. The Canadian FASD Diagnostic Guidelines were found to translate well for Aotearoa New Zealand (Chudley *et al.* 2005). The project evaluation showed that establishing multidisciplinary FASD diagnosis in Aotearoa New Zealand was feasible, justified and urgently needed (Rogan 2010).

Building capacity

The success of the initial investigation led to further opportunities whereby the now experienced core group of clinicians agreed to train other teams to integrate FASD assessment into their services. The first wave of training provided teams operating in three District Health Boards (DHBs) with training in the application of diagnostic tools and protocols (Rogan 2011).

The next part of this chapter describes the experience of one of those teams and how this work contributed to building a community of care for the people of their region.

Hawke's Bay

Hawke's Bay is situated on the east coast of the North Island of Aotearoa New Zealand. It is a region which receives one of the highest numbers of sunshine hours in Aotearoa New Zealand and has fantastic growing conditions for crops such as fruit, vegetables, olives and grapes. The population of Hawke's Bay stands at 156,000 (Central Region District Health

Boards 2011) of which 69 per cent are Pakeha (European descent), 24 per cent are Maori, 4 per cent are Pacific Nation and 3 per cent are Asian (Statistics New Zealand 2006). The local iwi, Ngati Kahungunu,[1] is Aotearoa New Zealand's third largest and traditionally centred in the Hawke's Bay, Tararua and Wairārapa regions.

Given the abundant food production and the sunny climate we might expect a healthy child population. However, this is not the case. Population health indicators in Hawke's Bay show that child and youth health is worse than the national average (e.g. breast fed rate, hearing, oral health, avoidable hospitalizations and immunization rates). Many of these outcomes are related to the social and physical environments that children and youth live in (e.g. poverty, overcrowding, parental smoking and reduced educational opportunities) (HBDHB 2009, 2010). In addition, many families have high levels of alcohol and drug abuse which may continue throughout pregnancy. In Hawke's Bay, 24.8 per cent of all adults have hazardous drinking patterns (HBDHB 2010). Hawke's Bay therefore has a population of children who have been prenatally exposed to alcohol and are at risk of having an FASD.

The Developmental Assessment Programme (DAP)

The Child Development Service (CDS) is a department of the Hawke's Bay District Health Board (HBDHB) that provides services to children with moderate to severe physiological, neurological, developmental and behavioural difficulties. Within the CDS is a Developmental Assessment Programme (DAP) which specializes in assessing children who have complex development, behavioural and learning problems such as autism spectrum disorders, attention deficit disorder, attachment issues and more recently FASDs. The DAP is run by a multidisciplinary team including a pediatrician, psychologists, an occupational therapist, a speech and language therapist, and social workers. Typically children are seen by each discipline across all settings (e.g. home, school and clinic). Information from all disciplinary assessments is integrated at a formulation meeting, and then provides the basis for an interdisciplinary assessment report. This is shared with the family, school and appropriate community agencies. A comprehensive referral plan is established, and children are often followed up by the pediatrician.

The need in our community

In the past, the DAP team would often see children who had been prenatally exposed to alcohol. These children would be referred for cognitive assessment only where intellectual disability was suspected, and did not receive an interdisciplinary assessment. It was noticed that the children with prenatal alcohol exposure often had unusual cognitive profiles with large deficiencies in some areas of functioning while other areas remained intact. These children were impulsive and often had attention difficulties. Interestingly, they enjoyed social interactions, but had a paucity of social skills. They presented with a social naivety which meant they were vulnerable in the community.

Prior to training in FASDs, interdisciplinary assessments would have described their cognitive, motor, speech and language strengths and difficulties, as well as psycho-social issues that were contributing to their presentation. However, this did not result in recommendations for specific strategies that are important for children with FASDs. The children were grouped into a broad category of FAE; or FAS if they presented with the facial features and growth impairments. Many professionals – clinicians, teachers, social workers – were involved in these children's care and education, but none understood the extent and specific characteristics of a child with an FASD. Everyone needed to *understand* and *learn* more about FASDs to help families, schools and their community understand these children better.

Upskilling in FASDs

In early 2010 the service drove its own review of the literature and started using the Canadian guidelines to assess Hawke's Bay children who had had prenatal alcohol exposure. The Alcohol Healthwatch task force became aware of our team's work through families who had recently been diagnosed. Subsequently one pediatrician and two psychologists were invited to be part of a national training programme in multidisciplinary FASD assessment. This training comprised two one-day workshops in Aotearoa New Zealand, one of which was facilitated by Dr Albert Chudley, lead author of the Canadian Guidelines. Following these workshops the team was sent to Vancouver, Canada, to attend the 4th International Conference on FASD and complete training at the Asante Centre, a Centre of Excellence for FASD diagnosis and assessment. Right from the beginning, diagnosis was a way of connecting key families, clinicians, health professionals and organizations.

New practices for our service

Once the DAP team was trained, it was clear that new pathways for FASD assessments needed to be developed within current service resources. No additional funding was available and therefore the team needed to be pragmatic and provide service where it would be most effective. We agreed that these children required a multidisciplinary assessment to address the complexity of their developmental, behavioural and psycho-social issues, and explored how best to maximize the assessment opportunity.

With FASDs, difficulties increase as children age and some of the key areas of deficit such as executive functioning, social abilities and self-care skills do not become apparent until middle childhood (Anderson 2002). Our service did not have the capacity to repeatedly assess children, and therefore we agreed we would not formally assess for a diagnosis of FASDs until a child reached the age of eight years. However we had a number of children who were identified as being 'at risk' and potentially having an FASD prior to eight years of age, and therefore we needed a pathway for providing support while they waited for assessment. The DAP neurodevelopmental pediatrician, Dr Kate Robertshaw, developed a pathway for the pediatric service which comprised a two-stage assessment model outlined below (Robertshaw 2011).

Stage 1 – screening and information collection

This stage is completed by pediatricians for children already in the service and new referrals to pediatrics or CDS where a suspected FASD is the referral basis. Pediatricians complete an FASD proforma which captures a detailed history of prenatal alcohol exposure alongside data about growth, sentinel facial features and learning and behavioural problems. Pediatricians have been trained to measure and document FASD facial features according to the Washington

4-Digit Diagnostic Code. Although it is understood that complete information is not always available, FASD referrals are based around a documented concern of prenatal alcohol exposure rather than on suspicion only. Children who have been prenatally exposed to alcohol but have no evidence of central nervous system dysfunction are not assessed. Following a positive pediatric screen the child is then referred to CDS for a clinical DAP assessment deferred until the child is at least eight years. Children over eight years are put on our DAP waiting list. Once accepted onto the waiting list all children are visited by the DAP social worker, who considers their needs and support while on the waiting list. Families are given:

- basic information about FASDs;
- advice on eligibility for Child Disability Allowance;
- advice on eligibility for a service through Options Hawke's Bay (a needs assessment coordination service) and Tautoko Services (a non-governmental organization that provides behaviour support to children and adults with intellectual disability);
- information on other support services (e.g. CCS Disability Action);
- involvement of the Ministry of Education Special Education where appropriate;
- involvement with the Child Adolescent and Family Service (the HBDHB service for children and adolescents with mental health issues) if required.

The social worker may need to work with the referring pediatrician to provide this package of care.

Stage 2 – definitive interdisciplinary assessment

The DAP team then provides an assessment in accordance with the Canadian guidelines which consists of:

- neuropsychological assessment of the key domains of central nervous system dysfunction: cognition, academic achievement, adaptive functioning, executive functioning, memory and attention;
- speech and language assessment including assessment of the social use of language and problem solving for the domains of language and executive functioning;
- occupational therapy assessment of the motor and sensory domains of central nervous system dysfunction;
- social work assessment to obtain important information regarding the home environment and any factors that may affect development;
- school observation and discussion with the teacher to add context and provide information about functional/academic difficulties;
- further pediatric assessment if required.

Once information is collected it is formulated by the team, and the psychologist coordinates all input into the report. Families are given feedback about the outcomes of the assessment and are given a draft copy of the report. Recommendations, referrals and possible resources are suggested and discussed with the family. They are then able to comment on the report and clarify any information if required. Once families are satisfied with the report, the school is visited to talk through supports and strategies that would be most appropriate for the neurobehavioural profile of the child. Children are then followed up by the pediatrician.

Diagnosis using the FASD pathway raises understanding about the child's needs and points the way for tailored intervention. However diagnosis is only part of the process. What happens before diagnosis, and more importantly after, is key.

Implications of changes to our practice

Through this new diagnostic practice, a greater understanding of the child, which has been hugely appreciated by families and schools, can be provided. Creating understanding and changing expectations has a positive effect on the environment and therefore on the behaviour of the child. These children are now receiving a holistic assessment from multiple disciplines at one time, which is important because of the pervasiveness of impairment found within FASDs.

However, an increase in FASD referrals has occurred, which is why it is extremely important for pediatricians to screen these children carefully so that only appropriate referrals are made for DAP assessment. The workload has increased. Whereas before, these children may have received only a stand-alone cognitive assessment by the psychologist, now they require a full interdisciplinary assessment including a complete neuropsychological examination. Despite this increase, this work is now core to our service. The outcomes of collaboration by all professional disciplines is valued by our families, teachers and supporting organizations. An interdisciplinary team is analogous to a small community where the sum is greater than its individual parts.

The importance of sharing knowledge

As learning increased so did the need to enskill important sectors of our community. Since the training began in 2010, the DAP team has shared its FASD knowledge through formal presentations to resource teachers of learning and behaviour (RTLBs), special needs coordinators (SENCOs) in schools, after-school programmes for children with special needs, non-governmental organizations providing social work input, police, correction services, public health nurses, child, adolescent and family services (CAFS) and community youth workers. It is important to note that this training is not for diagnosis, but to raise the understanding that difficult behaviour may, but not always, be symptomatic of an underlying FASD.

The team spends time enskilling clinicians, support staff, social workers and specialist teachers in the use of frameworks and strategies to intervene and manage learning and behaviour for children with FASDs. Resources are passed on, and the service offers a point of contact for consultation and education about FASDs. The education focus is part of the DAP remit and is considered imperative so that those working in our community have an increased awareness about FASDs and know how to recognize, relate to and respond to those affected. Diagnosis must be substantiated by raising awareness and knowledge in the community.

Future directions

The DAP team is committed to increasing knowledge in our community through (1) supporting individual cases, (2) specific knowledge sharing presentations, and (3) consultation as required. Data is captured to highlight the presence and effects of FASDs in our community and to explore whether current health screening programmes are identifying all children who are exhibiting behaviour that may be consistent with an FASD diagnosis.

Aotearoa New Zealand needs to develop better pathways for identification of these vulnerable children with FASDs and for supporting them and their families as they move along the developmental trajectory of a child with an FASD. Diagnosis brings recognition of problems from prenatal alcohol use in our community so it can be more effectively prevented. At the national level, consistent diagnostic practice is needed. The DAP is thankful and commend Alcohol Healthwatch's initiative to train clinicians. Change is going to occur only when it is possible to prove how prevalent FASDs are. The team supports future training projects and participates within a national clinical network to discuss and share ideas. Consultation and building community never stops: it just keeps evolving.

Conclusion

Working across clinical and non-clinical contexts to improve FASD diagnosis has been a very positive experience overall. Though not without challenges, its success has been built on cooperation, clarity and trust, together with a shared commitment to improve outcomes for affected children. It is recognized that diagnosis alone is insufficient and that integration must include supportive follow-up and outreach into the community. When the diagnostic process is comprehensive, it can prevent the 'revolving door' series of partial assessments which are equally time consuming, often duplicated and costly.

The shift that has occurred since setting out on this journey has opened doors previously closed to us. While these changes have yet to manifest into systemic health policy and planning, it has proven extremely worthwhile for those most closely involved. Clinical teams from other regions are expressing interest in enhancing their diagnostic practice and care of children with suspected FASDs. As one of our trainers described it, 'We had to get the train moving out of the station for people to start thinking they should be on it!'

Alcohol Healthwatch will continue to play its part. This collaborative approach is not only beneficial for those born affected by FASDs, but it is a critical pathway toward its prevention in the longer term.

Note

1 Ngati Kahungunu Incorporated: www.kahungunu.iwi.nz. In Māori society, the iwi (which can translate as 'tribe') are the largest social group, and each is descended from a common named ancestor or ancestors. An iwi is made up of hapū (clans or descent groups), which defend land and provide support for members.

References

Alcohol Healthwatch (2007) *Fetal Alcohol Spectrum Disorder: Activating the awareness and intervention continuum*, Auckland: Alcohol Healthwatch.
Anderson, P. (2002) 'Assessment and development of executive function (EF) during childhood', *Child Neuropsychology*, 8(2): 71–82.
Central Region District Health Boards (2011) *Regional Services Plan 2011–2012*, Wellington: Central Region's Technical Advisory Services Limited.
Centre for Addiction and Mental Health (2012) *Economic Impact of Fetal Alcohol Syndrome (FAS) and Fetal Alcohol Spectrum Disorder (FASD): A systematic literature review*, Toronto: Health Canada.

Chudley, A., Conry, J., Cook, J.L., Loock, C., Rosales, T. and LeBlanc, N. (2005) 'Fetal alcohol spectrum disorder: Canadian guidelines for diagnosis', *Canadian Medical Association Journal* 172(5 Suppl): S1–21.

Connor, J. (2012) 'Measuring alcohol harm to children in NZ', plenary presentation at the third annual conference of Alcohol Action New Zealand (AANZ), 'Babies, Children and Alcohol', Wellington, New Zealand, 22 March [online at: www.youtube.com/watch?v=w_JLCN0EmO0&list=PL9125 EDCCEABC7708&index=2&feature=plpp_video; accessed: 13 November 2012].

Fast, D.K., Conry, J. and Loock, C. (1999) 'Identifying fetal alcohol syndrome among youth in the criminal justice system', *Developmental and Behaviour Pediatrics*, 20(5): 370–2.

HBDHB (Hawke's Bay District Health Board) (2009) *Healthy Populations Plan July 2009–30 June 2012*, Hastings: HBDHB.

HBDHB (Hawke's Bay District Health Board) (2010) *Healthy People, Healthy Places: Hawke's Bay District Health Board Health Status Review 2010: risk and protective factors*, Hastings: HBDBH.

Ho, R. and Jacquemard, R. (2009) 'Maternal alcohol use before and during pregnancy among women in Taranaki', *New Zealand Medical Journal*, 122(1306): 20–32 [online at: www.nzma.org.nz/journal/122-1306/3883/; accessed: 13 November 2012].

Law Commission (2010) *Alcohol in Our Lives: Curbing the harm*, report of the Review of the Regulatory Framework for Alcohol, Wellington: Law Commission.

Leversha, A.M. and Marks, R.E. (1995) 'The prevalence of fetal alcohol syndrome in New Zealand', *New Zealand Medical Journal*, 108(1013): 502–5.

May, P.A. and Gossage, J.P. (2001) 'Estimating the prevalence of fetal alcohol syndrome: a summary', *Alcohol Research & Health*, 25(3): 159–67.

May, P.A., Fiorentino, D., Coriale, G., Kalberg, W.O., Hoyme, E.H., Aragón, A.S., Buckley, D., Stellavato, C., Gossage, J.P., Robinson, L.K., Lyons Jones, K., Manning, M. and Ceccanti, M. (2011) 'Prevalence of children with severe fetal alcohol spectrum disorders in communities near Rome, Italy: new estimated rates are higher than previous estimates', *International Journal of Environmental Research and Public Health*, 8(6): 2331–51 [online at: www.ncbi.nlm.nih.gov/pmc/articles/PMC3138028/pdf/ijerph-08-02331.pdf; accessed: 25 September 2011].

Ministry of Health (2008) 'Fetal alcohol spectrum disorder and youth justice', paper prepared by the Ministry of Health for the 18 June 2008 Youth Justice Minister's Group meeting.

Petition of Haimona te Aotearangi and 167 Others (1874) Presented to the House of Representatives on 18 August 1874, *Appendix to the Journals of the House of Representatives, 1874 Session, I – J 01* [online at: http://atojs.natlib.govt.nz/cgi-bin/atojs?a=d&d=AJHR1874-I.2.2.6.1; accessed: 15 November 2012].

Robertshaw, K. (2011) *Pathway for the Assessment of Fetal Alcohol Spectrum Disorders (FASD)*, Hawke's Bay: Hawke's Bay District Health Board.

Rogan, C. (2010) *Toward Multidisciplinary Diagnostic Services for Fetal Alcohol Spectrum Disorder*, Auckland: Alcohol Healthwatch.

Rogan, C. (2011) *Final Report Summary on FASD Diagnostic Training Project*, Auckland: Alcohol Healthwatch.

Statistics New Zealand (2006) *Quick Stats about Hawke's Bay Region*, Wellington: Statistics New Zealand.

Streissguth, A., Barr, H., Kogan, J. and Bookstein, F. (1996) *Understanding the Occurrence of Secondary Disabilities in Clients with Fetal Alcohol Syndrome (FAS) and Fetal Alcohol Effects (FAE): Final report*, Washington, DC: University of Washington, School of Medicine, Department of Psychiatry and Behavioural Sciences.

World Health Organization (1986) 'Ottawa Charter for Health Promotion (1986)', presented at the first International Conference on Health Promotion, Ottawa, Canada, 21 November.

Wartnik, A.P. (2007) 'Fetal alcohol spectrum disorder: what juvenile/youth court professionals need to know', presented at the Ministries of Justice, Social Development, Education, Health and the New Zealand Police conference on 'Working Together: A Practical Conference on Offending by Young People in New Zealand', Wellington, 28 November.

Wouldes T. (2012) *What's Mum Been Smoking? Methamphetamine, Mental Illness and Addiction: Early cross-cultural results from the Infant Development, Environment and Lifestyle (IDEAL) Longitudinal Study comparing US and NZ women who use methamphetamine 'P' during pregnancy*. Auckland: Department of Psychological Medicine, Auckland University.

15

THE BABY BUNDLE PROJECT

Midwives on the front line of fetal alcohol spectrum disorders prevention

Susan Fleisher

FASD training for midwives: the journey

The journey that led to the Baby Bundle Training for Midwives and the founding of the charity, the National Organisation for Fetal Alcohol Syndrome UK (NOFAS-UK), began when I adopted my very special daughter, Addie, 20 years ago. When Addie was ten years old, I learned that she had alcohol-related brain damage known as fetal alcohol spectrum disorder (FASD).[1]

I acquired my first knowledge of FASDs when I attended a conference for adoptive parents in 1999. When a doctor at the conference described all the traits of a child with fetal alcohol syndrome (FAS), it sounded as if he was describing Addie. He said that alcohol killed brain cells in the developing fetus and that, as a result, the brain and the head circumference were smaller in children exposed to alcohol *in utero* (see Figure 15.1).

When I heard this, alarm bells went off for me. I had been to every bicycle shop in my neighbourhood, and no one had a child's bicycle helmet small enough for my ten-year-old daughter. We had to put padding inside her helmet.

I immediately took Addie to Great Ormond Street Children's Hospital in London, and they confirmed my suspicion. My daughter had FAS, one of the conditions in the group of FASDs. I knew that my daughter's birth mother was an alcoholic, but little had I realized that this would affect my child for the rest of her life. This new knowledge changed the course of Addie's life as well as mine.

I looked around for support and information in the UK, only to find that very little existed. There was practically no information about FASDs in the UK. There was minimal support for children and families who struggled every day with the wide range of FASDs. All sources of information seemed to be in the USA and Canada. To learn more, I began attending conferences in America and meeting every doctor and expert I could find.

At that time, the owners of the AVENT baby bottle company, Celia and Edward Atkin, stepped in. They knew my daughter and had watched her struggle. As they had an interest in baby nutrition, they asked me to produce an educational film to teach teenagers about the risks of drinking alcohol during pregnancy. Edward and Celia's funding produced our DVD,

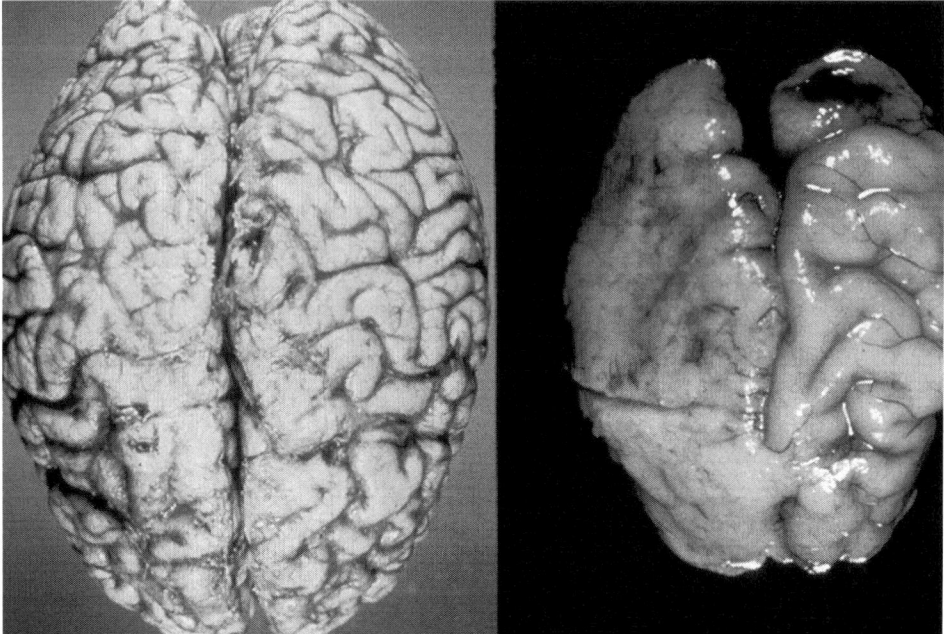

FIGURE 15.1 Comparison between the brain of a typically developing baby and that of a baby with FAS (photograph courtesy of Dr Sterling Clarren).

A Child for Life, which the company distributed to all 4,609 secondary schools in the UK. This eventually led to my establishing NOFAS-UK, the International FASD Medical Advisory Panel and, in 2009, the Baby Bundle Training for Midwives.

When I founded NOFAS-UK, my two main objectives were:

1. To support everyone born with and affected by FASDs.
2. To provide education to prevent more babies being born with FASDs.

The impact of prenatal alcohol

How many disabilities are preventable? Very few. FASDs are 100 per cent preventable if pregnant women *do not* drink alcohol. We can guarantee that *every* pregnant woman who does *not* drink any alcohol (*any* brand, *any* amount) will have a child born *without* alcohol-related brain damage, although some studies have found that not all children of women who drink during pregnancy are affected. Nothing is predictable. However, there is *no* evidence of a 'safe' level of alcohol during pregnancy. There is *no* evidence to predict when alcohol will or will not affect a baby. Since there is no known safe amount of alcohol consumption during pregnancy, the only way to be 100 per cent certain is to abstain from drinking alcohol during pregnancy. In 2007 the UK Department of Health updated its short guideline on the safe use of alcohol in pregnancy to recommend that: 'pregnant women or women trying to conceive should avoid drinking alcohol' (House of Commons Science and Technology Committee 2011: Ch. 3 para. 32).

Reports of drinking among pregnant women, however, are worrying. The 2005 Infant Feeding Survey (Bolling *et al.* 2007), revealed that over half (54 per cent) of the mothers who took part in the survey drank alcohol during pregnancy, and 15 per cent of these (8 per cent of all mothers) drank more than two units of alcohol per week. Professor Terence Stephenson, president of the Royal College of Paediatrics and Child Health, states that 18 per cent of women binge drink during pregnancy, consuming six units or more in a single drinking session (Campbell 2011).

The effect of alcohol on the fetus will last the lifetime of the child because alcohol permanently kills brain cells. Studies have found sections of the brain missing or even misplaced within the brain. Missing brain cells means missing out on normal functions and abilities for life. Addressing a conference in 2002, Dr Sterling Clarren, an international authority on FASDs, stated, 'What does alcohol do to the brain? Anything it wants. What systems does it disrupt? All of them!' (Clarren 2002).

The power of a midwife's influence

Although midwives are not always involved at the very beginning of a woman's pregnancy, they can support women to avoid alcohol at any point. It is never too late to stop drinking. The heart, the lungs and other organs form in the first trimester. However, the brain and central nervous system develop throughout all three trimesters (see Figure 15.2). Alcohol consumed in the third trimester will continue to damage the brain and nervous system. This is when learning, memory and social behaviours are affected. At any time during her pregnancy, if a pregnant woman stops drinking alcohol, it will reduce the risk and improve the outcome for her baby.

How can we prevent FASDs? By educating, informing and supporting all pregnant women. Who are some of the most influential people who work with pregnant women? Midwives!

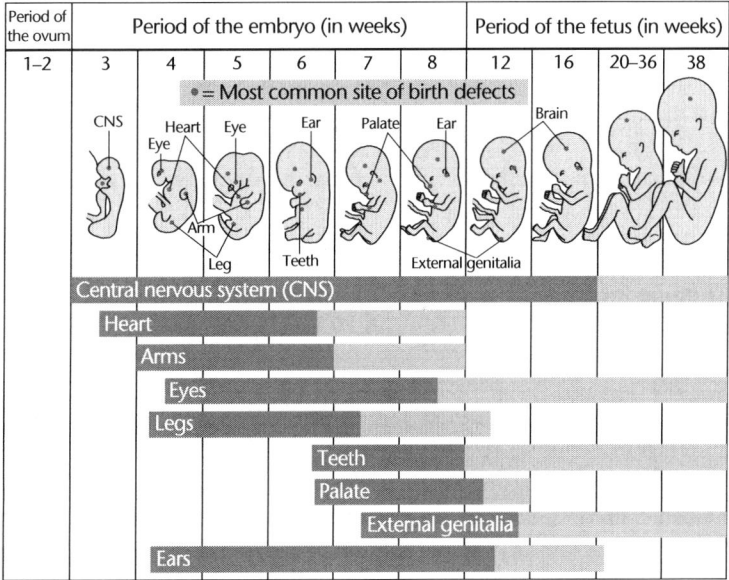

FIGURE 15.2 The impact of alcohol consumption on the fetus throughout pregnancy.

Midwives, general practitioners and obstetricians are the first and early points of medical contact for pregnant women, and midwives are arguably best placed to advise pregnant women on alcohol consumption during pregnancy, in terms of numbers, role, knowledge, skills and opportunities (de Crespigny *et al.* 2003). Midwives deliver 63 per cent of the babies born in Britain (Griggs *et al.* 2007). They are on the frontline – educating and supporting pregnant women. They have responsibility for providing up-to-date information and advice to their clients and their clients' partners. In the NOFAS-UK *No Alcohol, No Risk: FASD information for midwives* video (see www.nofas-uk.org), Dr Raja Mukherjee, lead clinician at a UK FASD specialist clinic, states: 'Midwives are key. By intervening and giving the right advice, the midwife has a chance to prevent a disorder which causes significant, lifelong damage to a child.'

According to the 2005 Infant Feeding Survey (Bolling *et al.* 2005), 89 per cent of expectant mothers had received advice from midwives, compared with 32 per cent gaining information from literature, and 20 per cent from doctors. Three-quarters had been given general information about the effects of drinking alcohol on their baby, almost half had been advised to limit intake, and less than a quarter had been advised to stop drinking alcohol.

Advice given by midwives has a powerful impact on pregnant women and helps them to avoid risks. Women are most motivated to reform their alcohol habits during pregnancy for the sake of their baby. They see midwives as a source of expert advice during pregnancy (Jones *et al.* 2011; Jonsson *et al.* 2009), and are more likely to confide in midwives than other health professionals.

Although Bolling *et al.* (2005) reported that advice on alcohol during pregnancy had little effect on mothers' drinking behaviour, this may reflect the quality of the advice. Midwives and pregnant women interviewed for research by Jones *et al.* (2011) said that the discussions they had had were ineffective – 'generally limited to brief screening questions at the first visit, and the risks were rarely discussed or explained' (p. 489). A birth mother of two sons with FASDs, who did not receive alcohol advice while she was pregnant, emphasizes how essential clear advice is: '[Midwives] should stop being so reluctant to raise [the question of mothers' alcohol intake]. Women need to realise that it's like Russian roulette: if you drink a certain amount you could be putting your baby at risk' (Campbell 2011: 24).

In NOFAS-UK's *No Alcohol, No Risk* film, Melissa, a young mother who has been limiting her alcohol intake to recommended low levels during her pregnancy, states: 'If this is true, and they are saying that if you drink anything your child is at risk of developing any of these things then there's got to be an absolute zero policy when it comes to drinking.'

What midwives know about FASDs

In 2009, NOFAS-UK developed the Baby Bundle Project in collaboration with doctors, FASD experts and the Royal College of Midwives to increase midwives' awareness of the impact of alcohol on the unborn child, and prepare them to inform and support families. Through a three-year intensive programme of training funded by Diageo, the project aims to reach 10,000 midwives, who in turn will advise at least one million pregnant women. For the first time, midwives in the UK have access to specialist education about the effects of alcohol on the fetus including face-to-face training, an online course and a distance-learning package.

One aim of the Baby Bundle Training was to increase the quality of information about alcohol in pregnancy given by midwives to pregnant women. When the Baby Bundle

Project began, the subject of FASDs was not a part of the standard curriculum for student midwives. Although midwives knew it was not a good idea for a woman to drink while she was pregnant, many of them said they were unaware of the severe consequences for babies who had been exposed to alcohol *in utero*. They had not been given in depth information or evidence about the consequences later in life.

Many midwives knew that smoking while pregnant was dangerous for their unborn child. Until recently, it was assumed that smoking was more dangerous than alcohol. It was also assumed that hard drugs such as cocaine and heroin were more dangerous. Of course hard drugs are harmful to the mother and will cause the baby to suffer trauma and withdrawal at birth. Smoking may affect newborns' birth weight. Despite this, in fact, *alcohol is the most harmful drug a pregnant woman can ingest*. A midwife interviewed for the *No Alcohol, No Risk* video (NOFAS-UK/Mencap 2012) observed:

> With smoking we have to discuss the risks, and we have to sign and date [our records] to say [we have covered] all the different effects, but with alcohol we don't have to do that ... if we were to do that, [pregnant mothers] could go away with the knowledge that alcohol causes long term effects on their baby.

At the moment, there is no consistent guidance about what advice midwives should offer mothers-to-be on alcohol intake. The midwives who attended the Baby Bundle Training for Midwives, told us that a lot of the information they received from the Project was new to them. The purpose of the training is to equip midwives to inform and support the mothers and fetuses in their care. The training introduces midwives to:

- the impact of maternal alcohol consumption on the fetus;
- common false beliefs about consuming alcohol during pregnancy;
- how to talk to mothers about alcohol usage;
- possible early indicators of FAS in babies;
- supporting mothers whose baby has been diagnosed with FAS.

During training, midwives shared some of the false beliefs they had held about mothers drinking alcohol in pregnancy. Through the evidence they were given during the Baby Bundle Training, they were able to dismiss some of the following myths:

MYTH 1:

✗ 'Guinness is good for pregnant mothers because of the iron content.' During the 1935 'Guinness is good for you' campaign, pregnant women were advised to drink Guinness.

✓ Today, Diageo, the distributors of Guinness, back the campaign for 'zero alcohol in pregnancy'. The potential damage that alcohol can do to the brain and other organs of the fetus outweigh any benefits from the iron content of Guinness, which can be found in other healthy sources. The damage caused by alcohol to the unborn child is irreversible and permanent.

MYTH 2:

✗ 'Moderate drinking after the first trimester of pregnancy is risk-free.' In 2007, the National Institute for Health and Clinical Excellence (NICE) advised pregnant women that the main risk of damage was only during the first trimester. They suggested that women could begin drinking moderately in the second and third trimesters.[2]

✓ In fact the fetus is vulnerable throughout the entire pregnancy. In the first trimester, in addition to the risk of miscarriage, the organs are forming. Towards the end of pregnancy, during the third trimester, the disruption to the final development of the brain and nervous system can affect learning, memory and nervous disorders.

MYTH 3:

✗ 'FASDs are genetic – they can be inherited.'

✓ FASDs are *not* genetic and cannot be inherited. If a woman does not consume *any* alcohol in pregnancy her child will *not* have an FASD. Even if a mother has FAS herself, she will not pass it on to her children if she does not drink any alcohol in her pregnancy. However, there are studies in progress researching the genetic components from both the mother and father that could influence the vulnerability of the fetus to alcohol.

MYTH 4:

✗ 'Heroin, cocaine, cannabis and hard drugs are more damaging to the fetus than alcohol.'

✓ Alcohol is *more* damaging than any of these drugs. When a baby is born to a mother who has ingested hard drugs during pregnancy, at birth it undergoes withdrawal from hard drugs. Smoking by a mother during pregnancy can cause prematurity and low birth weight for her baby. However, the effects of alcohol are even more complex and severe because it permanently kills brain cells. There is no cure for Alcohol-Related Brain Damage. Children cannot outgrow Alcohol-Related Brain Damage. It will last a lifetime.

MYTH 5:

✗ 'Getting a diagnosis for an FASD is pointless; it only stigmatizes a child. Once the damage is done, there is nothing we can do about it.'

✓ Getting a diagnosis is useful and important. Early diagnosis is essential for both the child and the family because it allows for early intervention. The increased opportunity for appropriate treatment and support will improve a child's life outcome.

Without appropriate support services, people with FASDs have a high risk of developing secondary disabilities such as mental illness, getting into trouble with the law, unwanted pregnancies, alcohol and drug abuse. There is a lot that can be done to improve the life

> outcomes of people affected by FASDs. The benefits of getting a diagnosis will improve lives and far outweigh the drawbacks. A diagnosis is the first tool to put in place for support. We would not think of removing a wheelchair or crutches from a person who could not walk. Why would we not give people with FASDs the tools to improve their lives?

A UK survey of 29 midwives by Anne Marie Winstone (2009), which focused on the antenatal advice about FAS and alcohol intake given by these midwives to expectant mothers, found that their professional knowledge about FAS and practice in advising pregnant mothers varied. Midwives' responses to questions exploring their knowledge of FAS suggested that:

- 100 per cent agreed that educational resources on FAS should be readily available to midwives and mothers.
- 93 per cent believed that an early diagnosis would improve treatment plans.
- 90 per cent correctly agreed that FAS was a preventable condition.

but

- Only 10 per cent identified all four diagnostic characteristics of FAS (i.e. dysmorphic features, central nervous system abnormality, growth restriction and confirmed alcohol exposure).
- 0 per cent felt 'very prepared' to deal with the topic of FASDs.

Unless midwives know the key facts about the risks to the fetus from maternal alcohol use and the possible lifelong developmental effects, they lack the motivation to advise pregnant mothers, and the advice they do give is not effective (Gilinksy 2009; Riley et al. 2003). Midwives' reluctance to talk with pregnant women about their alcohol use can be due to feelings that:

> - They are prying into parents' private lives.
> - They are raising an issue which parents will not be expecting.
> - They do not know enough about alcohol use in pregnancy and its impact.
> - There is not enough time.
> - Only alcohol-addicted patients need support.
> - They will damage professional–patient trust.
> - Intervention will not make any difference.
> - They are compromised by their own life choices.
>
> *(de Crespigny et al. 2003; Gilinsky 2009)*

Scenarios for midwives

All midwives on the Baby Bundle Training agreed that asking anyone, especially a pregnant woman, about their drinking habits, is a delicate and often awkward challenge. The training provides discussions and workshops tackling the difficulties in asking 'The Alcohol Question'.

Here are two scenarios the midwives tackled in previous workshops written by Joanna Buckard of Red Balloon Training.[3] Read them and ask yourself what you would do.

Nicola's story

Nicola is 24 years old. She is 18 weeks pregnant for the fourth time and you have never cared for her before. She is under stress because she has had some difficult life experiences.

Nicola tells you that her first pregnancy was normal and that she has a seven-year-old son at home. Her next pregnancy resulted in the premature birth of her daughter at 23 weeks, and she died a few hours after birth. Her third pregnancy was a son born at 28 weeks. He is now three years old and has developmental delays. In her fourth pregnancy, Nicola has found it hard to cope with her losses and drinks heavily. Nicola lives with her partner, John, who has fathered her last three children. Neither of the couple work and the family live on benefits.

As Nicola's midwife, what support and advice are you going to offer her?

Sam's story

Sam is 32 years old and is 11 weeks pregnant. She lives with her partner Steve, who is 34 and works full-time running his own company. Sam works full-time as a solicitor and they are thrilled to be having their first child.

Sam thinks she became pregnant about eight weeks ago. She reports that she has a healthy diet with plenty of oily fish and vegetables and only eats organic food. She normally does a yoga class once a week and goes running three times a week.

Sam and Steve have their parents and some of their siblings fairly close by and they are all excited by the prospect of a new addition to the family.

Sam tells you that they have a good social life and usually go out drinking every weekend. Sam tells you that she has reduced her drinking to two glasses of red wine a week since she found out that she was pregnant. She reports that she is feeling well and has not suffered much with sickness.

As Sam's midwife what support and advice are you going to offer her?

Overcoming the barriers

To overcome the barriers to talking with mothers about alcohol use, midwives need training so that they realize their advice is critical to protecting the fetus, and the child it will become. With knowledge of:

- what to tell a pregnant woman about alcohol;
- whether it is it safe to drink during pregnancy;
- how alcohol might affect the baby;
- common attitudes regarding alcohol use and FASDs;
- effective ways of discussing alcohol consumption with a pregnant woman;
- how to screen for alcohol consumption in pregnancy (e.g. using T-ACE, Tweak, Audit-C);
- how to prompt appropriately to gain a full alcohol intake history from mothers;

- how to identify those at high risk from alcohol use in pregnancy, and recognize alcohol issues;
- how to maintain open, non-judgemental dialogue and action with parents;
- access and referral routes to support services for mothers (e.g. counselling, rehabilitation).

(Drug and Alcohol Services South Australia 2006; Jones et al. 2011; Riley et al. 2003), midwives are able to overcome reluctance they personally feel in raising what is often regarded as a taboo subject (e.g. de Crespigny et al. 2003; Jonsson et al. 2009).

The Baby Bundle Training provides midwives with key messages to share with mothers-to-be about the effects of drinking alcohol during pregnancy. For example:

- When a pregnant woman consumes alcohol, she does not drink alone. Whatever she drinks she shares with her unborn child.
- There is no known safe level for alcohol consumption in pregnancy.
- Though not all women who consume alcohol in pregnancy will affect their child, drinking during pregnancy is never risk-free.
- Every woman is different. Every fetus is different. There is no way to predict who is vulnerable and at what point during fetal development brain damage may occur.
- Alcohol can cause lifelong mental and physical disabilities, cot death and miscarriage.

Conversations with mothers about alcohol use during their pregnancy should not be one-off. At every monitoring appointment between a midwife and an expectant mother, conversations about alcohol consumption need to take place and a detailed record should be transferred to *both* the mother and child's medical records. Accurate information taken by midwives during a mother's pregnancy is crucial if a diagnosis of FAS is to be established. Without this, there can be no FAS diagnosis. Without diagnosis, the child and parents will not have access to the support they need to protect them from poor life outcomes.

In Winstone's survey, none of the midwives provided advice to expectant mothers that was entirely consistent with the UK's 2008 NICE pregnancy guidelines:

- 100 per cent advised that pregnant women should consider not drinking at all (in line with the British Medical Association guidelines).
- 100 per cent routinely asked pregnant women about their alcohol use.
- 55 per cent provided information on the consequences of antenatal alcohol use.
- 14 per cent asked about risk factors often associated with alcohol use (e.g. drugs).
- 10 per cent advised women not to become intoxicated.
- 3 per cent recommended drinking according to NICE guidelines.
- 0 per cent advised women not to binge drink.

As a result of her research, Winstone concluded that, if best clinical practice was to be achieved, midwives and their clients would benefit from readily available information and resources, and specialist training for midwives should be considered, with particular focus on the most up-to-date prenatal alcohol advice, how to diagnose FAS, and how to effectively approach expectant mothers about their alcohol consumption.

Recognizing the signs of FAS

Early recognition of FAS is important. It can pave the path to early intervention which will improve the life of every baby born with FAS.

Before birth

Doctors and midwives can detect, from scans of the fetus, whether a mother has drunk even low levels of alcohol during pregnancy. The Baby Bundle Training includes a film by Professor Peter Hepper containing footage of a fetus in the womb whose mother had ingested alcohol. This fetus shows a significantly increased number of spontaneous 'startle effects' compared with fetuses whose mothers had not consumed alcohol.

In typically developing fetuses who have not been exposed to alcohol, at 18 weeks gestation the primitive startle reflex disappears. However, for those fetuses whose mothers drank one to four units of alcohol per week, the startle reflex remained throughout pregnancy (Hepper 1998). Scans show periods of fetal quiescence punctuated by sudden, whole-body animations, instead of the constant, specific motor movements of a fetus who has not been exposed to low levels of alcohol. Hepper reported that, even at low levels, this suggested that the fetus had central nervous system damage.

Immediately after birth

Midwives may recognize the signs of FAS during the first days of life. At birth *some* of the following signs may indicate that the baby has been prenatally exposed to alcohol:

- the mother was intoxicated while giving birth;
- the baby has distinctive FAS facial features (see Figure 15.3);
- the baby's low birth weight and under normal percentile size;
- the baby's unusual, tremulous, irritable behaviour;
- the baby's continuous crying, becoming inconsolable;
- the baby's weak sucking reflexes, which may make it difficult for them to feed and nurse normally;
- the baby's over-reaction to normal sounds;
- the baby's extremely erratic sleep patterns;
- the baby's failure to thrive;
- bonding problems between mother and baby.

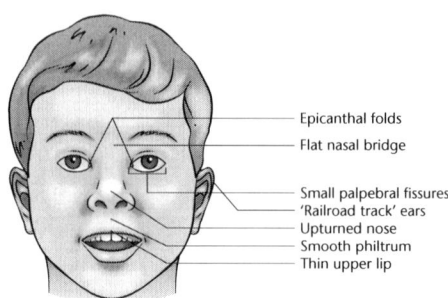

FIGURE 15.3 Characteristic facial features in FAS.

If a baby is born with FAS, a midwife has the opportunity to see and assess the facial and physical features associated with it. However, without the features midwives may not be able to predict that the baby may have the other conditions under the umbrella of FASDs. The adverse behaviours and learning disabilities of FASDs will not become apparent until later in life. For this reason it is important for midwives to record the alcohol history. Without the alcohol history or physical features a child may be deprived of a correct diagnosis.

Midwives may also see other signs of disabilities at birth. However, sadly, if alcohol kills the relevant brain cells it can actually cause a number of the overlapping disabilities shown in Table 15.1 in childhood.

TABLE 15.1 Overlapping behavioural characteristics and related mental health diagnoses in children

Overlapping Characteristics & Mental Health Diagnoses	FASD	ADD/ADHD	Sensory Int. Dys.	Autism	Bi-Polar	RAD	Depression	ODD	Trauma	Poverty
	Organic	Organic	Organic	Organic	Mood	Mood	Mood	Mood	Environ	Environ
Easily distracted by extraneous stimuli	X	X	X							
Developmental dysmaturity	X			X						
Feels different from other people	X			X						
Often does not follow through on instructions	X	X					X	X	X	X
Often interrupts/intrudes	X	X	X	X	X		X			X
Often engages in activities without considering possible consequences	X	X	X	X	X					X
Often has difficulty organizing tasks and activities	X	X		X	X		X			X
Difficulty with transitions	X		X	X	X					
No impulse control, acts hyperactive	X	X	X		X	X				
Sleep disturbance	X				X		X		X	
Indiscriminately affectionate with strangers	X		X		X	X				
Lack of eye contact	X		X	X	X	X				
Not cuddly	X			X	X	X				
Lying about the obvious	X				X	X				
Learning lags: 'Won't learn, some can't learn'	X		X			X			X	X
Incessant chatter, or abnormal speech patterns	X		X	X	X	X				
Increased startle response	X		X						X	
Emotionally volatile, often exhibits wide mood swings	X	X	X	X	X	X	X	X	X	
Depression develops, often in teen years	X	X				X			X	
Problems with social interactions	X			X	X		X			
Defect in speech and language, delays	X			X						
Over/under-responsive to stimuli	X	X	X	X						
Perseveration, inflexibility	X			X	X					
Escalation in response to stress	X		X	X	X		X		X	
Poor problem solving	X			X	X		X			
Difficulty seeing cause and effect	X			X						
Exceptional abilities in one area	X			X						
Guess at what 'normal' is	X			X						
Lies when it would be easy to tell the truth	X				X	X				
Difficulty initiating, following through	X	X			X		X			
Difficulty with relationships	X		X	X	X	X	X			
Manages time poorly/lack of comprehension of time	X	X			X		X			X
Information processing difficulties speech/language: receptive vs. expressive	X			X						
Often loses temper	X		X		X		X	X	X	
Often argues with adults	X				X			X		
Often actively defies or refuses to comply	X				X			X		
Often blames others for his or her mistakes	X	X			X		X	X		
Is often touchy or easily annoyed by others	X				X		X	X		
Is often angry and resentful	X						X	X		

Source: Cathy Bruer-Thompson, Adoption Training Coordinator, Hennepin County, MN. cathy.bruer-thompson @co.hennepin.mn.uk, 2006. With much appreciation to the many who edited and contributed.

Breaking the news

If midwives are involved in telling a mother that her newborn has FAS, following diagnosis by a clinician with expertise in FASDs, the midwife should be prepared with information to help the mother cope with her guilt and grief. The Baby Bundle Project provides tools and strategies for midwives to provide support, help and hope for mothers. The outcome does not have to be all doom and gloom.

The Baby Bundle Training advises women who have newly discovered their child's diagnosis *not* to surf the internet, where they will find over three million websites, *all* with the same frightening facts. Since all sites repeat this information, we suggest that pregnant women and their partners limit their research to no more than three to four reputable sites. As their children grow, NOFAS-UK and other reputable FASD charities will be able to provide them with positive support.

The passionate presenters on the training days

Though the content of the course is based on evidence from over 4,000 international studies, the Baby Bundle Training for Midwives does not rely solely on research. The presenters are the experts and the real people who have first-hand experience diagnosing and living with FAS.

At the face-to-face trainings:

- **Birth mothers** who are raising their own children with FAS explain the circumstances that caused them to drink when they were pregnant. They discuss their experience with the midwives attending the trainings and how it might have been different.
- **Specialist midwives** speak to their colleagues and present their specialist experience.
- **Expert doctors** explain FAS and FASD diagnosis, the physical characteristics, the learning disabilities, developmental delays, behavioural challenges and the expected life outcomes.
- **Adoptive mothers and foster carers** present their experience and the challenges of raising a child with FASDs.
- **Young adults with FASDs** speak for themselves and explain what it is like to live with their disability.

The training also includes powerful stories on film. Midwives are shown films of children and adults with FAS with their mothers. A prison officer breaks down after he finds out that his adopted son has FAS and realizes he has been blaming and punishing prisoners in his care who may have had FAS like his son.

What about fathers?

Whenever possible, midwives should also talk to fathers and supportive family members. (There is a NOFAS-UK booklet for fathers; see Figure 15.4.) Although science tells us that *only* the mother's alcohol intake during pregnancy can affect the fetus, a father can play a major role in protecting his and his partner's child from lifelong alcohol-related brain damage. The father can support the mother to avoid alcohol for her entire pregnancy. For example,

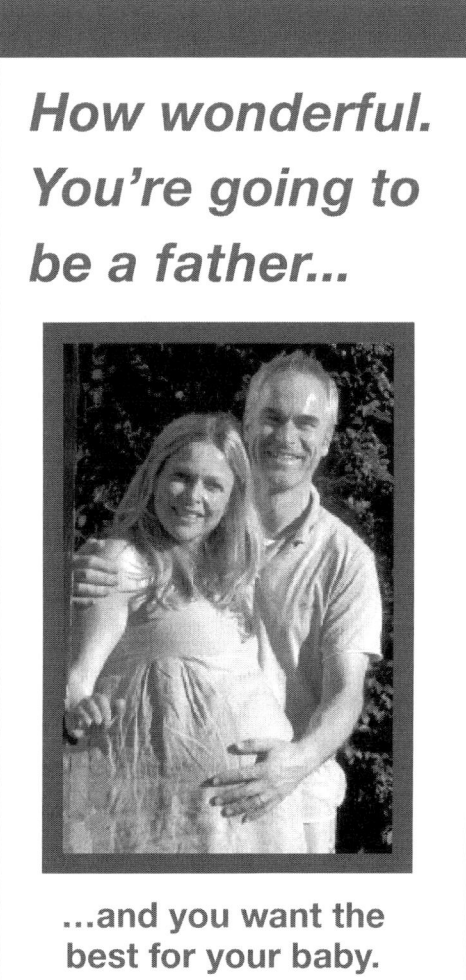

FIGURE 15.4 National Organisation on Fetal Alcohol Syndrome UK (NOFAS-UK) booklet for fathers.

if the father is not informed, he may unknowingly encourage his pregnant wife to join him at the pub or for a nightcap at home.

At the end of the Baby Bundle Training...

Many midwives said that although they had known that pregnant women should not drink alcohol, the training had explained *why* and how serious and sometimes life-threatening it can be. They had been surprised to learn that alcohol is more dangerous than other drugs. Midwives said they felt empowered with the information, evidence and the tools they were given. A summary is written in NOFAS-UK's *Alcohol and Pregnancy: Information for midwives* leaflet (see Figure 15.5; NOFAS-UK 2010).

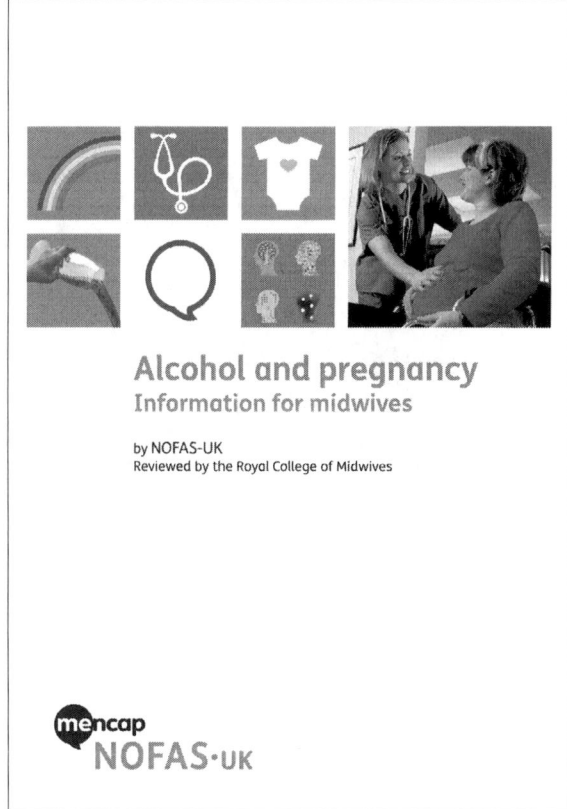

FIGURE 15.5 NOFAS-UK information booklet for midwives.

Alcohol is the most teratogenic drug a pregnant woman can ingest. As a result of their training, midwives said:

- ✓ They would put alcohol at the top of their list of teratogens (a substance that can damage and disrupt the developing embryo).
- ✓ They would tell pregnant mothers alcohol is a high-risk substance … ahead of soft cheese, sushi and smoking.

Midwives' feedback on the Baby Bundle Training day told us that their enhanced knowledge had given them new confidence to raise the subject of alcohol with pregnant women. They were asked to give feedback about the Baby Bundle Training. These are some of their responses:

- Very stimulating and thought-provoking study day. I shall certainly strengthen my advice to pregnant women.
- I am full of admiration for what you do… Numerous other midwives told me how valuable the day was and how they're taking away important information to use… Know that you have achieved so much, however much more there always seems still to be done!
- A brilliant study day! I am spreading the word…

- Thank you all for a fantastic and very worthwhile study day ... I am so passionate about this topic after learning so much from your training day! ... Would it ever be possible for you to arrange a training day in Wales?

Video highlights of the training days can be seen on YouTube.[4]

What we can all do about fetal alcohol prevention

Through the Baby Bundle Project in the UK, at last mothers-to-be will be provided with accurate information so that they can make informed choices about drinking alcohol. Most importantly, FASD training will empower midwives with evidence and confidence to support pregnant women to avoid alcohol and reduce the number of babies born with lifelong FASD disabilities.

Although the Baby Bundle Project has focused primarily on midwives, because midwives play an important role and can advise a pregnant woman, one must look at the broader picture. The majority of the world enjoys alcohol and drinks by choice. It is ultimately the choice of a mother whether she drinks or does not drink while she is pregnant. The responsibility of providing her with all the right information so that she can make an informed choice, lies with not just the midwife, but with every one of us – men and women, teenagers, adults, teachers, social workers, all medical professionals. We can *all* inform others about the effects of alcohol in pregnancy. As Joanna Buckard, FASD trainer and consultant, says in the *No Alcohol, No Risk* video (NOFAS-UK/Mencap 2012): 'Women want to have healthy babies, and by understanding the risks of low level drinking it could make all the difference.'

I will end this chapter as we do after each training day, with a quote from the late Eleanor Roosevelt:

> Yesterday is history,
> Tomorrow is a mystery,
> Today is a gift ... That is why they call it the 'Present'.

I hope you take the knowledge of today as a gift to improve the lives of our children tomorrow.

I want to give our thanks and acknowledge the generous support we receive from Celia Atkin and Lord and Lady Mitchell. I would like to thank Diageo for making the Baby Bundle Training for Midwives possible with funding and for giving our medical advisors complete control of all the course content. We would also like to thank our medical advisors and midwives who verified all the course content. The materials for the training were reviewed by the Royal College of Midwives.

Notes

1. Fetal Alcohol Spectrum Disorders is an umbrella term covering Fetal Alcohol Syndrome (FAS), Partial Fetal Alcohol Syndrome (pPFAS), Fetal Alcohol Effects (FAE), Alcohol-Related Birth Defects (ARBD) and Alcohol-Related Neurodevelopmental Disorders (ARND).
2. NICE Guidelines, 2008:
    1.3.9.1 Pregnant women and women planning pregnancy should be advised to avoid drinking alcohol in the first 3 months of pregnancy if possible, because it may be associated with an increased risk of miscarriage.

1.3.9.2 If women choose to drink alcohol during pregnancy they should be advised to drink no more than 1 to 2 UK units once or twice a week ... Although there is uncertainty regarding a safe level of alcohol in pregnancy, at this low level there is no evidence of any to their unborn baby.

1.3.9.3 Women should be informed that getting drunk or binge drinking during pregnancy (six units of alcohol on a single occasion) may be harmful to the unborn baby.

3 www.redballoontraining.co.uk
4 See www.youtube.com/watch?v=tvwW5IEjOws

References

Bolling, K., Grant, C., Hamlyn, B. and Thornton, A. (2007) *Infant Feeding Survey 2005: A survey conducted on behalf of The Information Centre for health and social care and the UK Health Departments by BMRB Social Research*, London: The Information Centre/Leeds: NHS Information Centre.

Campbell, D. (2011) 'Smoking and drinking in pregnancy "harms 10,000 babies in UK each year"', *The Guardian*, 12 November, 24 [online at: www.guardian.co.uk/society/2011/nov/11/smoking-drinking-pregnancy-harms-babies#history-link-box; accessed: 13 October 2012].

Clarren, S. (2002) 'Keynote address' to the Prairie Northern Conference on Fetal Alcohol Syndrome, 'A Lifetime of Solutions', Whitehorse, Yukon, 8 May [online at: http://come-over.to/FAS/Whitehorse/WhitehorseArticleSC1.htm; accessed: 15 June 2013].

de Crespigny, C., Talmet, J., Modystack, K., Cusack, L. and Watkinson, J. (2003) *Alcohol, Tobacco and Other Drugs: Clinical guidelines for nurses and midwives*, Version 2, Adelaide: Flinders University and Drug and Alcohol Services Council, South Australia [online at: www.dassa.sa.gov.au/webdata/resources/files/ATOD_Clinical_Guidelines-book2.pdf; accessed: 14 October 2012].

Drug and Alcohol Services South Australia (2006) *Fetal Alcohol Spectrum Disorders: A guide for midwives*, Government of South Australia/Southern Adelaide Health Service [online at: www.dassa.sa.gov.au/webdata/resources/files/FASD_resource.pdf; accessed: 13 October 2012].

Gilinsky, A. (2009) *Alcohol-Related Health Promotion in Maternity Services: Factors associated with midwifery practice in NHS Tayside*, Dundee: NHS Tayside.

Griggs, I., Hodgson, M. and Owen, J. (2007) 'Birth in Britain: too few midwives, too many risks', *Independent on Sunday*, 4 March: 8–9.

Hepper, P. (1998) *Report on Prenatal Exposure to Alcohol: Final report*, Belfast: University of Belfast.

House of Commons Science and Technology Committee (2011) *Alcohol Guidelines*, London: House of Commons/Science and Technology Committee [online at: www.publications.parliament.uk/pa/cm201012/cmselect/cmsctech/1536/153602.htm; accessed: 14 June 2013].

Jones, S.C., Telenta, J., Shorten, A. and Johnson, K. (2011) 'Midwives and pregnant women talk about alcohol: what advice do we give and what do they receive?' *Midwifery*, 27(4): 489–96.

Jonsson, E., Dennett, L. and Littlejohn, G. (2009) *Fetal Alcohol Spectrum Disorder (FASD): Across the Lifespan: Proceedings from an IHE Consensus Development Conference 2009*, Edmonton, AB: Institute of Health Economics.

National Organisation for Fetal Alcohol Syndrome UK (NOFAS-UK) (2010) *Alcohol and Pregnancy: Information for midwives* (booklet), London: NOFAS-UK.

National Organisation for Fetal Alcohol Syndrome UK (NOFAS-UK)/Mencap (2012) *No Alcohol, No Risk: FASD information for midwives* (video), London: Mencap/NOFAS-UK.

NICE (National Institute for Health and Clinical Excellence) (2008) *Antenatal Care: Routine Care for the Healthy Pregnant Woman (Guideline 6)*, London: NICE [online at: www.nice.org.uk/nicemedia/pdf/CG062NICEguideline.pdf; accessed: 14 June 2013].

Riley, E.P., Guerri, C., Calhoun, F., Charness, M.E., Foroud, T.M., Li, T.-K., Mattson, S.N., May, P.A. and Warren, K.R. (2003) 'Prenatal alcohol exposure: advancing knowledge through international collaborations', *Alcoholism: Clinical and Experimental Research*, 27(1): 118–35.

Winstone, A.M. (2009) *Addenbrookes Hospital Fetal Alcohol Syndrome (FAS) Research Study and Pocket Guide Project* (MSc dissertation), Cambridge: Anglia Ruskin University [summary report online at: www.alcohollearningcentre.org.uk/LocalInitiatives/projects/projectDetail/?cid=6345; accessed: 13 October 2012].

16

FETAL ALCOHOL SPECTRUM DISORDERS AND CRIMINAL RESPONSIBILITY

Julian Killingley

In this chapter, I propose to consider some of the problems facing those who have fetal alcohol spectrum disorders (FASDs) when their conduct brings them into conflict with the law. Even this limited objective is too broad to be adequately covered here, so I shall begin by outlining likely problems that may arise during the investigative stage of criminal proceedings before moving on to a more detailed examination of ways in which diagnosis of the condition might be relevant to post-conviction proceedings.

The law and diminished responsibility

The law has long recognized that certain cognitive deficits and mental disturbances may affect the way society should treat those who have such conditions. In particular, the law has immunized those suffering from substantial intellectual disabilities against criminal responsibility for their actions. It has held them to be *doli incapax* in the same way that young children are also held incapable of forming the necessary criminal intent to commit crimes. This has been part of English common law since at least the eighteenth century[1] and the position regarding liability for criminal acts committed by the 'insane' was established in the mid-nineteenth century.[2]

This seemingly humane concern for the offender has not always found favour with juries and legislatures. British readers will recall that Peter Sutcliffe, the so-called 'Yorkshire Ripper', unsuccessfully asserted a defence of diminished responsibility under Section 2 of the Homicide Act 1957 and was convicted of several murders. However, after his initial incarceration in Parkhurst prison in 1981, he was later transferred to Broadmoor High Security Psychiatric Hospital where he has remained ever since – it was only politics that kept him out of hospital from the moment of his conviction. American readers will recall that John Hinckley Jr, who attempted to assassinate President Ronald Reagan in 1981, was found not guilty by reason of insanity and, like his contemporary Sutcliffe, has remained in secure psychiatric care since.

In Britain, the tabloid press has ensured that public interest in paranoid schizophrenic Peter Sutcliffe has never died down. In America, an immediate legislative backlash followed

Hinckley's acquittal. Public and congressional sentiment was so outraged that Congress passed the Insanity Defense Reform Act 1984 which made it significantly more difficult to successfully plead an insanity defence. Idaho, Montana and Utah abolished the insanity defence in its entirety, while other states substituted verdicts of 'guilty but mentally ill' for verdicts of 'not guilty by reason of insanity'.

Vulnerability and the justice system

As the term suggests, FASDs cover a range of disorders, and some may have a greater propensity to lead to criminal conduct than others. The American consulting group FASD Experts[3] has suggested that certain behaviours are commonly associated with FASDs; these include: being easily led by more sophisticated peers; frequent arrests for multiple low-grade offences committed with others during adolescence; committing offences that 'do not make sense'; commission of impulsive crimes; a tendency to 'fight or flight' behaviour in high-stress situations; and an over-reaction with aggressive 'fight' responses to perceived imminent threats. It is apparent from this that those affected by FASDs can be implicated in almost any kind of criminal behaviour from the relatively trivial to homicide.

Psychiatrist Dr Stephen Greenspan has noted that all humans can behave foolishly, but has characterized FASD sufferers (among others suffering intellectual disabilities) as behaving 'foolishly more frequently and in situations where danger signs are evident to most individuals, and their foolish actions are more likely to have serious life-altering consequences' (Greenspan 2008: 151). He defines 'foolish action' as 'behavior that has a high likelihood of backfiring, sometimes with disastrous consequences, because of a failure to attend to risks that are obvious to most people' (Greenspan 2008: 149). Stratton *et al.* (1996: 169) noted that 'those persons with FAS show impaired judgment, lability, poor impulse control, and deficits in social and adaptive functioning similar to the kinds of problems seen in patients who have frontal lobe injuries'.

In a study from British Columbia, Fast *et al.* (1999) determined the incidence of fetal alcohol syndrome (FAS) and fetal alcohol effects (FAE) in all juveniles remanded for a psychiatric/psychological assessment to a forensic psychiatric inpatient assessment unit. The subjects were evaluated for FAS/FAE and it was found that 23.3 per cent had an alcohol-related diagnosis with 1 per cent having a diagnosis of FAS and 22.3 per cent a diagnosis of FAE. They concluded this group was disproportionately represented in the juvenile justice system.

In England and Wales, all juveniles suspected of crimes must be interviewed in the presence of a person called the 'appropriate adult' (usually a parent or social worker) and are offered the benefit of free legal advice. This reduces the risk of juveniles acting in a way that is not in their best interests. However, the position is more problematic for adults. In their presentations given at the 2010 Capital Defense Conference at Airlie House, Warrenton, Virginia, Drs Richard Adler and Natalie Novick Brown suggested that those with FASDs were more likely to waive their rights on arrest, make guileless confessions (including false confessions), show no apparent guilt or remorse, and were unable to appreciate the seriousness of the offences they were suspected of committing.

If it becomes apparent to investigating police officers that a person has, or may have, a learning disability, then the Police and Criminal Evidence (PACE) Code C (Home Office 2008: 1.4, 1.7) requires that an 'appropriate adult' must be appointed to look after the interests of the suspect whether or not he has a legal representative. This was the case in the high profile murder case of Fred West where, from an abundance of caution, the police appointed Janet Leach as West's appropriate adult lest he should subsequently have been declared to be a vulnerable person. If the investigating police officers know that an adult suspect has an FASD then they would be obliged to appoint an appropriate adult. The problem is that many people with FASDs are undiagnosed with the condition and may exhibit few outward signs that they are 'vulnerable' adults. Although many with FASDs may also have learning disabilities that satisfy the DSM-V (American Psychiatric Association 2013) diagnostic criteria, some do not and may be processed through police interviews without the benefit of the protections to be afforded vulnerable adults.

The consequences for suspects with FASDs may be profound. They may decline the services of the Duty Solicitor – the police do not press suspects who decline the offer to think again. They may confess, whether truthfully or falsely, to committing a crime but later, after taking advice, seek to retract their confessions. Greenspan (2008: 156) explains how individuals with mild intellectual disabilities are especially susceptible to social influence because of their social neediness and because of the tendency of individuals with more severe learning disabilities to use others as models. Such individuals are said to have an 'external' orientation, in which they look to others for clues as to how to avoid looking foolish. This can lead to their being encouraged by police questioning to confess in circumstances where they would be best advised to say nothing. Such apparently voluntary confessions are prized by the police and attempts to retract them, often after taking legal advice at a later stage, are frequently not believed by juries (Baldwin and McConville 1980).

Brown *et al.* (2011) report a study that suggests that persons with FASDs may be highly suggestible in interrogative situations, which appears to stem from a combination of neurologically based tendencies to acquiesce to leading questions and change their responses to questions as a function of negative feedback. Again, their apparent lack of affect can help confirm investigating officers' suspicions of their guilt and, if shown in court on video-recorded interviews, may not play well with judge and jury. Above all, their lack of awareness of the seriousness of their situation may lead to displays of bravado or insouciance that are detrimental to their interests.

Obtaining a forensic diagnosis

While these problems are foreseeable, there are no easy solutions to them. Although the law provides protections, these are dependent upon the condition being known or the individual behaving in such a manner as to lead the investigating officers to believe he has a learning disability. In practice it is likely that many individuals with FASDs may be interviewed without the required protections being in place and may go on to be prosecuted, convicted and sentenced without anybody in the criminal justice system being any the wiser. In minor cases this may lead to little or no hardship, but in more serious cases it may mean serious injustice being done. This may only, if ever, come to light if it becomes apparent that a miscarriage of justice has occurred and a referral to the Court of Appeal is sought by the Criminal Cases Review Commission.

It should be noted that awareness of FASDs and use of the term in mitigation in criminal proceedings is far better established in the United States (US) than it is in England and Wales. A search of the Westlaw database revealed mentions of FAS or FASDs in more than 100 reported federal criminal decisions, and numerous mentions in state decisions. In contrast, in England and Wales there were a mere two reported decisions where FAS was mentioned – and neither of these was a criminal case. Mentions of FAS or FASDs occur widely in American state-reported decisions dealing with children and social services and, from this, we can expect that many probation or social inquiry reports in American criminal proceedings will routinely report these earlier diagnoses and use may be made of them by defence attorneys. The National Organization on Fetal Alcohol Syndrome in the US seeks, in appropriate cases, to intervene in appeals to provide information on the syndrome's effects.[4]

A small number of American psychiatrists and psychologists have made it their business to give presentations at legal conferences with a view to widening awareness of the condition and its effects.[5] The cost of evaluating a defendant with a view to producing a diagnosis of FASD to forensic standards is considerable. The consulting group of FASD Experts provides guidelines as to likely fees,[6] which are typically around $25,000 plus expenses and with additional fees if neuro-imaging is required. Establishing FASDs requires a complex interdisciplinary medical diagnosis, and there is no reason to believe it would be any less costly to establish such a diagnosis to forensic standards in Britain. The American public criminal defence system is run on a shoestring budget compared with its British counterpart, and the cost of such an evaluation is beyond reach in all but the most serious cases. In practice, defence-requested FASD diagnoses in criminal cases are most frequently encountered in capital cases.

In the US, the judiciary has far less discretion in sentencing than it does in Britain because of complex federal and state statutory sentencing guidelines. In capital trials the only discretion lies with the jury which, if it convicts of a capital offence, has to consider in penalty phase proceedings whether to sentence the defendant to death or life imprisonment. In many cases where the defendant's guilt is something of a foregone conclusion, the defence will devote its greatest efforts to persuading the jury to impose a life sentence. American capital penalty jurisprudence has developed in a way that has created certain constitutionally mandated categorical exemptions from the death penalty, including exemptions for those who become insane post-conviction[7] and for those suffering from learning disabilities[8] as described in DSM-V or similar standards.

Individuals with FASDs who are able to convince the jury that they also satisfy the DSM-V standards for intellectual disability or equivalent may not be sentenced to death. However, not all of those with FASDs also suffer from learning disabilities, and in their cases their claims of FASDs form part of a general mitigating narrative where the jury is called upon to assess whether the aggravating features of their conduct are outweighed by the mitigating features. Sandys *et al.* (2008) and others have argued that unfortunately all too often what should be seen as a mitigating circumstance is viewed by the jury as an aggravating circumstance and an informal indicator of future dangerousness. Accordingly, a number of American lawyers with an interest in the welfare of those with cognitive disabilities are currently seeking appropriate vehicles to bring before the appellate courts the question of whether those with FASDs who commit capital crimes should also be entitled to the benefit of a categorical exemption from capital punishment.

The impact of a diagnosis of FASD on justice outcomes

What part might a claim of FASD play in proceedings before a British court? In most cases it is unlikely that the condition alone could allow the sufferer to claim a general defence to a crime, like *M'Naghton* insanity, or even a limited defence such as that of diminished responsibility.[9] Its role is likely to be confined to mitigating circumstances pleaded with a view to persuading a judge to exercise her discretion to reduce a sentence. In both Britain and the US the defence has great latitude in what it can say in mitigation on behalf of a defendant. Generally, mitigating speeches are just that – they are not usually supported by evidence subjected to cross-examination, but are often just a series of unproven factual assertions. Defence counsel may refer to independent assertions of fact and opinion made by probation officers or occasionally call character witnesses, but for the most part in less serious cases pleas in mitigation are formulaic.

Anyone familiar with the workings of our criminal courts recognizes a regular pattern of social background in many offenders. Wilson and Killingley (2004) described the social backgrounds of a cohort of 12 substance-abusing recidivists aged under 25 undergoing training. Three of these former offenders presented as having suffered the death of one of their parents. Three had been physically or sexually abused by one, or both, of their parents. Five came from backgrounds where parents or elder siblings were drug abusers. Five had been raised in children's homes, foster care or residential schools. Ten had been abandoned or disowned by one, or both, of their parents. Three had been categorized as 'special needs pupils' at their secondary schools; five had failed to complete their secondary education either through an exclusion order, persistent truanting, or simple withdrawal. All were poly-substance abusers and had served at least one prison sentence. While it is not difficult to see how an advocate can fashion such histories of deprived backgrounds into mitigating narratives for offenders, such circumstances are so common that judges and magistrates have heard it all before and many believe that, just as such narratives are routinely deployed in speeches in mitigation, they are just as routinely ignored or discounted by case-hardened courts.

Clearly it is open to advocates who are aware of a prior-diagnosis of FASDs to use that information in mitigation. However, awareness of FASDs is low in the legal profession in Britain and, unless brought to the advocate's attention, is unlikely to be something for which the defence will actively seek a forensic evaluation. Where an evaluation would be speculative, this could not be justified in all but the most serious cases because of attendant costs.

Without further research it is difficult to say to what extent Ministry of Justice evaluations test for FASDs. Every person convicted of murder is subject to a mandatory sentence of life imprisonment. While on remand awaiting trial or sentence, every such offender is subjected to psychiatric and psychological evaluations conducted on behalf of the state, in addition to any evaluations made on behalf of the defence. While there are a number of references to FAS and FASDs in American and Canadian reported cases, there are none reported from Britain. It is unlikely that the prevalence of FASDs is any lower in Britain than it is in the US and Canada and so the absence of references to FAS or FASDs suggest that its presence may not be routinely evaluated.

I suggest that such an evaluation would be helpful in Britain for sentencing in two circumstances: minimum term fixing under Section 225 of the Criminal Justice Act 2003 as amended in connection with mandatory sentences of life imprisonment and, in respect of lesser offences, for discretionary indeterminate sentences passed for public protection. In these cases the court is required to fix a minimum term of imprisonment which must be served before the prisoner is eligible for parole or release. The minimum term is meant to represent the element of punishment to be inflicted for the offence committed and is imposed to meet the needs of retribution and deterrence. Any subsequent period of detention is based upon an evaluation of the continuing risk the offender may pose to the public. There are guidelines to assist judges when fixing minimum terms but, compared with their American counterparts, they have considerable latitude in sentencing. Courts may depart from the guidelines subject to explaining their reasons for doing so.[10] The current guidelines are set out in Schedule 21 of the Criminal Justice Act 2003 which lists aggravating factors and some mitigating factors. Paragraph 11 of Schedule 21 includes among mitigating factors, 'offender suffering from mental disorder or disability'. Although some might quibble as to whether FASDs are a 'mental disorder or disability', it matters not because the Paragraph 11 factors are illustrative and not exhaustive as mitigating factors.

In an adversarial system of justice like the Anglo–American one, the prosecution has little interest in minimizing the culpability of defendants. It is the role of the defence to put the best possible construction on the defendant's actions and to seek out appropriate mitigating evidence. Special factors in the US, which are not present in the United Kingdom, have resulted in greatly heightened defence community awareness of FASDs. In its 1984 decision in *Strickland v Washington*, 466 U.S. 668, the US Supreme Court interpreted the requirement of the Sixth Amendment to the US Constitution that '[i]n all criminal prosecutions, the accused shall enjoy the right… to have the Assistance of Counsel for his defence' in such a way that the 'assistance' provided had to be 'effective'. The Court laid down a two-part test for establishing 'ineffective assistance of counsel' (IAC) claims – the defendant had to show first that his counsel's performance in proceedings fell short of an objective standard of reasonableness and, second, that had counsel performed adequately the result of the proceedings would have led to a different outcome.

One result of *Strickland* is that IAC claims have burgeoned in capital appeals and that national Bar guidelines (ABA 2003) for good practice have been promulgated which place a heavy emphasis on adequate preparation for mitigation. Guideline 10.1 states that counsel 'at every stage of the case have a continuing duty to investigate issues bearing upon penalty and to seek information that supports mitigation or rebuts the prosecution's case in aggravation' (ABA 2003: 1055). One aspect of that duty is that counsel should pay heed to the potential for categorical exemption from execution by seeking any evidence of the defendant's intellectual disability. The search for such evidence might reveal the presence of FASDs with or without attendant intellectual disabilities. As awareness of FASDs is spread through the defence community, failure to seek evidence of FASDs might be indicative of counsel's failure to meet objectively reasonable standards of practice.

The English approach bears similarities to that in *Strickland*. In *R. v. Clinton* (1993) 97 Cr.App.R. 320, the Court of Appeal held that the approach to be adopted in cases where it was alleged that solicitors and counsel inadequately prepared and presented the defence case was that the proper inquiry is not whether there has been a material irregularity, but rather whether the conviction was unsafe and unsatisfactory within the meaning of Section 2(1)(a) of the Criminal Appeal Act 1968. The degree of ineptitude displayed by a defendant's trial lawyers was less important than the effect of the ineptitude on the fairness of the trial. There is no equivalent to IAC claims in English practice and the circumstances in which a defendant can appeal his conviction or sentence based upon negligent preparation and presentation of the defence case are more limited than in America where IAC claims are routinely pursued in criminal appeals.

Conclusion

I suggest that the English legal profession deserves a greater awareness of FASDs and their potential for mitigating culpability in appropriate cases, particularly those involving indeterminate sentences. The defence advocate's principal task in mitigating such cases is to minimize the minimum term to be served. This presents us with a chicken and egg problem. The ability to gather and present evidence of the condition is reliant upon the development of multidisciplinary teams in Britain like those in the US. Without robust evidence prepared by such teams the existence of FASDs in a defendant cannot be demonstrated to forensic standards. However, such teams are unlikely to form unless there is a demand for their services created within the legal profession. Awareness is best raised through conferences, training, continuing professional education programmes and publications.

More research is needed to determine awareness of FASDs and their effects among the judiciary, the legal profession and the National Offender Management Service. Although FASDs are conditions that cannot be cured, the effects may be ameliorated if a diagnosis is made. Since rehabilitation is one of the aims of the criminal justice system, we owe it to those suffering from the effects of FASDs and serving custodial or community sentences to ensure that they receive the best help we can provide to help them manage their condition and reduce the circumstances in which they are likely to reoffend.

Notes

1 See Blackstone, W. (1769) *Commentaries on the Laws of England: volume IV* (p. 24).
2 See M'Naghton's Case, 8 Eng. Rep. 718 (1843).
3 See www.fasdexperts.com.
4 See e.g. motion for leave to file amicus curiae brief in Holmes v Louisiana, 130 S.Ct. 70 (2009).
5 For example, Drs Richard Adler and Natalie Novick Brown gave presentations at the 2010 Capital Defense Conference at Airlie House, Warrenton, VA, organized by the NAACP. They are part of a multidisciplinary team that work together and provide diagnostic services under the name FASD Experts – see www.fasdexperts.com.
6 See www.fasdexperts.com/Hours.shtml and the associated retainer agreements.
7 See Ford v Wainwright, 477 U.S. 399 (1986).
8 See Atkins v. Virginia, 536 U.S. 302 (2002). Note that the American medico-legal literature is replete with references to 'mental retardation' or 'intellectual and developmental disabilities' rather than our term 'learning difficulties'.
9 A plea of diminished responsibility under s.2 Homicide Act 1957 as amended by s. 52 Coroners and Justice Act 2009, if accepted, would reduce a charge of guilty of murder to guilty of manslaughter by reason of diminished responsibility.
10 See R v Jones 2006 2 Cr. App. R. (S) 19.

References

ABA (American Bar Association) (2003) 'Guidelines for the appointment and performance of defense counsel in death penalty cases', *Hofstra Law Review*, 31: 913.
American Psychiatric Association (2013) *Diagnostic and Statistical Manual of Mental Disorders*, 5th edition, (DSM-V), Washington, DC: American Psychiatric Press.
Baldwin, J. and McConville, M. (1980) *Confessions in Crown Court Trials*, London: The Stationery Office.
Brown, N.N., Gudjonsson, G. and Connor, P. (2011) 'Suggestibility and fetal alcohol spectrum disorders: I'll tell you anything you want to hear', *Journal of Psychiatry and the Law*, 39(1): 39–71.
Fast, D.K., Conry, J. and Loock, C. (1999) 'Identifying fetal alcohol syndrome among youth in the criminal justice system', *Journal of Developmental and Behavioral Pediatrics*, 20(5): 370–2.

Greenspan, S. (2008) 'Foolish action in adults with intellectual disabilities: the forgotten problem of risk unawareness', *International Review of Research in Mental Retardation*, 36: 147–94.

Home Office (2008) *Police and Criminal Evidence (PACE) Act 1984 Code C: Code of Practice for the Detention, Treatment and Questioning of Persons by Police Officers*, London: Home Office [online at: www.homeoffice.gov.uk/publications/police/operational-policing/pace-codes/pace-code-c; accessed: 13 January 2013].

Sandys, M., Trahan, A. and Pruss, H. (2008) 'Taking account of the "diminished responsibilities of the retarded": are capital jurors up to the task?', *DePaul Law Review*, 57: 679.

Stratton, K., Howe, C. and Battaglia, F. (eds) (1996) *Fetal Alcohol Syndrome: Diagnosis, epidemiology, prevention, and treatment,* Washington, DC: National Academy Press.

Wilson, D. and Killingley, J. (2004) *Voices of Desistance: An ethnographic study of the C-FAR training programme*, Birmingham: Centre for Applied Criminology, University of Central England, Birmingham [online at: www.professorwilson.com/filestore/CFarFinal2.pdf; accessed: 13 January 2013].

17
SOCIAL CARE AND FETAL ALCOHOL SPECTRUM DISORDERS IN THE UK

Alison McCormick

How effective is the UK Social Care system in meeting the needs of families with children who have been prenatally exposed to alcohol? In this chapter I will briefly review the legal framework and how local authorities are reported to have met their responsibilities in delivering their Social Care role for these families.

Substance misuse is a key feature in social work with children and families across the UK. The 2008 Northern Ireland Department of Health, Social Services and Public Safety report, *Responding to the Needs of Children Born to and Living with Parental Alcohol and Drug Misuse in Northern Ireland*, states that 70 per cent of the Looked After Children in Northern Ireland are living away from home as a direct result of parental substance abuse (see also www.fasaonline.org). Of the different forms of substance misuse, alcohol misuse is arguably the least understood area, especially in terms of its long-term effects on families.

Hidden Harm (ACMD 2003), published by the Home Office, was the first major UK attempt to look at the impact of drug and alcohol misuse on children. It has been estimated that while between 250,000 and 350,000 children in England and Wales lived in families where one or both parents had a serious drug problem (ACMD 2003), around 900,000 children are thought to be affected by alcohol misuse (Brisby *et al.*, in Forrester *et al.* 2006). The *Munro Review of Child Protection* (Munro 2010: 12) emphasizes the importance of Social Care professionals maintaining a focus on such children:

> The biennial reviews of SCRs [serious case reviews] report recurrent problems in practice, e.g. children being invisible to professionals because the focus is on the parents, inadequate assessment of the dangers of parental problems of substance misuse, domestic violence, and mental illness, and fixed judgments not being challenged and revised.

There appears to be a discrepancy in the level of Social Care response for children affected by family drug misuse compared with those living in families who misuse alcohol; those cases involving alcohol typically come to the attention of Social Services later and follow a different pathway through Social Care (Adamson and Templeton 2012). The facts that (1) misused drugs are often illegal and alcohol is legal, and (2) the recommendations for screening and assessment in *Models of Care for Alcohol Misusers* (Department of Health and National Treatment Agency for Substance Misuse 2006) do not extend to their children (Cleaver *et al.* 2011), perhaps account for this. However, Forrester and Harwin (2004: 126) found that:

> Children are far more likely to have already experienced harm at the point of allocation if their parents misused alcohol and, worryingly, the harm was often more serious in nature. By contrast, most children affected by parental drug misuse were identified at an early stage and strong and co-ordinated protective action was taken before harm had set in.

Research in the USA found that cases involving alcohol misuse were given more chances of rehabilitation, although they were less likely to succeed than any other type of case (Murphy *et al.* 1991). A retrospective review of the social work cases in the study exposed a worrying trend of leaving vulnerable children at home in an over-optimistic belief that the mother would overcome her difficulties. Placing the child out of home was more typical in situations of drugs misuse.

Children with fetal alcohol syndrome disorders (FASDs)

The United States Department of Health and Human Services report to Congress (Substance Abuse and Mental Health Services Administration 2002: 46) states that: 'Of all the substances of abuse, including heroin, cocaine and marijuana, alcohol produces by far the most serious neurobehavioral effects in the fetus'. Based on a widely accepted prevalence for FASDs of one in 100 live births (Sampson *et al.* 1997), it is estimated that over 7,000 babies with FASDs are born in the UK every year to families where the mother drinks during pregnancy. However, this figure is believed to be conservative (May 2009).

Many of these children need permanent substitute families. Alarmingly, findings from the Foetally Affected Children's Team (FACT) study of children placed by Parents for Children (a specialist FASD adoption, fostering and family support agency now merged with TACT[1]) (see Williams, Chapter 8, this publication) highlighted huge areas of unmet need and a lack of understanding of these children's functional deficits (Brocklesby *et al.* 2009). The project found that many children placed by Social Care had never had their needs comprehensively assessed in the context of their probable, hidden, prenatal alcohol damage. Local authorities appeared reluctant to fund assessments for these children, perhaps fearing, with some justification, that the identification of long-term support needs for the children could prove to be costly and complex. Families had not been given essential background information and so were struggling to access resources from education, health and social services systems. Prospective carers had been told they had to 'live with uncertainty' without any explanation of what this 'uncertainty' might mean or what services were in place to help. As the complexity of the child's problems emerged, they were often left struggling to cope alone. As Cousins and Wells (2005: 381) state: 'It is unfair to expect families to take on the challenges and responsibilities of caring for a child affected by FAS [fetal alcohol syndrome] without a clear idea of what this may involve.'

The lack of knowledge of FASDs among Social Care professionals was the most consistent feedback from parents involved in Dumont's (2011) research into strategies developed by parents to support their adopted children with FASDs. Parents felt unsupported by Social Care's lack of understanding of the complexities of FASDs, reporting that they had had to waste energy and time continuously fighting – for their children's diagnosis, for professionals' awareness and support, and for adequate resources to meet their children's needs. Most parents stated that they had to explain to professionals what FASDs were, and that they were not always believed. Some were told by a range of professionals that there was nothing wrong with their children, and that they were fantasizing. Others explained that their children's so-called 'bad behaviour' had been perceived as due to poor parenting rather than as organic brain damage. While involvement with professionals who had an understanding of FASDs led to better support for their children, most participants expressed anger and disappointment at the lack of provision and support for their children, as well as at the lack of awareness of how FASDs impacted on their children and their families.

Similar findings emerged from Turney *et al.*'s (2011) study, *Social Work Assessment of Children in Need – What Do We Know?*, and McCormick (2010) reported that, among 42 parents responding to her *Adoption Now* article, 91 per cent of adoptive parents felt professionals lacked awareness of their child's FASD disability and services required. This is a situation that needs urgently addressing.

The duties of the UK Social Care system and children with FASDs

Research among families of children with FASDs has uncovered apparent failure by Social Care to follow legislation, regulations and policy, including the Children Act 1989, The Adoption Act 2004 and The Adoption Support Services Regulations, and has found discrepancies between placing and receiving local authorities (Brocklesby *et al.* 2009).

Local authorities, via Social Care, have a duty to safeguard and promote the welfare of children under the Children Act 1989 and to recognize the needs of carers under the Carers (Recognition and Services) Act 1995. According to the Children Act 1989 (Section 17 (10)), a child is taken to be 'in need' if they require services to achieve or maintain a reasonable standard of health or development and would suffer significant impairment without them. Once a child is identified as 'in need', they have an initial meeting with a social worker, following which the child and family are assessed and offered services (e.g. from Social Services, Health, Education or voluntary organizations) to help them resolve any problems or difficulties they are experiencing.

Section 10 of the Children Act 2004[2] states that services should:

- enable families and carers to effectively support their children;
- intervene before a crisis necessitates statutory intervention;
- urgently resolve weak accountability and poor relationships between agencies;
- value, train and support all those working with children and young people so they can carry out their work competently and confidently.

For those children who need to be placed with adoptive families, Regulation 3 of *The Adoption Support Regulations 2005* outlines a comprehensive range of support services to be offered to meet the needs of adoption. Regulation 4 states that a local authority must carry out an assessment of their needs for adoption support services. Despite this, 90 per cent of 42 families who responded to McCormick's (2010) *Adoption Now* article reported that their children with FASDs had not been properly assessed or had been placed for adoption without a diagnosis or an appropriate support package.

The tragic abuse and death of Victoria Climbié (age eight years) at the hands of her relatives, and the subsequent Laming inquiry (Laming 2003), highlighted the failure of the services involved to communicate with each other and intervene to protect her. Developed in response to the inquiry findings, the Every Child Matters strategy (Department for Education and Skills 2004) was intended to fuel a radical reform of public services in England, and to address the inadequacies revealed in how different services dealt with children at risk or in need. In England, the strategy was quickly enshrined in the Children Act 2004, and was described as 'one of the most significant changes in local children's services in living memory' (Lownsbrough and O'Leary 2005: 11). It prompted the development of integrated, accessible, personalized, child-centred services. The government's aim was for every child from birth to age 19 years, whatever their background or their circumstances, to have the support they needed to make progress against five key outcomes: to be healthy; stay safe; enjoy and achieve; make a positive contribution; and achieve economic well-being.

Although *Every Child Matters* offered a sweeping vision about children and young people's entitlements, full accountability for the delivery of the services that enable children, young people and their parents/carers to achieve these entitlements is delegated to local public services (Munro 2010). Difficulties arise because of the different laws and policies across counties in the UK, and prevent uniform practice and entitlement to services.

The need for professional training

Unbelievably, there is currently no requirement for social workers studying for a social work degree to learn about substance misuse (Forrester and Harwin 2004), although the awareness of this need is growing. Galvani and Hughes (2010), in an exploration of social work students' knowledge and attitudes about substance use, found that 96 per cent of students thought that training on substance use was very or extremely relevant to their practice, but that 69 per cent had not received any. They concluded that alcohol and drug education needs to be included in social work training. (For training resources developed, see: Galvani and Forrester 2008 2010; Forrester *et al.* 2006; McCarthy and Galvani 2010.) The Office of the Children's Commissioner of England (Adamson and Templeton 2012) also noted the lack of, and necessity for, pre- and post-qualification training.

However, while there is plentiful information in the Social Care literature on illegal drugs and how they may compromise parenting, there is comparatively little about alcohol misuse in pregnancy, the prevention, assessment and awareness of FASDs, and the complex impact that FASDs may have on children and their carers. There is also little information regarding good social work practice specific to FASDs, whether this be policy interpretation, management strategies or ways to enhance practice, assessment or support of families.

The FACT project (Brocklesby *et al.* 2009) noted a lack of understanding of FASDs and all its complexities, implications and stages among professionals, and the families involved disclosed that social workers, midwives, health visitors and teachers did not have enough insight or training regarding the long-term consequences of alcohol misuse. Forrester and Harwin (2004) in their study of children exposed to parental substance misuse found that social workers were often isolated and ill prepared, and that 71 per cent of these families had no professional trained in substance misuse working with them. This resulted in the use of inadequate conceptual frameworks and a lack of understanding of how to help families.

The FACT study found that many social workers working with families of children with FASDs:

- undertook only superficial case histories;
- accepted information given by birth parents about maternal prenatal alcohol consumption at face value even when contradicted by other evidence on file (e.g. alcohol-induced antisocial behaviour and witness statements);
- wrongly attributed children's complex problems to other difficulties (e.g. attachment disorders, post-traumatic stress disorders or poor parental coping);
- had not identified developmental discrepancies (e.g. between a child's expressive and receptive language) and their likely impact.

Assessment and diagnosis

The significance of obtaining accurate information to maximize the child's outcomes in life for both diagnosis and prognosis is poorly understood (Brocklesby *et al.* 2009). Families of children with FASDs are often passed from professional to professional, accumulating diagnoses, none of which fully addresses the young person's complexity.

Good assessment has a critical role to play in early intervention strategies, contributing to the effective and timely targeting of interventions. As Turney *et al.* (2011: 4) write:

> The importance of timely assessment is reflected in the current concern with very early or 'earlier' intervention… The rationale for this approach – that it is better to intervene before difficulties become established and potentially more severe – is hard to challenge.

A good Social Care assessment can improve home stability for children by preventing delay and helping to ensure the provision of appropriate and adequate support (Wade *et al.* 2010). However, there are many ways that a child with an FASD can 'slip through the net' of commonly used assessment tools, and their support needs are often not picked up. For the Common Assessment Framework to have effective service provision outcomes for children with FASDs, those assessing will require an in-depth understanding of the FASD-associated 'hidden' developmental disabilities (Armistead and McCormick 2011); also many FASD issues and complexities cannot be identified through generic 'tick box' formats (Cleaver *et al.* 2004, 2007; Mitchell and Sloper 2008; Munro 2010). FASD professionals, parents and researchers agree that most local authorities are not in a position to accurately assess and identify the needs of a child with an FASD (Armistead and McCormick 2011; Dumont 2011; McCormick 2010; Turney *et al.* 2011). Turney *et al.* (2011: 14) caution:

> Barriers to quality in assessment… can operate at a number of levels… including whether or not the practitioner is competent, has the appropriate knowledge and confidence to carry out the required task and has the scope to do so within their individual caseload.

There are also concerns about the usefulness of existing assessment formats for recording the views of young people with FASDs (Mitchell and Sloper 2008). While these young people may appear to the uninitiated to be articulate, intelligent and able to converse appropriately, this often masks developmental and cognitive delays and a very uneven neurological profile (Brocklesby et al. 2009). Their language and comprehension difficulties impact on their social functioning and capacity for judgment (Brocklesby et al. 2009). An assessor unsensitized to FASDs may not be able to recognize or gather evidence pointing to the young person's lack of understanding, inability to differentiate between fact and fantasy, or the fragmented logic they use to interpret the world. With an unusually strong desire to please, many young people with FASDs hide their poor memory recall by confabulating – inventing very inaccurate stories according to what they think the assessor wants to hear. They have no understanding of the consequences of what they may be saying. For example, they may unwittingly trigger Child Protection alarm bells. Inexperienced professionals may find it difficult to comprehend FASD issues, and may even hold parents responsible for the child's difficulties (Armistead and McCormick 2011; Brocklesby et al. 2009; Dumont 2011; McCormick 2010; Turney et al. 2011).

The FASAware UK (www.fasaware.co.uk) survey of 38 parents (a 71 per cent response rate from 52 approached) revealed their perceptions and experiences of the Social Care system (Armistead and McCormick 2011):

- lack of appropriate understanding of FASDs and the associated, complex, invisible impact on families;
- unwillingness to seek information from parents, FASD charities or medical personnel;
- refusals to assess children;
- stressful and time-consuming assessment processes;
- serious inaccuracies in records and assessments leading to unhelpful recommendations;
- unwillingness to correct inaccuracies.

Inaccurate recording and assessments have serious implications. All the studies reported in this chapter found significant errors in children's files and no means of amending them. The *Every Child Matters* drive towards joined-up services has led to the indiscriminate sharing of confidential and sensitive information via joined-up databases. If this information is inaccurate, it can damage innocent people seeking help for their disabled child.

In the course of the FACT study (Brocklesby et al. 2009), researchers designed an assessment which took account of the issues and needs associated with FASDs. As part of this assessment, a specialist social worker with knowledge of the family and child undertook a comprehensive assessment backed up by validated psychometric screening tests appropriate to the child's age and development. Wherever possible, the child was assessed in a familiar and local environment either at home or at school. The services of an occupational therapist, a psychiatrist, a paediatrician, a speech and language therapist, an education consultant and an advocate were also engaged where appropriate. A summary report was then sent to the main carers, and also to the local authority or the court. The multidisciplinary assessment was linked to an annual review and FACT's ongoing support system involving specialists suitable for the child's needs. The FACT multidisciplinary assessment provided ample evidence of the need for specialist services for children and young people with FASDs, particularly special school placements, respite care and more information and support for carers.

Families' experiences of service provision

Increasingly, children fetally affected by alcohol are permanently placed out of their family or find themselves living with extended family members, including aging grandparents. This can be an issue. Children and young adults with FASDs have a spectrum of complex hidden needs and disabilities, and can be very challenging and exhausting to care for, sometimes resulting in parent/carer exhaustion and burnout. Brocklesby *et al.* (2009) found very high levels of carer stress and distress due to huge barriers in identifying and supporting fetally affected children, and to the extreme levels of supervision and care-giving skills they demand – emotionally, physically and mentally – 24 hours a day, 7 days a week, 52 weeks a year. In some situations, the demands of children with FASDs may make them vulnerable to further abuse and secondary disabilities.

The British Medical Association report on FASDs (2007: 32) unequivocally identifies the service implications: 'Treatment for FASD requires the implementation of tailored management programmes and specialized support in the provision of healthcare, education and social services.'

However, from Armistead and McCormick's (2011) survey of 38 UK parents/carers with parental responsibility[3] for 57 young people with a diagnosed FASD, it was clear that many parents found themselves battling for services. These parents reported: fraught and hostile relationships with agencies; failure by Social Care to provide support and respond to parents' requests for help; and unwillingness by Social Care to seek information from parents, FASD charities or medical personnel. The survey highlighted the following issues:

- Evidence of enormous disparity between government agencies' understanding of FASDs as 'disabilities' in relation to government definitions. Only three of 57 children met Social Care's disabled children's services threshold criteria, yet 51 out of 57 children had been awarded high rate Disability Living Allowance (DLA). Twenty received some form of support via Social Care, mainly via Direct Payments.
- None of the children had received respite care provided directly by Social Care post-adoption, even though some had previously received it when fostered.
- Only one family (two children out of 57), who did not live on the UK mainland, reported receiving Social Care support services suitable for their needs.

When Social Care support was provided, parents/carers reported that it was often inadequate; for example, insufficient Direct Payments for families to organize their own appropriate help. One family was offered 90 minutes respite funding a month – equating to approximately £15 – to be shared between their three children with FASDs (Armistead and McCormick 2011). The family declined the payment saying that this would not cover even one hour's care for one child and, rather than supporting the family, would hinder them due to the time taken to manage the Direct Payments. In the FACT study (Brocklesby *et al.* 2009), two families each with three children with FASDs reported that the only resolution offered by Social Care to the repeated challenging behaviour of one of their children, was to place them back into care without trying out any practical support or innovative thinking. While this may have alleviated the families' immediate stress, in the long term it would have compounded the relationship and attachment issues for their already complex adopted children.

Adopters were often expected to navigate their own way through disability and medical services to get their own and their child's needs met (McCormick 2010). Families reported that their child with an FASD fell between two categories: respite care was judged by Social Services to be inappropriate and was usually inaccessible via adoption support budgets; yet, because the children lacked a 'visible disability', they were rarely classified as disabled therefore adoptive families were unable to access the short-break care funded through *Aiming High* (Department for Children, Schools and Families 2007).

Both Armistead and McCormick (2011) and Brocklesby *et al.* (2009) reported cases where requests by parents/carers for respite care had been misinterpreted by local authorities and child and adolescent mental health services resulting in parents/carers being blamed and isolated. In some cases, professionals had questioned parents'/carers' commitment or ability to parent their children, and a few had culminated in Child Protection investigations. Four families from four different areas, each caring for three children with FASDs, described how they had been accused by social workers (who were unqualified in medicine or mental health) of fabricating their situation and of having unresolved mental health issues themselves (Armistead and McCormick 2011). The allegations made by Social Care professionals against one mother following 'unreasonable requests for help' resulted in extended court proceedings, a major psychiatric assessment, financial hardship and nearly cost her home and marriage. (This needless, traumatic process ended with her being judged as fit to adopt the three children with FASDs who had been placed with her family.)

An informal survey of responses from 42 adoptive families following the author's *Adoption Now* article (McCormick 2010; see also Figure 17.1) revealed that:

- 80 per cent of families responding had not been able to access respite care despite their requests, even when this had been in place previously for their child's foster carers.
- More than half the adoptive parents/carers had either had children removed or feared their removal.
- More than a third had had child protection allegations made against them, allegedly due to Social Care's misunderstanding of the nature of FASDs (i.e. children's concrete thinking, tendency to fantasize or to confabulate memories to please listeners, and their lack of understanding of consequences).
- Half of the carers confided they had had a relationship breakdown or partial breakdown within their own family which they attributed to the stresses of the placement and lack of support and understanding from agencies.

Finally, the studies found a lack of understanding within Social Care about the development of FASDs across the lifespan. This has led to failures by Social Care professionals to put in place, prior to children's adoption, appropriate long-term intervention and support plans which would prevent the later serious secondary disabilities associated with FASDs (Brocklesby *et al.* 2009). While very young children may present with near typical development at the point of adoption, as these children grow older their difficulties become increasingly acute and challenging. McCormick (2010) found that most adoptive carers responding to her article had not been offered any post-adoption support because their child had been classified as having 'no problems' early on. There has to be acknowledgement by Social Care that families of children with FASDs may need to access services post-adoption.

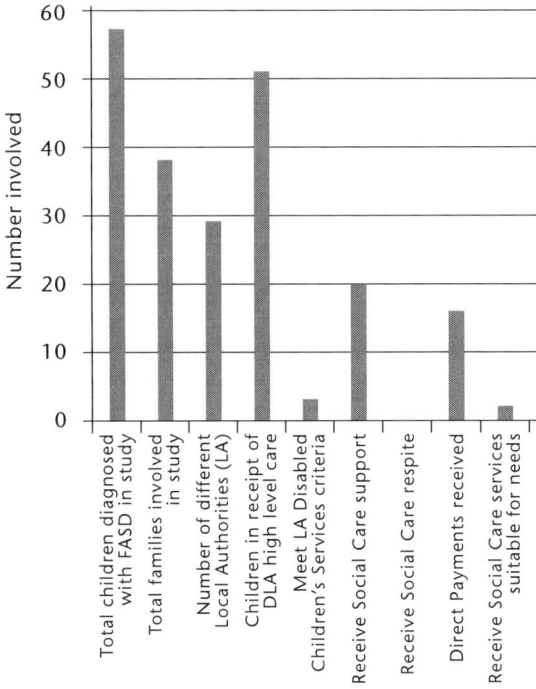

FIGURE 17.1 Perceptions and experiences of the 38 parents of 57 children with FASDs of the Social Care support they received.

Currently, once an adoption order is granted, funding or access to an appropriate assessment is near impossible (Brocklesby *et al.* 2009). Families of children with FASDs should not be abandoned with the sole, permanent responsibility for managing their children's acute problems for which most have been woefully ill prepared.

Summary and conclusion

Most people with FASDs feel like a 'square peg in a round hole', no service or facility fits their requirements, and they are grossly misunderstood. People with FASDs, due to their inherent invisible brain dysfunction and disability, place demands on each of their environments – family, school and the wider community. If their needs are not understood and met, their behaviours can become out of control, bizarre, desperate, unpredictable, impulsive and dysfunctional. Many find themselves in corrective institutions and/or with poor mental health (Streissguth *et al.* 1997).

The compelling evidence outlined in this chapter suggests that the UK's Social Care model is not robust enough to prevent an avalanche of innocent children being born every year with FASDs or to provide adequately educated professionals and appropriate support services for fetally affected individuals and their families. The families of all studied children reported Social Care's resistance to recognizing FASDs as disabilities according to the government's definition and the Children in Need criteria, and to providing appropriate services and support as laid down by *Every Child Matters*. This is contrary to both national guidance and accepted good practice. Many families have had to go to significant lengths and through great crisis to care for their complex disabled child with minimal support.

It is vital that Social Care practitioners, management and strategic decision makers address the systemic denial of FASDs and take action on alcohol misuse seriously, especially in pregnancy where there is a chance to alleviate the risks of having a child, or further children, with an FASD and the impact of possible secondary disabilities for the person, their agency and society. Social Care needs to take a positive lead on FASDs – obtaining fully evidenced facts and recording accurate data; sending out strong messages regarding alcohol misuse; maximizing training on FASDs; and developing effective and supportive policies (Munro 2010). It needs to improve outcomes for families by: raising awareness of how to prevent and detect FASDs; obtaining accurate multidisciplinary assessments; accessing funding for effective personalized support packages; and understanding the enormous lifelong impact this disability has on the person, their family, carers and society.

Alcohol consumption is a major problem for Social Care. Many cases tend to be 'top end' involving Care Proceedings or Child Protection. The costs are high, complex and involve a large amount of interagency liaison (often by professionals with insufficient FASD training and awareness) with very vulnerable and often disabled children (Forrester and Harwin 2004). In Yukon, Canada, the government found that children with FASDs from the care system are approximately four times more costly to care for, both financially and in care time, and are significantly more likely to require additional education, health and support than other adoptive children who do not have FASDs (Alton and Evenson 2006).

However, if the government does nothing to support families of children with FASDs, the costs are likely to spiral in adulthood. In an American study, Streissguth *et al.* (1997) found that children with FASDs were likely to be vulnerable to life events and to develop secondary disabilities in adulthood: out of a cohort of 415 individuals with FASDs, 90 per cent had needed long-term support in the transition to adulthood; 60 per cent were or had been confined in mental health and criminal justice situations; and 50 per cent exhibited some form of sexually inappropriate behaviour. Children with FASDs are therefore a group whom it is worth understanding and making an investment in at an early stage to reduce costs to society.

This is a large agenda, especially in a time of great cutbacks, but alcohol misuse in the UK is out of control. It is one of the most important challenges and areas of future expenditure facing Social Care's policymakers, budget holders and practitioners this century. Tackling the UK's drinking culture will need an engaged, sustained and appropriately complex response to change attitudes, knowledge and behaviour (Stead *et al.* 2009). Young women who binge drink play 'Russian Roulette' with their pregnancies, while children with preventable and lifelong disabilities are born in enormous numbers every year. Multi-targeted actions at policy and service level are needed to support people in making changes.

In the UK there is still no legal requirement to notify and centrally record if a child is diagnosed with FASDs (Adamson and Templeton 2012). This lack of central recording is failing our children by preventing them getting the support they rightly require and feeding systemic denial in services. Until this and our alcohol culture are addressed, children will continue to be born with a devastating and preventable disability. Ensuring a good childhood is hard enough (Layard and Dunn 2009), but for the increasing numbers of children born fetally affected in 'Binge Britain', Social Care needs to take action to optimize the long-term well-being of an ever-increasing number of innocent people and to provide services for a hidden section of society crying out for practical help with one of the most frustrating and complex conditions to manage.

Notes

1 www.tactcare.org.uk
2 www.legislation.gov.uk/ukpga/2004/31/section/10
3 That is, adoptive, birth and extended families only; no feedback was requested from carers of accommodated children.

Bibliography

Adamson, J. and Templeton, L. (2012) *Silent Voices: Supporting children and young people affected by parental alcohol abuse*, London: The Office of the Children's Commissioner.
AMCD (Advisory Council on the Misuse of Drugs) (2003) *Hidden Harm: Responding to the needs of children of problem drug users*, London: Home Office.
Alton, H. and Evenson, D. (2006) *Making a Difference: Working with students who have Fetal Alcohol Syndrome*, Whitehorse, Yukon: Yukon Education, Government of Yukon.
Armistead, G. and McCormick, A. (2011) 'FASAwareUK study of social care support' (unpublished).
British Medical Association (2007) *Fetal Alcohol Spectrum Disorders: A guide for healthcare professionals*, London: British Medical Association.
Brocklesby, E., Le Vaillant, J., McCormick, A., Mandelli, D. and Mather, M. (2009) 'Substance misuse in pregnancy: an unrecognised and misdiagnosed problem for a child', *Seen and Heard*, 19(1): 22–32.
Cleaver, H., Unell, I. and Aldgate, J. (2011) *Children's Needs – Parenting Capacity: Child Abuse: Parental mental illness, learning disability, substance misuse and domestic violence* (2nd edition), London: The Stationery Office.
Cleaver, H., Walker, S. and Meadows, P. (2004) *Assessing Children's Needs and Circumstances: The impact of the Assessment Framework*, London: Jessica Kingsley.
Cleaver, H., Nicholson, D., Tarr, S. and Cleaver, D. (2007) *Child Protection, Domestic Violence and Parental Substance Misuse: Family experiences and effective practice*, London: Jessica Kingsley.
Cousins, W. and Wells, K. (2005) '"One more for my baby": foetal alcohol syndrome and its implications for social workers', *Child Care in Practice*, 11(3): 375–83 [online at: http://ulster.academia.edu/WendyCousins/Papers/271217/One_More_for_My_Baby_Foetal_Alcohol_Syndrome_and_Its_Implications_for_Social_Workers; accessed: 6 October 2012].
Department for Children, Schools and Families (2007) *Aiming High for Disabled Children: better support for families*, London: HM Treasury.
Department for Education and Skills (2004) *Every Child Matters: change for children*, Annesley: DfES Publications.
Department of Health and National Treatment Agency for Substance Misuse (2006) *Models of Care for Alcohol Misusers (MoCAM)*, London: Department of Health.
Dumont, L. (2011) *Exploring Strategies Developed by Parents to Support their Adopted Children with Foetal Alcohol Spectrum Disorder*, London: Goldsmiths University.
FASA (2008–2012) 'Family matters' [online at: www.fasaonline.org/young-people/services/family-matters/; accessed: 1 October 2012].
Forrester, D. and Harwin, J. (2004) 'Social work and parental substance misuse', in R. Phillips (ed.) *Children Exposed to Parental Substance Misuse: Implications for family placement*, London: British Association for Adoption and Fostering.
Forrester, D., McCambridge, J., Rollnick, S., Strang, J. and Waissbein, C. (2006) *Child Risk and Parental Resistance: Can motivational interviewing improve the practice of child and family social workers in working with parental alcohol misuse?*, London: Alcohol Research UK.
Galvani, S. and Forrester, D. (2008) *What Works in Training Social Workers about Drug and Alcohol Use? A survey of student learning and readiness to practice*, Coventry: University of Warwick/University of Bedfordshire.

Galvani, S. and Forrester, D. (2010) *Social Work and Substance Use: Teaching the basics*, Southampton: Higher Education Academy, Subject Centre for Social Policy and Social Work (SWAP).

Galvani, S. and Hughes, N. (2010) 'Working with alcohol and drug use: exploring the knowledge and attitudes of social work students', *British Journal of Social Work*, 40(3): 946–62.

Laming, Lord (2003) *The Victoria Climbié Inquiry: Report of an Inquiry by Lord Laming*, Norwich: HMSO.

Layard, R. and Dunn, J. (2009) *A Good Childhood,* London: The Children's Society.

Lownsbrough, H. and O'Leary, D. (2005) *The Leadership Imperative: Reforming children's services from the ground up*, London: Demos.

May, P. (2009) 'Prevalence and incidence internationally', in E. Jonsson, L. Dennett and G. Littlejohn (eds) *Fetal Alcohol Spectrum Disorder (FASD): Across the lifespan (proceedings from an IHE Consensus Development Conference 2009)*, Edmonton, AB: Institute of Health Economics.

McCarthy, T. and Galvani, S. (2010) *Alcohol and Other Drugs: Essential information for social workers*, Luton: University of Bedford.

McCormick, A. (2010) 'Caring for children with foetal alcohol syndrome', *Adoption Now*, 3: 26–29.

Mitchell, W. and Sloper, P. (2008) 'The Integrated Children's System and disabled children', *Child and Family Social Work*, 13(3): 274–85.

Munro, E. (2010) *The Munro Review of Child Protection: Part 1 – A systems analysis*, Norwich: The Stationery Office.

Murphy, J.M., Jellinek, M., Quinn, D., Smith, G., Poitrast, F.G. and Goshko, M. (1991) 'Substance abuse and serious child mistreatment: prevalence, risk, and outcome in a court sample', *Child Abuse and Neglect*, 15(3): 197–211.

Sampson, P.D., Streissguth, A.P., Bookstein, F.L., Little, R.E., Clarren, S.K., Dehaene, P., Hanson, J.W. and Graham, J.M. Jr (1997) 'Incidence of fetal alcohol syndrome and prevalence of alcohol-related neurodevelopmental disorder', *Teratology*, 56(5): 317–26.

Stead, M., Gordon, R., Holme, I., Moodie, C., Hastings, G. and Angus, K. (2009) *Changing Attitudes, Knowledge and Behaviour: A review of successful initiatives*, London: Joseph Rowntree Foundation.

Stratton, K., Howe, C. and Battaglia, F. (1996) *Fetal Alcohol Syndrome: Diagnosis, epidemiology, prevention, and treatment*, Washington, DC: Institute of Medicine, National Academy Press.

Streissguth, A., Barr, H., Kogan, J. and Bookstein, F. (1997) 'Primary and secondary disabilities in fetal alcohol syndrome', in A. Streissguth and J. Katner (eds) *The Challenge of Fetal Alcohol Syndrome: Overcoming secondary disabilities,* Washington, DC: University of Washington Press.

Substance Abuse and Mental Health Services Administration (2002) *Report to Congress on the Prevention and Treatment of Co-occurring Substance Abuse Disorders and Mental Disorders.* Washington, DC: United States Department of Health and Human Services.

Turney, D., Platt, D., Selwyn, J. and Farmer, E. (2011) *Social Work Assessment of Children in Need – What Do We Know?: Messages from research,* Bristol: School for Policy Studies, University of Bristol.

Wade, J., Biehal, N., Farrelly, N. and Sinclair, I. (2010) *Outcomes for Children Looked After for Reasons of Abuse or Neglect: The consequences of staying in care or returning home*, report to Department for Education, York: University of York.

18

THE EFFECTS OF PRENATAL ALCOHOL EXPOSURE ON BRAIN AND BEHAVIOUR

Tanya T. Nguyen and Edward P. Riley

Introduction

Alcohol is a potent teratogen, impacting the developing fetus and leading to both physical and behavioural deficits. Prenatal exposure to alcohol can adversely impact fetal development, resulting in growth retardation, physical anomalies, facial dysmorphology, and central nervous system (CNS) dysfunction, including brain damage and cognitive impairment. Of these potential consequences, alterations to the developing brain and resulting neurobehavioural impairments are the most devastating. Since the earliest reports on fetal alcohol syndrome (FAS) in the 1970s (Jones and Smith 1973; Jones *et al.* 1973), research has consistently documented damage to brain structure and function among individuals with FAS. Early autopsy reports of infants with FAS revealed widespread and severe brain damage (Clarren 1986; Coulter *et al.* 1993; Jones and Smith 1973, 1975). Nevertheless, the abnormalities reported in autopsy cases tend to be of greater severity and may not be representative of most individuals exposed to alcohol *in utero*. Prenatal alcohol exposure is now understood to produce a continuum of effects and result in a spectrum of disorders referred to as fetal alcohol spectrum disorders (FASDs). Individuals along this spectrum display varying degrees of anomalies, including neurological alterations and neurobehavioural deficits. Through the use of sophisticated brain imaging techniques such as magnetic resonance imaging (MRI), functional magnetic resonance imaging (fMRI), magnetic resonance spectroscopy (MRS) and diffusion tensor imaging (DTI), researchers have gained tremendous insight into CNS abnormalities in FASDs. These techniques have enabled researchers to analyse the size and volume of the overall brain and specific brain regions, examine the integrity of white matter tracts, detect changes in metabolite levels and biochemical brain processes, and investigate relationships between brain function and behaviour. This chapter summarizes some of the most salient neuroimaging and neuropsychological research findings related to FASDs and discusses the neurobehavioural correlates of structural as well as functional brain abnormalities in individuals with FASDs.

Structural brain abnormalities in FASDs

Global brain

Microcephaly, or abnormally small brain size, is one of the most consistent findings in brain imaging studies of individuals with FASDs. Early post-mortem studies revealed that severely affected children with heavy prenatal alcohol exposure had smaller head and brain sizes (Clarren and Smith 1978; Jones and Smith 1973; Jones et al. 1973; Wisniewski et al. 1983). More recent MRI studies have supported these findings, reporting simultaneous volumetric reductions of the cranial vault along with reduced total brain volume (Archibald et al. 2001; Astley et al. 2009; Coles et al. 2011; Johnson et al. 1996; Lebel et al. 2008; Nardelli et al. 2011; Roussotte et al. 2012; Sowell et al. 2001a; Swayze et al. 1997), cerebral volume (Archibald et al. 2001; Mattson and Riley 1996; Mattson et al. 1992), and cerebellar volume (Archibald et al. 2001; Astley et al. 2009; Mattson and Riley 1996; Mattson et al. 1992; O'Hare et al. 2005; Riikonen et al. 1999; Sowell et al. 1996). Among these studies, children with a diagnosis of FAS tended to have greater impairments than those exposed prenatally to alcohol but who lacked sufficient alcohol-related facial features for an FAS diagnosis (Archibald et al. 2001; Mattson and Riley 1996; Mattson et al. 1992).

Cerebral cortex

Prenatal alcohol exposure does not uniformly affect brain development. While certain brain regions and tissue are particularly vulnerable to alcohol teratogenesis, others are relatively spared. Furthermore, nondysmorphic individuals appear less affected than those with a full diagnosis of FAS. Within the cerebral cortex, the parietal lobe – a region typically associated with visual–spatial functioning, attention and mathematics processing – is among the most susceptible to developmental alcohol exposure. After controlling for total brain volume, the parietal lobe is disproportionately reduced (Archibald et al. 2001), and prominent differences are seen in grey and white matter densities (Archibald et al. 2001; Sowell et al. 2001b, 2002a), specifically increases in grey matter and decreases in white matter (Sowell et al. 2001b, 2002a). Moreover, individuals with FASDs demonstrate increased cortical thickness (Figure 18.1) in the parietal lobe (Sowell et al. 2008b; Yang et al. 2012). These differences may be the result of excessive grey matter due to a lack of normal synaptic pruning of neurons or decreased myelination of axons that subsequently appear as grey matter on an MRI (Sowell et al. 2002a). Additionally, the temporal lobe – a region integral for learning and memory as well as language comprehension – also shows structural abnormalities. Similar to the parietal lobe, the temporal lobe shows increased grey matter and decreased white matter (Sowell et al. 2002b), as well as increased cortical thickness (Sowell et al. 2008b; Yang et al. 2012) in alcohol-exposed individuals. Finally, research has also reported changes in the frontal lobes – a region of the brain important for higher-order cognitive processes such as executive function. These changes include reduced total lobe volume (Astley et al. 2009; Sowell et al. 2002a), decreased grey and white matter volumes (Astley et al. 2009), and increased cortical thickness (Sowell et al. 2008b; Yang et al. 2012). Notably, abnormal cerebral development is closely associated with degree of facial dysmorphology, as frontal lobe volumes progressively vary with severity of FASD diagnostic group (Astley et al. 2009) and inferior frontal cortical thickness is correlated with palpebral fissure length (Yang et al. 2012).

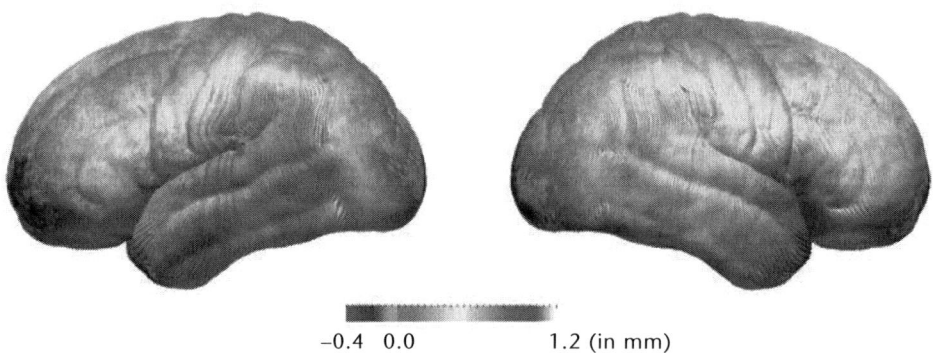

FIGURE 18.1 Maps of the mean difference in cortical thickness in the brains of subjects with FASDs compared to control subjects. Increases in cortical thickness of up to 1.2 mm were observed in subjects with FASDs in most regions of the lateral brain surface, including frontal, temporal, occipital and parietal cortices (Reprinted with permission from Sowell et al. 2008b).

Corpus callosum

The corpus callosum, a large bundle of white matter fibres connecting the left and right cerebral hemispheres, is the most examined brain structure in FASDs. Reports of callosal abnormalities in FASDs include complete absence (Astley et al. 2009; Johnson et al. 1996; Mattson et al. 1992; Riley et al. 1995; Swayze et al. 1997) and partial absence (Autti-Ramo et al. 2002; Johnson et al. 1996) as well as underdevelopment of the corpus callosum (Autti-Ramo et al. 2002; Mattson et al. 1992; Swayze et al. 1997). Significant reduction in volume (Riley et al. 1995) and displacement of the corpus callosum (Sowell et al. 2001a) have also been reported in alcohol-exposed individuals. Although abnormalities have been observed across the entire length of the corpus callosum, the posterior region appears to be most affected, both in terms of frequency and severity of abnormalities (Autti-Ramo et al. 2002; Riley et al. 1995; Sowell et al. 2001a). The corpus callosum also shows greater shape variability in alcohol-exposed children than typically developing children (Bookstein et al. 2001; Bookstein et al. 2002b), and variability in callosal shape has been used to distinguish children with heavy prenatal alcohol exposure from typically developing controls with some sensitivity and specificity (Bookstein et al. 2002a).

White matter microstructure

While structural MRI techniques have focused on macrostructural abnormalities of white matter, newer DTI technology, which assesses the integrity of white matter tracts, has revealed that prenatal alcohol exposure is also associated with significant microstructural abnormalities. DTI provides a measure of the magnitude and directionality of water diffusion in tissue. Unrestricted water diffusion in all directions is referred to as isotropic diffusion and indicated by mean diffusivity (MD); directional diffusion of water is referred to as anisotropic and measured by fractional anisotropy (FA). Highly ordered tissue, such as myelinated axon fibre bundles, is typically characterized by unrestricted diffusion in the principal direction of the axon and little diffusion in the perpendicular plane (i.e. high FA and low MD). Abnormal brain development can contribute to lower FA and higher MD values in white matter (Neil *et al.* 2002), and such effects are observed in prenatal alcohol exposure. Microstructural abnormalities are evident and range across the entire FASD continuum, even in individuals who do not meet full criteria for FAS (Li *et al.* 2009). Abnormalities of white matter integrity are seen within the corpus callosum of individuals with FASDs (Figure 18.2), most notably in the posterior regions, the isthmus and splenium (Lebel *et al.* 2008; Li *et al.* 2009; Ma *et al.* 2005; Sowell *et al.* 2008a; Wozniak *et al.* 2006, 2009). Studies have revealed higher MD and lower FA values (i.e. less white matter integrity) in the isthmus and splenium, the most posterior regions of the corpus callosum. Lower FA values in the splenium are also associated with poorer visual–motor integration in children with FASDs (Sowell *et al.* 2008a). Moreover, callosal fibres within the splenium, which project to cortical areas, display inter-hemispheric functional connectivity disturbances (Wozniak *et al.* 2011). On the other hand, results for the anterior regions of the corpus callosum are mixed. While one study found individuals with FAS to have lower FA and higher MD in the most anterior end of the corpus callosum (Ma *et al.* 2005), another examining individuals with FASDs revealed lower MD in this region, a finding that instead suggests a higher degree of fibre coherence and organization (Lebel *et al.* 2008). Microstructural abnormalities in white matter are also apparent in brain regions beyond the corpus callosum, including the temporal, frontal and occipital lobes, anterior-posterior fibre bundles, corticospinal tracts, cerebellum, thalamus and basal ganglia (Fryer *et al.* 2009; Lebel *et al.* 2010, 2008; Sowell *et al.* 2008a).

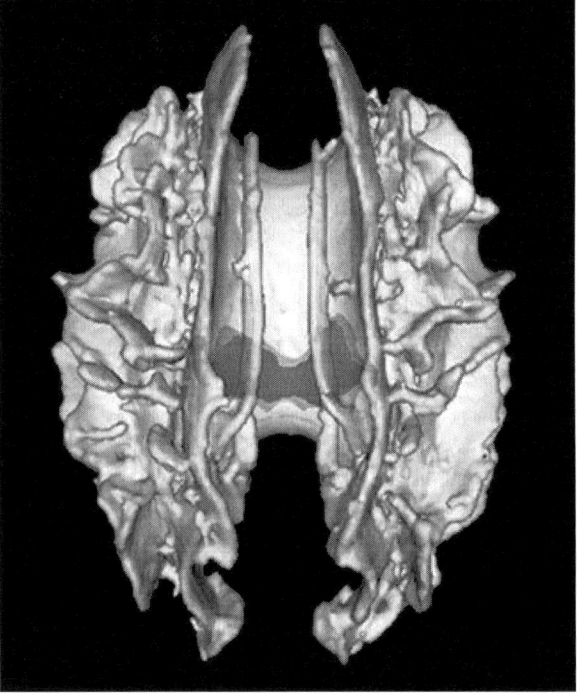

FIGURE 18.2 The isthmus of the corpus callosum in alcohol-exposed individuals with dysmorphic features showed significantly lower FA values than these of the control individuals (Reprinted with permission from Li *et al.* 2009).

Cerebellum

Another structure particularly sensitive to prenatal alcohol exposure is the cerebellum, a region of the brain best known for its involvement in motor coordination. Alcohol-exposed individuals show reductions in cerebellar volume and surface area (Archibald et al. 2001; Autti-Ramo et al. 2002; Mattson et al. 1994; Mattson and Riley 1996; Mattson et al. 1992). However, like the cerebral cortex, not all regions of the cerebellum are equally susceptible to alcohol-related damage. Specifically, the anterior cerebellar vermis, a narrow region connecting the two cerebellar hemispheres, is significantly reduced in area and displaced as a result of prenatal alcohol exposure (O'Hare et al. 2005; Sowell et al. 1996). Of note, displacement of the anterior cerebellar vermis is observed even in the absence of facial features required for a diagnosis of FAS, albeit to a lesser magnitude (O'Hare et al. 2005). The degree of vermal displacement is also negatively associated with verbal learning and memory performance, emphasizing the cerebellum's additional involvement in some cognitive processes (O'Hare et al. 2005).

Subcortical structure

Deep grey matter structures that lie beneath the cerebral cortex such as the basal ganglia and hippocampus also demonstrate substantial consequences of prenatal alcohol exposure. These structures, along with their projections to and from the prefrontal cortex of the frontal lobes, are important for complex cognitive processes such as learning and memory, executive function and attention. The basal ganglia are disproportionately smaller in children with FAS than typically developing children, even after controlling for overall brain volume (Archibald et al. 2001; Astley et al. 2009; Mattson et al. 1996c; Nardelli et al. 2011). Furthermore, when the basal ganglia are subdivided into components, the caudate nucleus, putamen, globus pallidus and lenticular nuclei are significantly reduced in alcohol-exposed individuals (Archibald et al. 2001; Astley et al. 2009; Mattson et al. 1996c; Nardelli et al. 2011; Riikonen et al. 2005; Roussotte et al. 2012). Once overall brain volume is taken into account, the caudate nucleus, putamen and globus pallidus remain significantly reduced in alcohol-exposed subjects (Archibald et al. 2001; Mattson et al. 1996c; Roussotte et al. 2012). Additionally, the hippocampus, a structure located inside the medial temporal lobe and important for consolidation of memory, demonstrates consequences of prenatal alcohol exposure. Smaller hippocampal volume has been observed after accounting for total brain volume in some studies (Autti-Ramo et al. 2002; Nardelli et al. 2011; Willoughby et al. 2008), and only before total brain correction in others (Archibald et al. 2001; Astley et al. 2009; Coles et al. 2011; Riikonen et al. 2005; Roussotte et al. 2012).

Human MRI studies on other deep grey matter structures in FASDs are mixed. Subcortical structures such as the diencephalon, thalamus and amygdala are either significantly smaller or unchanged beyond total alcohol-induced brain reduction, depending on the study (Archibald et al. 2001; Astley et al. 2009; Autti-Ramo et al. 2002; Nardelli et al. 2011; Riikonen et al. 2005; Roussotte et al. 2012). The nucleus accumbens, a brain region considered to mediate fear and reward, has only been measured in a single study and was not significantly affected by prenatal alcohol exposure (Archibald et al. 2001).

Neuropsychological and behavioural effects of FASDs

Exposure of the developing brain to alcohol during gestation results in a wide range of neurobehavioural effects. Children exposed prenatally to alcohol have an increased risk of cognitive impairment in various neuropsychological domains, including general intelligence, executive function, learning and memory, visuospatial abilities, language, motor function and attention.

General intelligence

One of the most common and robust neurocognitive findings among individuals exposed to alcohol during pregnancy is diminished intellectual function. FAS is considered one of the leading causes of intellectual disability (i.e. defined as overall IQ score <70 and adaptive disability) (Abel and Sokol 1987; Pulsifer 1996). However, it is important to note that the majority of individuals with FAS are not intellectually disabled, and intellectual disability is not required for a diagnosis of FAS. Impaired intellectual development is observed in alcohol-exposed individuals even in the absence of facial or growth features, though individuals without dysmorphological traits tend to be less affected (Chasnoff *et al.* 2010; Dalen *et al.* 2009; Mattson *et al.* 1997). That is, intelligence is inversely related to degree of physical dysmorphology (Ervalahti *et al.* 2007). The average IQ of individuals with prenatal alcohol exposure has been reported as in the low 70s for those with FAS (Mattson *et al.* 1997; Streissguth *et al.* 1991) and in the low 80s for those without alcohol-related facial features (Mattson *et al.* 1997).

Executive function

Executive functions encompass a variety of abilities such as planning, response inhibition, abstract reasoning, cognitive flexibility and working memory. These abilities rely on neural circuits connecting the frontal lobe and subcortical structures (Cummings 1993), regions susceptible to developmental alcohol exposure. Children with prenatal alcohol exposure show clinical impairment on a parent rating scale of executive function (i.e. the Behavior Rating Inventory of Executive Functioning, BRIEF) (McGee *et al.* 2008a; Rasmussen *et al.* 2006, 2007; Schonfeld *et al.* 2006). In addition, neuropsychological studies of individuals with FASDs demonstrate deficits in problem-solving, planning, response inhibition, concept formation and conceptual set-shifting, verbal and nonverbal fluency, and working memory.

Problem-solving and planning

Many studies have found that alcohol-exposed children have deficient problem-solving and planning skills (Figure 18.3). These children show impairment on a commonly used spatial planning task that requires subjects to mentally plan and execute a sequence of moves to reach a solution (e.g. Tower of Hanoi/London). Compared to typically developing subjects, children with FASDs make greater rule violations, perseverate longer on incorrect strategies, pass fewer items and spend less time on each item formulating a strategy (Aragon *et al.* 2008b; Green *et al.* 2009b; Kodituwakku *et al.* 1995; Mattson *et al.* 1999).

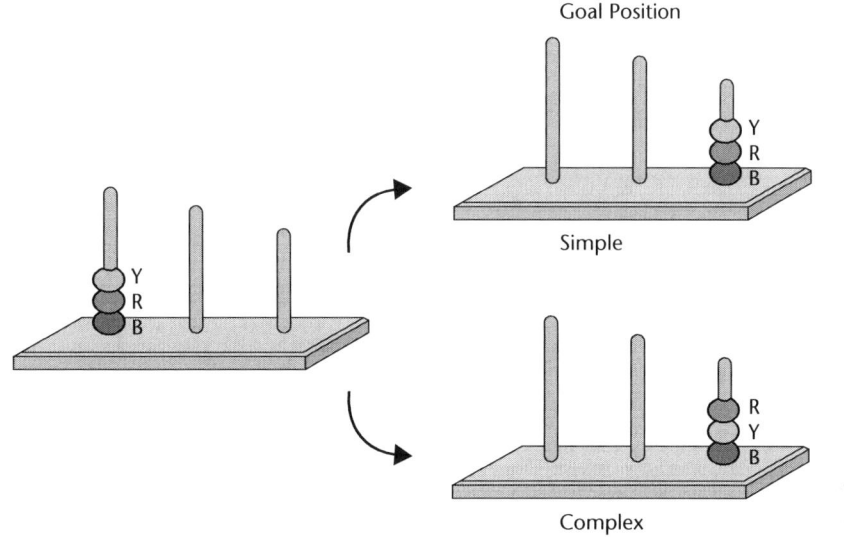

FIGURE 18.3 An illustration of a prototypical tower task commonly used to assess problem-solving and planning skills. The figure depicts two typical problems with different levels of complexity as administered as part of the Progressive Planning Test (PPT). In both instances the subject must move several beads from their initial positions to the goal position. When solving the problem, the subject can move only one bead at a time; once a bead has been moved from its initial position, it cannot be returned to that position. The problems shown here used three beads, each of a different colour: yellow (Y), red (R) and blue (B). The 'simple' problem has a straightforward solution that does not strain the subject's working memory. The subject must move the beads as follows: the yellow bead to peg # 2 (denoted as Y to 2), then R to 2, B to 3, R to 3, and Y to 3. In contrast, the 'complex' problem requires greater mental manipulation by the subject to reverse the order of the two beads (i.e. the Y and R beads) when placing them in the second position before moving the B bead to the goal position. Thus six steps are required to solve the problem: Y to 3, R to 2, Y to 2, B to 3, Y to 3, and R to 3. (*Source*: Kodituwakku *et al.* 2001).

Response inhibition

Likewise, these individuals exhibit poor inhibitory control. Tasks that assess response inhibition (e.g. Stroop Test) are particularly difficult for children with histories of prenatal alcohol exposure, especially when interference is introduced and when they are required to switch responses (Connor *et al.* 2000; Mattson *et al.* 1999). Response inhibition has more recently been evaluated in combination within functional brain activation, which is discussed later in this chapter.

Concept formation and set-shifting

Another area of weakness in alcohol-exposed individuals is abstract concept formation and conceptual set-shifting. Concept formation is the development of ideas or rules based on common properties of objects, events, or qualities using the processes of abstract reasoning and generalization. Conceptual set-shifting involves displaying flexibility of cognitive strategies in response to changes in the environment. Tasks that measure these domains require subjects to generate, recognize and shift categories (e.g. Wisconsin Card Sorting Task). When compared to typically developing children, children with prenatal alcohol exposure demonstrate greater difficulties forming and identifying abstract concepts and shifting to new categories in both verbal and nonverbal domains (Coles *et al.* 1997; Mattson *et al.* 1999; McGee *et al.* 2008b; Olson *et al.* 1998; Vaurio *et al.* 2008).

Fluency

Fluency is an executive function domain of cognitive flexibility and strategic thinking, which requires the generation of multiple responses under time constraints. Fluency tasks may be traditional (production of as many responses within a single category) or set-shifting (alternation of responses between two or more categories). Children with prenatal exposure to alcohol demonstrate deficits on both verbal and nonverbal measures of fluency, as well as on traditional and set-shifting measures. Compared to typically developing controls, alcohol-exposed children have difficulty generating words that begin with a specific letter (letter fluency) or belong in a particular category (category fluency) (Aragon *et al.* 2008b; Kodituwakku *et al.* 2006b; Mattson *et al.* 1999; Rasmussen and Bisanz 2009; Vaurio *et al.* 2008), and they are deficient at producing novel nonverbal responses (design fluency) (Schonfeld *et al.* 2001). Finally, individuals with prenatal alcohol exposure are impaired on set-shifting measures of fluency above and beyond those deficits accounted for by traditional measures as well as lower IQ (Schonfeld *et al.* 2001) (Figure 18.4).

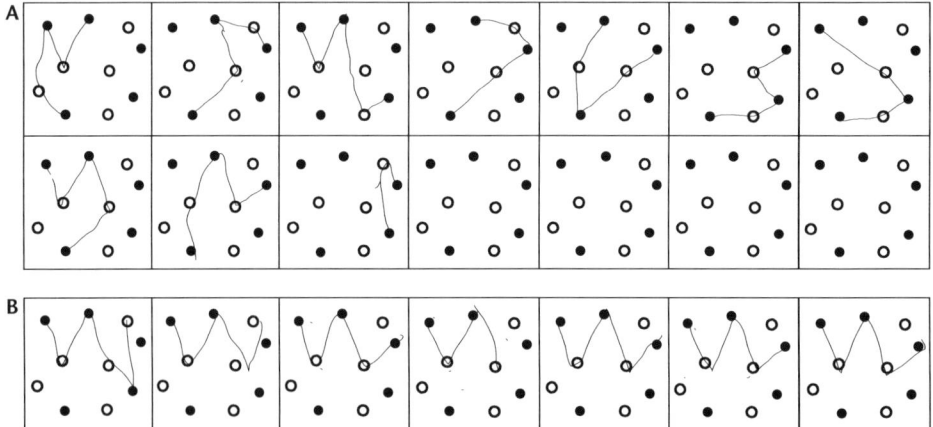

FIGURE 18.4 Representative designs on Delis–Kaplan Executive Function System (D-KEFS). Design Fluency Set-Shifting by two 15-year-old right-handed females, a typically developing control (A) and one with heavy prenatal exposure to alcohol (B). In this task examinees are presented with squares each containing five filled and five empty dots. Children must use only four straight lines to connect dots, switching between empty and filled dots for each line drawn to create as many distinct designs as possible within a one-minute time limit. Compared with the typically developing child (nine correct designs), the alcohol-exposed child produces fewer designs and, of those, makes a greater number of errors (only one correct design) (*Source*: Delis *et al.* 2001).

Working memory

Working memory is the ability to actively hold and manipulate information in the mind to perform more complex tasks such as reasoning, and is a notable area of weakness in individuals with FASDs. In the verbal domain, children prenatally exposed to alcohol recall fewer items when asked to repeat a series of digits in reverse order (digit-span backwards) (Aragon *et al.* 2008b; O'Hare *et al.* 2009; Olson *et al.* 1998), and they struggle on a verbal arithmetic task, which also engages working memory and the ability to recall and mentally manipulate numbers in order to produce a correct response (Streissguth *et al.* 1990). In addition, they show deficits in visual–spatial working memory (Green *et al.* 2009b), and these deficits persist even after IQ is statistically controlled (Burden *et al.* 2005). Working memory may be the cognitive process underlying executive functioning and attention skills that is most affected by prenatal alcohol exposure (Burden *et al.* 2005). Therefore, some researchers suggest working memory to be a core neuropsychological deficit of prenatal alcohol exposure (Rasmussen 2005).

Learning and memory

Prenatal alcohol exposure leads to a wide range of learning and memory deficits in both verbal and nonverbal domains. Children with and without the facial features of FAS are impaired in both learning and memory of verbal information (Roebuck *et al.* 1998). Children with FASDs not only remember less information in learning trials but also have greater difficulty recalling it in free recall and recognition trials (Crocker *et al.* 2011; Mattson *et al.* 1996b; Mattson and Roebuck 2002). However, these memory deficits appear to be a result of poor encoding processes rather than inadequate retention of information (Coles *et al.* 2010; Kaemingk *et al.* 2003; Mattson and Roebuck 2002; Roebuck-Spencer and Mattson 2004; Willoughby *et al.* 2008). Children with FASDs show improved learning and memory when verbal information is presented in a story rather than a word-list (Pei *et al.* 2008); however, although subjects recall more information, they also recount more inaccurate information. Two studies within the same cohort of children exposed to light to moderate levels of alcohol during pregnancy found that prenatal alcohol exposure predicted poor memory for stories at ten years of age (Richardson *et al.* 2002) but not at 14 years (Willford *et al.* 2004), suggesting a delay rather than persistent deficit in function, at least in less affected individuals.

A comparable pattern of deficits is also detected in the nonverbal domain, as children with FASDs have difficulty learning and recalling nonverbal information. However, it is unclear whether retention is spared in this domain after initial learning is accounted for, as results have not been consistent across studies (Aragon *et al.* 2008b; Kaemingk *et al.* 2003; Mattson and Roebuck 2002). Furthermore, prenatal alcohol exposure impairs visual–spatial memory abilities. Children with FASDs have difficulty processing, recalling and reproducing spatial information (Aragon *et al.* 2008b; Hamilton *et al.* 2003; Richardson *et al.* 2002; Uecker and Nadel 1996, 1998; Willoughby *et al.* 2008). Nevertheless, impairments in spatial memory may not be completely attributable to a material-specific memory deficit but rather accounted for by impairments in lower order processes such as visual perception and verbal memory (Kaemingk and Halverson 2000).

Visual–spatial ability

In comparison to other cognitive domains, less is known about visual–spatial processing in FASDs. Children prenatally exposed to alcohol demonstrate impairments on simple tasks of visual–spatial construction or visual–motor integration, in which they are asked to recreate a visual stimulus (Aronson and Hagberg 1998; Chiodo *et al.* 2009; Conry 1990; Janzen *et al.* 1995; Jirikowic *et al.* 2008; Korkman *et al.* 1998; Roebuck *et al.* 1998; Uecker and Nadel 1996). On a clock-drawing task, children with FAS display difficulty reproducing objects with spatial dimensions (Uecker and Nadel 1996). Despite understanding the essential elements of the clock to be replicated, they show a complete disregard for spacing of numbers (Figure 18.5). This visual–spatial distortion may signify a lack of planning or poor mental visual representation of the object. Some authors suggest that children with FAS may demonstrate a form of constructional apraxia (Uecker and Nadel 1996). Additionally, children with prenatal alcohol exposure do not process specific features of visual stimuli with the same capacity. Given a hierarchical stimulus (one that consists of a larger global feature made up of smaller local features), these children show greater difficulty processing the local aspects rather than global aspects of stimuli (Mattson *et al.* 1996a).

Language

Findings of language capabilities in individuals with FASDs have been mixed. Retrospective group studies consistently reveal observations of language deficits, such as word comprehension (Conry 1990; LaDue *et al.* 1992; Roebuck *et al.* 1998), naming ability (Roebuck *et al.* 1998), articulation (Becker *et al.* 1990; Kodituwakku *et al.* 2006a), grammatical and semantic abilities (Becker *et al.* 1990), pragmatics (Abkarian 1992), and expressive and receptive skills (Aragon *et al.* 2008a; Carney and Chermak 1991; Janzen *et al.* 1995; McGee *et al.* 2009). On the other hand, prospective studies are more ambiguous about language disabilities in this population. In a series of reports from a longitudinal prospective study of children prenatally exposed to alcohol, decreased language comprehension and expression were observed at 13 months

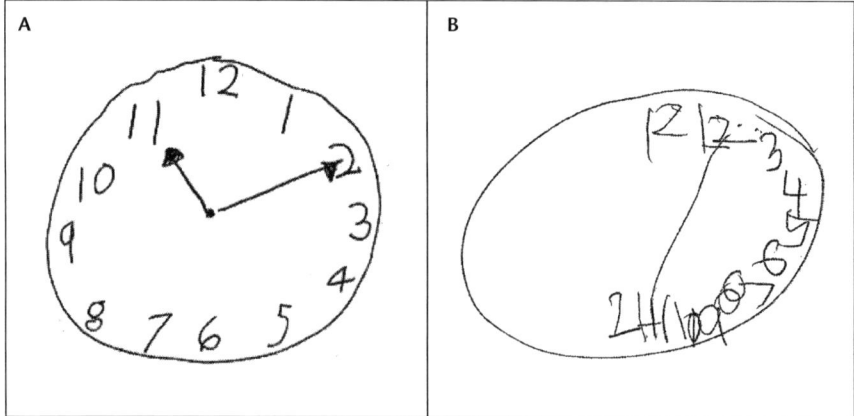

FIGURE 18.5 Responses of two nine-year-old children on a clock-drawing task. The typically developing child (A) draws a correctly numbered clock while the alcohol-exposed child (B) completes a distorted clock figure with incorrectly placed numbers.

(Gusella and Fried 1984), two years (Fried and Watkinson 1988) and three years (Fried and Watkinson 1990), but no longer at four (Fried and Watkinson 1990), five or six years (Fried et al. 1992), suggesting a developmental delay rather than persistent deficit in language abilities. Another longitudinal prospective study found prenatal alcohol exposure to be associated with phonological processing deficits at 14 years of age in a dose-dependent fashion (Streissguth et al. 1994a). Lastly, a separate, more recent study found no language delays in children exposed to low levels of alcohol (O'Leary et al. 2009). The nature of these discrepancies among studies may be attributed to varying levels of alcohol exposure; retrospective studies tend to focus on heavy prenatal exposure, while children in prospective studies are primarily exposed to low or moderate levels of alcohol.

While many of the early studies on language development in FASDs occurred primarily in standardized contexts, more recent studies have focused on how children use language to achieve communicative goals in a social environment. Coggins and colleagues (2003) argue that children with FASDs have difficulty balancing the linguistic challenges and social demands of a given social interaction in order to produce contextually integrated conversation. Alcohol-exposed children not only provide insufficient information and organization for listeners in their stories, but also are more likely to use ambiguous references and fail to appropriately distinguish concepts (Coggins et al. 2007; Thorne et al. 2007). Parents also report that children often fail to consider the listener's perspective in their interactions (Timler et al. 2005).

Motor function

Considering the degree of neural damage to brain regions in the CNS involved in motor control (such as the cerebellum and basal ganglia), combined with abnormalities in peripheral nerve development (Avaria Mde et al. 2004; Bradley et al. 1999; David and Subramaniam 2005; Heaton and Bradley 1995; Phillips et al. 1991; Stromland and Pinazo-Duran 2002), it is not surprising that children prenatally exposed to alcohol experience a number of motor impairments in both gross and fine motor skills. The earliest observations by Jones and Smith (1973) reported poor hand/eye coordination, weak grasp, tremors and balance/gait difficulties. More recent findings among children and adolescents with prenatal alcohol exposure include postural instability (Roebuck et al. 1998), atypical gait (Marcus 1987), delayed motor reaction time (Simmons et al. 2010; Simmons et al. 2002), increased motor timing variability (Simmons et al. 2009; Wass et al. 2002), atypical patterns of goal-directed arm movements (Domellof et al. 2011), poor sensorimotor performance (Jirikowic et al. 2008), poor bimanual coordination (Roebuck-Spencer et al. 2004), weak grasp (Conry 1990), poor hand/eye coordination (Adnams et al. 2001), fine motor speed and coordination (Chiodo et al. 2009; Roebuck et al. 1998), impaired oculomotor control (Green et al. 2009a), and poor isometric and isotonic force regulation (Nguyen et al. 2013; Simmons et al. 2012). On a parent questionnaire measure, young children with FAS show significantly greater delays on fine compared to gross motor skills (Kalberg et al. 2006). It is not yet clear whether the deficits seen early in development persist into adulthood. While one study found that group differences on a motor reaction time task previously observed in children (Simmons et al. 2002) are no longer apparent among adolescents (Simmons et al. 2006), another revealed that adults with FASDs continue to exhibit balance and fine motor impairments (Connor et al. 2006).

Attention and activity levels

Hyperactivity and attention deficits are frequently observed in individuals with FASDs. Children with prenatal alcohol exposure consistently show impairment on neuropsychological tasks of vigilance, reaction time and information processing (Burden et al. 2005; Jacobson et al. 1994; Jacobson et al. 1993; Streissguth et al. 1986; Streissguth et al. 1984; Streissguth et al. 1994b). Attention difficulties are also commonly described on parent (Janzen et al. 1995; Mattson and Riley 2000; Nash et al. 2006; Olson et al. 1992) and teacher (Aragon et al. 2008a; Brown et al. 1991) reports of attention. In fact, more than 60 per cent of children with FASDs display deficits in attention (LaDue et al. 1992), and this clinical population receives diagnoses of attention-deficit/hyperactive disorder (ADHD) (Fryer et al. 2007a) and hyperkinetic disorders (Steinhausen et al. 1993) at a significantly higher rate than typically developing children. Despite a frequent co-morbid diagnosis of ADHD among individuals with FASDs (Burd et al. 2003) and the degree of symptom overlap between ADHD and FASDs, the nature of attention deficits in FASDs and ADHD differ (Burden et al. 2010; Coles et al. 1997; Kooistra et al. 2010). While children with ADHD present with greater difficulty focusing and sustaining attention, children with FASDs are more impaired in shifting attention, encoding information and problem-solving (Coles et al. 1997). Still, within FASDs, impairments in visual and auditory attention are not equivalent, although studies have not been consistent regarding the direction of these deficits. Some studies report greater difficulties in visual sustained attention (Coles et al. 2002; Mattson et al. 2006), while another describes greater auditory attention deficits (Connor et al. 1999).

Functional brain abnormalities in FASDs

Given the known structural brain abnormalities and neuropsychological impairment due to prenatal alcohol exposure, researchers have been interested in measuring brain activation concurrent with cognitive processes. Using functional neuroimaging techniques, studies have investigated functional brain differences in individuals exposed to alcohol during gestation, further broadening our understanding of brain and behaviour relationships in FASDs. A review of these studies reveal some inconsistencies in outcomes, which may be due to a number of different factors, including group differences on behavioural performance, subject characteristics and task parameters. Although these discrepancies highlight the challenges involved in interpreting functional neuroimaging results, it is nevertheless apparent that prenatal alcohol exposure is associated with altered brain function.

Working memory

Malisza et al. (2005) were the first to report differences in fMRI activation between individuals with histories of prenatal alcohol exposure and controls. They used a spatial working memory task and reported that subjects with FASDs had greater activation than controls in the frontal and parietal cortices. Also, while control individuals showed greater activation with increases in task difficulty, this was not observed in the alcohol-exposed group, especially in younger subjects. A subsequent study replicated these findings and also reported greater activation in frontal brain regions of alcohol-exposed youths compared to controls (Spadoni et al. 2009; Figure 18.6). In contrast, Astley and colleagues (2009) reported working memory deficits to

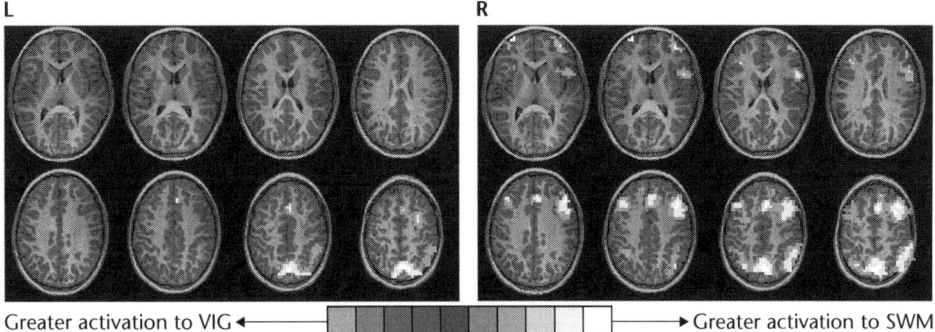

FIGURE 18.6 Regions of dorsolateral frontal parietal activation patterns during a spatial working memory task relative to vigilance: children in the alcohol exposed group (right) have relatively greater activation within the dorsolateral frontal parietal regions as well as in subcortical regions than the control group (left) (Reprinted with permission from Spandoni *et al.* 2009).

be correlated with decreased fMRI activation in the right posterior parietal lobe as well as the frontal and prefrontal cortices – all brain regions known to be involved in working memory. Importantly, neural activation in this study increased as severity of alcohol exposure decreased, suggesting that children across the entire spectrum of FASDs show working memory deficits that are correlated to abnormal brain activation.

Response inhibition

Several studies have investigated the neural bases that underlie poor inhibitory control seen in alcohol-exposed individuals. Measuring activation in frontal-striatal regions, Fryer *et al.* (2007b) reported increased fMRI activation compared to controls in prefrontal areas of the cortex and, interestingly, decreased activation in the caudate nucleus of the basal ganglia, despite equivalent performance among the groups. Similarly, another study revealed increased neural activation although groups did not differ in behavioural performance (Burden *et al.* 2009). These findings suggest that children with FASDs require greater cognitive effort to produce the same level of response inhibition.

Verbal learning and memory

Verbal learning is associated with increased fMRI activation in the frontal cortex but less activation in parts of the temporal lobe that were expected to be active during encoding and retrieval of verbal information (Sowell *et al.* 2007). It is possible that individuals with FASDs may be compensating for dysfunctional temporal memory systems and instead relying on frontal memory systems. A subsequent study examining verbal working memory revealed that despite equal performance between groups, the FASD group showed increased activation compared to controls in left frontal and left parietal cortices (O'Hare *et al.* 2009).

Mathematics processing

Finally, the relationship between functional brain abnormalities and mathematics ability in FASDs has also been examined. Parietal brain regions are believed to support mathematics abilities, such as arithmetic abilities and numerical processing (Dehaene et al. 2004; Dehaene et al. 2003). One study observed decreased neural activity in parietal and prefrontal regions during arithmetic processing (Santhanam et al. 2009) while another detected increased but more diffuse activation beyond the typically observed fronto-parietal network that is associated with maths processing in controls, suggesting that alcohol-exposed children require a broader range of cortical involvement to perform similar number processing tasks (Meintjes et al. 2010).

Together, these functional neuroimaging studies not only further replicate findings reported in the structural neuroimaging and neuropsychological literature but also illustrate that these brain and behavioural impairments temporally coincide with each other. To the extent that causal associations can be made with functional imaging techniques, these findings suggest that atypical brain functioning in FASDs is directly correlated with abnormal cognitive and behavioural functioning. Future neuroimaging and neuropsychological research through multimodal methods will continue to enhance our comprehension of the complex brain and behaviour relationships in FASDs.

Summary and conclusions

Since the initial reports of FAS in the 1970s, our knowledge of alcohol's effects on the developing brain and behaviour has grown immensely. *In utero* exposure to alcohol causes permanent damage to brain structure and function, which mediates alterations in cognition and behaviour. Modern imaging techniques have allowed for the detection of structural alterations as well as functional abnormalities. Documented brain changes include overall reduction in brain size, alteration in grey and white matter densities and integrity, volumetric reductions in the corpus callosum, cerebellum, basal ganglia and hippocampus, as well as regional displacement of the cerebellum and corpus callosum. These abnormalities highlight not only the pervasiveness but also specificity of alcohol's influence. Furthermore, these studies suggest that cognitive and behavioural deficits in FASDs are not global in nature but specific depending on affected brain regions. In fact, individuals with prenatal alcohol exposure present with a wide range of long-lasting impairments in a variety of neuropsychological domains, including diminished general intelligence, poor learning and memory, impaired executive and visual–spatial function, hyperactivity and attention deficits, and delayed motor and language development. An understanding of these brain–behaviour relationships in prenatal alcohol exposure is important in developing a reliable neurobehavioural profile of children with FASDs. Such a profile will aid in the diagnosis of individuals developmentally exposed to alcohol but who may not present with physical characteristics of FAS. A profile will also inform the development of targeted intervention programmes. Another primary goal of this research is to further identify and explore how risk factors moderate the relationship between alcohol exposure and the type and severity of brain and behavioural alterations. Knowledge of these relevant influences will further facilitate prevention and intervention strategies. Given that FASDs are a devastating yet preventable public health concern, developing safe and effective prevention and intervention techniques are among the most important challenges.

Acknowledgements

This research was supported by grants (T32 AA013525, R01 AA10417, and U24 AA014811) awarded by the United States National Institute on Alcohol Abuse and Alcoholism (NIAAA).

References

Abel, E.L. and Sokol, R.J. (1987) 'Incidence of fetal alcohol syndrome and economic impact of FAS-related anomalies', *Drug and Alcohol Dependence*, 19: 51–70.

Abkarian, G.G. (1992) 'Communication effects of prenatal alcohol exposure', *Journal of Communication Disorders*, 25: 221–40.

Adnams, C.M., Kodituwakku, P.W., Hay, A., Molteno, C.D., Viljoen, D. and May, P.A. (2001) 'Patterns of cognitive-motor development in children with fetal alcohol syndrome from a community in South Africa', *Alcoholism: Clinical and Experimental Research*, 25: 557–62.

Aragon, A.S., Coriale, G., Fiorentino, D., Kalberg, W.O., Buckley, D., Gossage, J.P., Ceccanti, M., Mitchell, E.R. and May, P.A. (2008a) 'Neuropsychological characteristics of Italian children with fetal alcohol spectrum disorders', *Alcoholism: Clinical and Experimental Research*, 32: 1909–19.

Aragon, A.S., Kalberg, W.O., Buckley, D., Barela-Scott, L.M., Tabachnick, B.G. and May, P.A. (2008b) 'Neuropsychological study of FASD in a sample of American Indian children: processing simple versus complex information', *Alcoholism: Clinical and Experimental Research*, 32: 2136–48.

Archibald, S.L., Fennema-Notestine, C., Gamst, A., Riley, E.P., Mattson, S.N. and Jernigan, T.L. (2001) 'Brain dysmorphology in individuals with severe prenatal alcohol exposure', *Developmental Medicine and Child Neurology*, 43: 148–54.

Aronson, M. and Hagberg, B. (1998) 'Neuropsychological disorders in children exposed to alcohol during pregnancy: a follow-up study of 24 children to alcoholic mothers in Goteborg, Sweden', *Alcoholism: Clinical and Experimental Research*, 22: 321–4.

Astley, S.J., Aylward, E.H., Olson, H.C., Kerns, K., Brooks, A., Coggins, T.E., Davies, J., Dorn, S., Gendler, B., Jirikowic, T., Kraegel, P., Maravilla, K. and Richards, T. (2009) 'Magnetic resonance imaging outcomes from a comprehensive magnetic resonance study of children with fetal alcohol spectrum disorders', *Alcoholism: Clinical and Experimental Research*, 33: 1671–89.

Autti-Ramo, I., Autti, T., Korkman, M., Kettunen, S., Salonen, O. and Valanne, L. (2002) 'MRI findings in children with school problems who had been exposed prenatally to alcohol', *Developmental Medicine and Child Neurology*, 44: 98–106.

Avaria Mde, L., Mills, J.L., Kleinsteuber, K., Aros, S., Conley, M.R., Cox, C., Klebanoff, M. and Cassorla, F. (2004) 'Peripheral nerve conduction abnormalities in children exposed to alcohol in utero', *Journal of Pediatrics*, 144: 338–43.

Becker, M., Warr-Leeper, G.A. and Leeper, H.A., Jr (1990) 'Fetal alcohol syndrome: a description of oral motor, articulatory, short-term memory, grammatical and semantic abilities', *Journal of Communication Disorders*, 23: 97–124.

Bookstein, F.L., Sampson, P.D., Streissguth, A.P. and Connor, P.D. (2001) 'Geometric morphometrics of corpus callosum and subcortical structures in the fetal-alcohol-affected brain', *Teratology*, 64: 4–32.

Bookstein, F.L., Sampson, P.D., Connor, P.D. and Streissguth, A.P. (2002a) 'Midline corpus callosum is a neuroanatomical focus of fetal alcohol damage', *The Anatomical Record*, 269: 162–74.

Bookstein, F.L., Streissguth, A.P., Sampson, P.D., Connor, P.D. and Barr, H.M. (2002b) 'Corpus callosum shape and neuropsychological deficits in adult males with heavy fetal alcohol exposure', *Neuroimage*, 15: 233–51.

Bradley, D.M., Beaman, F.D., Moore, D.B., Kidd, K. and Heaton, M.B. (1999) 'Neurotrophic factors BDNF and GDNF protect embryonic chick spinal cord motoneurons from ethanol neurotoxicity in vivo', *Brain Research: Developmental Brain Research*, 112: 99–106.

Brown, R.T., Coles, C.D., Smith, I.E., Platzman, K.A., Silverstein, J., Erickson, S. and Falek, A. (1991) 'Effects of prenatal alcohol exposure at school age II: attention and behavior', *Neurotoxicology and Teratology*, 13: 369–76.

Burd, L., Klug, M.G., Martsolf, J.T. and Kerbeshian, J. (2003) 'Fetal alcohol syndrome: neuropsychiatric phenomics', *Neurotoxicology and Teratology*, 25: 697–705.

Burden, M.J., Andrew, C., Saint-Amour, D., Meintjes, E.M., Molteno, C.D., Hoyme, H.E., Robinson, L.K., Khaole, N., Nelson, C.A., Jacobson, J.L. and Jacobson, S.W. (2009) 'The effects of fetal alcohol syndrome on response execution and inhibition: an event-related potential study', *Alcoholism: Clinical and Experimental Research*, 33: 1994–2004.

Burden, M.J., Jacobson, J.L., Westerlund, A., Lundahl, L.H., Morrison, A., Dodge, N.C., Klorman, R., Nelson, C.A., Avison, M.J. and Jacobson, S.W. (2010) 'An event-related potential study of response inhibition in ADHD with and without prenatal alcohol exposure', *Alcoholism: Clinical and Experimental Research*, 34: 617–27.

Burden, M.J., Jacobson, S.W., Sokol, R.J. and Jacobson, J.L. (2005) 'Effects of prenatal alcohol exposure on attention and working memory at 7.5 years of age', *Alcoholism: Clinical and Experimental Research*, 29: 443–52.

Carney, L.J. and Chermak, G.D. (1991) 'Performance of American Indian children with fetal alcohol syndrome on the test of language development', *Journal of Communication Disorders*, 24: 123–34.

Chasnoff, I.J., Wells, A.M., Telford, E., Schmidt, C. and Messer, G. (2010) 'Neurodevelopmental functioning in children with FAS, pFAS, and ARND', *Journal of Developmental and Behavioral Pediatrics*, 31: 192–201.

Chiodo, L.M., Janisse, J., Delaney-Black, V., Sokol, R.J. and Hannigan, J.H. (2009) 'A metric of maternal prenatal risk drinking predicts neurobehavioral outcomes in preschool children', *Alcoholism: Clinical and Experimental Research*, 33: 634–44.

Clarren, S.K. (1986) 'Neuropathology in fetal alcohol syndrome', in J.R. West (ed.) *Alcohol and Brain Development*, New York, NY: Oxford University Press.

Clarren, S.K. and Smith, D.W. (1978) 'The fetal alcohol syndrome', *The Lamp*, 35: 4–7.

Coggins, T.E., Olswang, L.B., Carmichael Olson, H. and Timler, G.R. (2003) 'On becoming socially competent communicators: the challenge for children with fetal alcohol exposure', *International Review of Research in Mental Retardation*, 27: 121–50.

Coggins, T.E., Timler, G.R. and Olswang, L.B. (2007) 'A state of double jeopardy: impact of prenatal alcohol exposure and adverse environments on the social communicative abilities of school-age children with fetal alcohol spectrum disorder', *Language, Speech, and Hearing Services in Schools*, 38: 117–27.

Coles, C.D., Goldstein, F.C., Lynch, M.E., Chen, X., Kable, J.A., Johnson, K.C. and Hu, X. (2011) 'Memory and brain volume in adults prenatally exposed to alcohol', *Brain and Cognition*, 75: 67–77.

Coles, C.D., Lynch, M.E., Kable, J.A., Johnson, K.C. and Goldstein, F.C. (2010) 'Verbal and nonverbal memory in adults prenatally exposed to alcohol', *Alcoholism: Clinical and Experimental Research*, 34: 897–906.

Coles, C.D., Platzman, K.A., Raskind-Hood, C.L., Brown, R.T., Falek, A. and Smith, I.E. (1997) 'A comparison of children affected by prenatal alcohol exposure and attention deficit, hyperactivity disorder', *Alcoholism: Clinical and Experimental Research*, 21: 150–61.

Coles, C.D., Platzman, K.A., Lynch, M.E. and Freides, D. (2002) 'Auditory and visual sustained attention in adolescents prenatally exposed to alcohol', *Alcoholism: Clinical and Experimental Research*, 26: 263–71.

Connor, P.D., Sampson, P.D., Bookstein, F.L., Barr, H.M. and Streissguth, A.P. (2000) 'Direct and indirect effects of prenatal alcohol damage on executive function', *Developmental Neuropsychology*, 18: 331–54.

Connor, P.D., Sampson, P.D., Streissguth, A.P., Bookstein, F.L. and Barr, H.M. (2006) 'Effects of prenatal alcohol exposure on fine motor coordination and balance: a study of two adult samples', *Neuropsychologia*, 44: 744–51.

Connor, P.D., Streissguth, A.P., Sampson, P.D., Bookstein, F.L. and Barr, H.M. (1999) 'Individual differences in auditory and visual attention among fetal alcohol-affected adults', *Alcoholism: Clinical and Experimental Research*, 23: 1395–402.

Conry, J. (1990) 'Neuropsychological deficits in fetal alcohol syndrome and fetal alcohol effects', *Alcoholism: Clinical and Experimental Research*, 14: 650–5.

Coulter, C.L., Leech, R.W., Schaefer, G.B., Scheithauer, B.W. and Brumback, R.A. (1993) 'Midline cerebral dysgenesis, dysfunction of the hypothalamic-pituitary axis, and fetal alcohol effects', *Archives of Neurology*, 50: 771–5.

Crocker, N., Vaurio, L., Riley, E.P. and Mattson, S.N. (2011) 'Comparison of verbal learning and memory in children with heavy prenatal alcohol exposure or attention-deficit/hyperactivity disorder', *Alcoholism: Clinical and Experimental Research*, 35: 1114–21.

Cummings, J.L. (1993) 'Frontal-subcortical circuits and human behavior', *Archives of Neurology*, 50: 873–80.

Dalen, K., Bruaroy, S., Wentzel-Larsen, T. and Laegreid, L.M. (2009) 'Cognitive functioning in children prenatally exposed to alcohol and psychotropic drugs', *Neuropediatrics*, 40: 162–7.

David, P. and Subramaniam, K. (2005) 'Prenatal alcohol exposure and early postnatal changes in the developing nerve-muscle system', *Birth Defects Research Part A: Clinical and Molecular Teratology*, 73: 897–903.

Dehaene, S., Molko, N., Cohen, L. and Wilson, A.J. (2004) 'Arithmetic and the brain', *Current Opinion in Neurobiology*, 14: 218–24.

Dehaene, S., Piazza, M., Pinel, P. and Cohen, L. (2003) 'Three parietal circuits for number processing', *Cognitive Neuropsychology*, 20: 487–506.

Delis, D.C., Kaplan, E. and Kramer, J.H. (2001) *Manual for the Delis-Kaplan Executive Function System*, San Antonio, TX: Psychological Corporation.

Domellof, E., Fagard, J., Jacquet, A.Y. and Ronnqvist, L. (2011) 'Goal-directed arm movements in children with fetal alcohol syndrome: a kinematic approach', *European Journal of Neurology*, 18: 312–20.

Ervalahti, N., Korkman, M., Fagerlund, A., Autti-Ramo, I., Loimu, L. and Hoyme, H.E. (2007) 'Relationship between dysmorphic features and general cognitive function in children with fetal alcohol spectrum disorders', *American Journal of Medical Genetics Part A*, 143A: 2916–23.

Fried, P.A., O'Connell, C.M. and Watkinson, B. (1992) '60- and 72-month follow-up of children prenatally exposed to marijuana, cigarettes, and alcohol: cognitive and language assessment', *Journal of Developmental and Behavioral Pediatrics*, 13: 383–91.

Fried, P.A. and Watkinson, B. (1988) '12- and 24-month neurobehavioural follow-up of children prenatally exposed to marihuana, cigarettes and alcohol', *Neurotoxicology and Teratology*, 10: 305–13.

Fried, P.A. and Watkinson, B. (1990) '36- and 48-month neurobehavioral follow-up of children prenatally exposed to marijuana, cigarettes and alcohol', *Journal of Developmental and Behavioral Pediatrics*, 11: 49–58.

Fryer, S.L., McGee, C.L., Matt, G.E., Riley, E.P. and Mattson, S.N. (2007a) 'Evaluation of psychopathological conditions in children with heavy prenatal alcohol exposure', *Pediatrics*, 119: e733–41.

Fryer, S.L., Schweinsburg, B.C., Bjorkquist, O.A., Frank, L.R., Mattson, S.N., Spadoni, A.D. and Riley, E.P. (2009) 'Characterization of white matter microstructure in fetal alcohol spectrum disorders', *Alcoholism: Clinical and Experimental Research*, 33: 514–21.

Fryer, S.L., Tapert, S.F., Mattson, S.N., Paulus, M.P., Spadoni, A.D. and Riley, E.P. (2007b) 'Prenatal alcohol exposure affects frontal-striatal BOLD response during inhibitory control', *Alcoholism: Clinical and Experimental Research*, 31: 1415–24.

Green, C.R., Mihic, A.M., Brien, D.C., Armstrong, I.T., Nikkel, S.M., Stade, B.C., Rasmussen, C., Munoz, D.P. and Reynolds, J.N. (2009a) 'Oculomotor control in children with fetal alcohol spectrum disorders assessed using a mobile eye-tracking laboratory', *European Journal of Neuroscience*, 29: 1302–9.

Green, C.R., Mihic, A.M., Nikkel, S.M., Stade, B.C., Rasmussen, C., Munoz, D.P. and Reynolds, J.N. (2009b) 'Executive function deficits in children with fetal alcohol spectrum disorders (FASD) measured using the Cambridge Neuropsychological Tests Automated Battery (CANTAB)', *Journal of Child Psychology and Psychiatry*, 50: 688–97.

Gusella, J.L. and Fried, P.A. (1984) 'Effects of maternal social drinking and smoking on offspring at 13 months', *Neurobehavioral Toxicology and Teratology*, 6: 13–17.

Hamilton, D.A., Kodituwakku, P., Sutherland, R.J. and Savage, D.D. (2003) 'Children with fetal alcohol syndrome are impaired at place learning but not cued-navigation in a virtual Morris water task', *Behavioural Brain Research*, 143: 85–94.

Heaton, M.B. and Bradley, D.M. (1995) 'Ethanol influences on the chick embryo spinal cord motor system: analyses of motoneuron cell death, motility, and target trophic factor activity and in vitro analyses of neurotoxicity and trophic factor neuroprotection', *Journal of Neurobiology*, 26: 47–61.

Jacobson, S.W., Jacobson, J.L. and Sokol, R.J. (1994) 'Effects of fetal alcohol exposure on infant reaction time', *Alcoholism: Clinical and Experimental Research*, 18: 1125–32.

Jacobson, S.W., Jacobson, J.L., Sokol, R.J., Martier, S.S. and Ager, J.W. (1993) 'Prenatal alcohol exposure and infant information processing ability', *Child Development*, 64: 1706–21.

Janzen, L.A., Nanson, J.L. and Block, G.W. (1995) 'Neuropsychological evaluation of preschoolers with fetal alcohol syndrome', *Neurotoxicology and Teratology*, 17: 273–9.

Jirikowic, T., Olson, H.C. and Kartin, D. (2008) 'Sensory processing, school performance, and adaptive behavior of young school-age children with fetal alcohol spectrum disorders', *Physical and Occupational Therapy in Pediatrics*, 28: 117–36.

Johnson, V.P., Swayze, V.W., II, Sato, Y. and Andreasen, N.C. (1996) 'Fetal alcohol syndrome: craniofacial and central nervous system manifestations', *American Journal of Medical Genetics*, 61: 329–39.

Jones, K.L. and Smith, D.W. (1973) 'Recognition of the fetal alcohol syndrome in early infancy', *Lancet*, 302: 999–1001.

Jones, K.L. and Smith, D.W. (1975) 'The fetal alcohol syndrome', *Teratology*, 12: 1–10.

Jones, K.L., Smith, D.W., Ulleland, C.N. and Streissguth, P. (1973) 'Pattern of malformation in offspring of chronic alcoholic mothers', *Lancet*, 1: 1267–71.

Kaemingk, K.L. and Halverson, P.T. (2000) 'Spatial memory following prenatal alcohol exposure: more than a material specific memory deficit', *Child Neuropsychology*, 6: 115–28.

Kaemingk, K.L., Mulvaney, S. and Halverson, P.T. (2003) 'Learning following prenatal alcohol exposure: performance on verbal and visual multitrial tasks', *Archives of Clinical Neuropsychology*, 18: 33–47.

Kalberg, W.O., Provost, B., Tollison, S.J., Tabachnick, B.G., Robinson, L.K., Eugene Hoyme, H., Trujillo, P.M., Buckley, D., Aragon, A.S. and May, P.A. (2006) 'Comparison of motor delays in young children with fetal alcohol syndrome to those with prenatal alcohol exposure and with no prenatal alcohol exposure', *Alcoholism: Clinical and Experimental Research*, 30: 2037–45.

Kodituwakku, P., Coriale, G., Fiorentino, D., Aragon, A.S., Kalberg, W.O., Buckley, D., Gossage, J.P., Ceccanti, M. and May, P.A. (2006a) 'Neurobehavioral characteristics of children with fetal alcohol spectrum disorders in communities from Italy: preliminary results', *Alcoholism: Clinical and Experimental Research*, 30: 1551–61.

Kodituwakku, P.W., Adnams, C.M., Hay, A., Kitching, A.E., Burger, E., Kalberg, W.O., Viljoen, D.L. and May, P.A. (2006b) 'Letter and category fluency in children with fetal alcohol syndrome from a community in South Africa', *Journal of Studies on Alcohol*, 67: 502–9.

Kodituwakku, P.W., Handmaker, N.S., Cutler, S.K., Weathersby, E.K. and Handmaker, S.D. (1995) 'Specific impairments in self-regulation in children exposed to alcohol prenatally', *Alcoholism: Clinical and Experimental Research*, 19: 1558–64.

Kodituwakku, P.W., Kalberg, W. and May, P.A. (2001) 'The effects of prenatal alcohol exposure on executive functioning', *Alcohol Research and Health*, 25: 192–8.

Kooistra, L., Crawford, S., Gibbard, B., Ramage, B. and Kaplan, B.J. (2010) 'Differentiating attention deficits in children with fetal alcohol spectrum disorder or attention-deficit-hyperactivity disorder', *Developmental Medicine and Child Neurology*, 52: 205–11.

Korkman, M., Granstrom, M.L., Appelqvist, K. and Liukkonen, E. (1998) 'Neuropsychological characteristics of five children with the Landau-Kleffner syndrome: dissociation of auditory and phonological discrimination', *Journal of the International Neuropsychological Society*, 4: 566–75.

LaDue, R.A., Streissguth, A.P. and Randels, S.P. (1992) 'Clinical considerations pertaining to adolescents and adults with fetal alcohol syndrome', in T.B. Sonderegger (ed.) *Perinatal Substance Abuse: Research findings and clinical implications*, Baltimore, MD: Johns Hopkins Press.

Lebel, C., Rasmussen, C., Wyper, K., Andrew, G. and Beaulieu, C. (2010) 'Brain microstructure is related to math ability in children with fetal alcohol spectrum disorder', *Alcoholism: Clinical and Experimental Research*, 34: 354–63.

Lebel, C., Rasmussen, C., Wyper, K., Walker, L., Andrew, G., Yager, J. and Beaulieu, C. (2008) 'Brain diffusion abnormalities in children with fetal alcohol spectrum disorder', *Alcoholism: Clinical and Experimental Research*, 32: 1732–40.

Li, L., Coles, C.D., Lynch, M.E. and Hu, X. (2009) 'Voxelwise and skeleton-based region of interest analysis of fetal alcohol syndrome and fetal alcohol spectrum disorders in young adults', *Human Brain Mapping*, 30: 3265–74.

Ma, X., Coles, C.D., Lynch, M.E., Laconte, S.M., Zurkiya, O., Wang, D. and Hu, X. (2005) 'Evaluation of corpus callosum anisotropy in young adults with fetal alcohol syndrome according to diffusion tensor imaging', *Alcoholism: Clinical and Experimental Research*, 29: 1214–22.

Malisza, K.L., Allman, A.A., Shiloff, D., Jakobson, L., Longstaffe, S. and Chudley, A.E. (2005) 'Evaluation of spatial working memory function in children and adults with fetal alcohol spectrum disorders: a functional magnetic resonance imaging study', *Pediatric Research*, 58: 1150–7.

Marcus, J.C. (1987) 'Neurological findings in the fetal alcohol syndrome', *Neuropediatrics*, 18: 158–60.

Mattson, S.N. and Riley, E.P. (1996) 'Brain anomalies in fetal alcohol syndrome', in E.L. Abel (ed.) *Fetal Alcohol Syndrome: From mechanism to prevention*, Boca Raton, FL: CRC Press.

Mattson, S.N. and Riley, E.P. (2000) 'Parent ratings of behavior in children with heavy prenatal alcohol exposure and IQ-matched controls', *Alcoholism: Clinical and Experimental Research*, 24: 226–31.

Mattson, S.N. and Roebuck, T.M. (2002) 'Acquisition and retention of verbal and nonverbal information in children with heavy prenatal alcohol exposure', *Alcoholism: Clinical and Experimental Research*, 26: 875–82.

Mattson, S.N., Calarco, K.E. and Lang, A.R. (2006) 'Focused and shifting attention in children with heavy prenatal alcohol exposure', *Neuropsychology*, 20: 361–9.

Mattson, S.N., Goodman, A.M., Caine, C., Delis, D.C. and Riley, E.P. (1999) 'Executive functioning in children with heavy prenatal alcohol exposure', *Alcoholism: Clinical and Experimental Research*, 23: 1808–15.

Mattson, S.N., Gramling, L., Delis, D.C., Jones, K.L. and Riley, E.P. (1996a) 'Global-local processing in children prenatally exposed to alcohol', *Child Neuropsychology*, 2: 165–75.

Mattson, S.N., Jernigan, T.L. and Riley, E.P. (1994) 'MRI and prenatal alcohol exposure: images provide insight into FAS', *Alcohol Health and Research World*, 18: 49–52.

Mattson, S.N., Riley, E.P., Jernigan, T.L., Ehlers, C.L., Delis, D.C., Jones, K.L., Stern, C., Johnson, K.A., Hesselink, J.R. and Bellugi, U. (1992) 'Fetal alcohol syndrome: a case report of neuropsychological, MRI and EEG assessment of two children', *Alcoholism: Clinical and Experimental Research*, 16: 1001–3.

Mattson, S.N., Riley, E.P., Delis, D.C., Stern, C. and Jones, K.L. (1996b) 'Verbal learning and memory in children with fetal alcohol syndrome', *Alcoholism: Clinical and Experimental Research*, 20: 810–16.

Mattson, S.N., Riley, E.P., Sowell, E.R., Jernigan, T.L., Sobel, D.F. and Jones, K.L. (1996c) 'A decrease in the size of the basal ganglia in children with fetal alcohol syndrome', *Alcoholism: Clinical and Experimental Research*, 20: 1088–93.

Mattson, S.N., Riley, E.P., Gramling, L., Delis, D.C. and Jones, K.L. (1997) 'Heavy prenatal alcohol exposure with or without physical features of fetal alcohol syndrome leads to IQ deficits', *Journal of Pediatrics*, 131: 718–21.

McGee, C.L., Bjorkquist, O.A., Riley, E.P. and Mattson, S.N. (2009) 'Impaired language performance in young children with heavy prenatal alcohol exposure', *Neurotoxicology and Teratology*, 31: 71–5.

McGee, C.L., Fryer, S.L., Bjorkquist, O.A., Mattson, S.N. and Riley, E.P. (2008a) 'Deficits in social problem solving in adolescents with prenatal exposure to alcohol', *American Journal of Drug and Alcohol Abuse*, 34: 423–31.

McGee, C.L., Schonfeld, A.M., Roebuck-Spencer, T.M., Riley, E.P. and Mattson, S.N. (2008b) 'Children with heavy prenatal alcohol exposure demonstrate deficits on multiple measures of concept formation', *Alcoholism: Clinical and Experimental Research*, 32: 1388–97.

Meintjes, E.M., Jacobson, J.L., Molteno, C.D., Gatenby, J.C., Warton, C., Cannistraci, C.J., Hoyme, H.E., Robinson, L.K., Khaole, N., Gore, J.C. and Jacobson, S.W. (2010) 'An FMRI study of number processing in children with fetal alcohol syndrome', *Alcoholism: Clinical and Experimental Research*, 34: 1450–64.

Nardelli, A., Lebel, C., Rasmussen, C., Andrew, G. and Beaulieu, C. (2011) 'Extensive deep gray matter volume reductions in children and adolescents with fetal alcohol spectrum disorder', *Alcoholism: Clinical and Experimental Research*, 35: 1404–17.

Nash, K., Rovet, J., Greenbaum, R., Fantus, E., Nulman, I. and Koren, G. (2006) 'Identifying the behavioural phenotype in fetal alcohol spectrum disorder: sensitivity, specificity and screening potential', *Archives of Women's Mental Health*, 9: 181–6.

Neil, J., Miller, J., Mukherjee, P. and Huppi, P.S. (2002) 'Diffusion tensor imaging of normal and injured developing human brain: a technical review', *NMR in Biomedicine*, 15: 543–52.

Nguyen, T.T., Levy, S.S., Riley, E.P., Thomas, J.D. and Simmons, R.W. (2013) 'Children with heavy prenatal alcohol exposure experience reduced control of isotonic force', *Alcoholism: Clinical and Experimental Research*, 37: 315–24.

O'Hare, E.D., Kan, E., Yoshii, J., Mattson, S.N., Riley, E.P., Thompson, P.M., Toga, A.W. and Sowell, E.R. (2005) 'Mapping cerebellar vermal morphology and cognitive correlates in prenatal alcohol exposure', *NeuroReport*, 16: 1285–90.

O'Hare, E.D., Lu, L.H., Houston, S.M., Bookheimer, S.Y., Mattson, S.N., O'Connor, M.J. and Sowell, E.R. (2009) 'Altered frontal-parietal functioning during verbal working memory in children and adolescents with heavy prenatal alcohol exposure', *Human Brain Mapping*, 30: 3200–8.

O'Leary, C., Zubrick, S.R., Taylor, C.L., Dixon, G. and Bower, C. (2009) 'Prenatal alcohol exposure and language delay in 2-year-old children: the importance of dose and timing on risk', *Pediatrics*, 123: 547–54.

Olson, H.C., Feldman, J.J., Streissguth, A.P., Sampson, P.D. and Bookstein, F.L. (1998) 'Neuropsychological deficits in adolescents with fetal alcohol syndrome: clinical findings', *Alcoholism: Clinical and Experimental Research*, 22: 1998–2012.

Olson, H.C., Sampson, P.D., Barr, H., Streissguth, A.P. and Bookstein, F.L. (1992) 'Prenatal exposure to alcohol and school problems in late childhood: a longitudinal prospective study', *Developmental Psychopathology*, 4: 341–59.

Pei, J.R., Rinaldi, C.M., Rasmussen, C., Massey, V. and Massey, D. (2008) 'Memory patterns of acquisition and retention of verbal and nonverbal information in children with fetal alcohol spectrum disorders', *Canadian Journal of Clinical Pharmacology/Journal Canadien de Pharmacologie Clinique*, 15: e44–56.

Phillips, D.E., Krueger, S.K. and Rydquist, J.E. (1991) 'Short- and long-term effects of combined pre- and postnatal ethanol exposure (three trimester equivalency) on the development of myelin and axons in rat optic nerve', *International Journal of Developmental Neuroscience*, 9: 631–47.

Pulsifer, M.B. (1996) 'The neuropsychology of mental retardation, *Journal of the International Neuropsychological Society*, 2: 159–76.

Rasmussen, C. (2005) 'Executive functioning and working memory in fetal alcohol spectrum disorder', *Alcoholism: Clinical and Experimental Research*, 29: 1359–67.

Rasmussen, C. and Bisanz, J. (2009) 'Executive functioning in children with fetal alcohol spectrum disorders: profiles and age-related differences', *Child Neuropsychology*, 15: 201–15.

Rasmussen, C., Horne, K. and Witol, A. (2006) 'Neurobehavioral functioning in children with fetal alcohol spectrum disorder', *Child Neuropsychology*, 12: 453–68.

Rasmussen, C., McAuley, R. and Andrew, G. (2007) 'Parental ratings of children with fetal alcohol spectrum disorder on the Behavior Rating Inventory of Executive Functioning (BRIEF)', *Journal of FAS International*, 5: 1–8.

Richardson, G.A., Ryan, C., Willford, J., Day, N.L. and Goldschmidt, L. (2002) 'Prenatal alcohol and marijuana exposure: effects on neuropsychological outcomes at 10 years', *Neurotoxicology and Teratology*, 24: 309–20.

Riikonen, R., Salonen, I., Partanen, K. and Verho, S. (1999) 'Brain perfusion SPECT and MRI in foetal alcohol syndrome', *Developmental Medicine and Child Neurology*, 41: 652–9.

Riikonen, R.S., Nokelainen, P., Valkonen, K., Kolehmainen, A.I., Kumpulainen, K.I., Kononen, M., Vanninen, R.L. and Kuikka, J.T. (2005) 'Deep serotonergic and dopaminergic structures in fetal alcoholic syndrome: a study with nor-beta-CIT-single-photon emission computed tomography and magnetic resonance imaging volumetry', *Biological Psychiatry*, 57: 1565–72.

Riley, E.P., Mattson, S.N., Sowell, E.R., Jernigan, T.L., Sobel, D.F. and Jones, K.L. (1995) 'Abnormalities of the corpus callosum in children prenatally exposed to alcohol', *Alcoholism: Clinical and Experimental Research*, 19: 1198–202.

Roebuck, T.M., Simmons, R.W., Richardson, C., Mattson, S.N. and Riley, E.P. (1998) 'Neuromuscular responses to disturbance of balance in children with prenatal exposure to alcohol', *Alcoholism: Clinical and Experimental Research*, 22: 1992–7.

Roebuck-Spencer, T.M. and Mattson, S.N. (2004) 'Implicit strategy affects learning in children with heavy prenatal alcohol exposure', *Alcoholism: Clinical and Experimental Research*, 28: 1424–31.

Roebuck-Spencer, T.M., Mattson, S.N., Marion, S.D., Brown, W.S. and Riley, E.P. (2004) 'Bimanual coordination in alcohol-exposed children: role of the corpus callosum', *Journal of the International Neuropsychological Society*, 10: 536–48.

Roussotte, F.F., Sulik, K.K., Mattson, S.N., Riley, E.P., Jones, K.L., Adnams, C.M., May, P.A., O'Connor, M.J., Narr, K.L. and Sowell, E.R. (2012) 'Regional brain volume reductions relate to facial dysmorphology and neurocognitive function in fetal alcohol spectrum disorders', *Human Brain Mapping*, 33: 920–37.

Santhanam, P., Li, Z., Hu, X., Lynch, M.E. and Coles, C.D. (2009) 'Effects of prenatal alcohol exposure on brain activation during an arithmetic task: an fMRI study', *Alcoholism: Clinical and Experimental Research*, 33: 1901–8.

Schonfeld, A.M., Mattson, S.N., Lang, A.R., Delis, D.C. and Riley, E.P. (2001) 'Verbal and nonverbal fluency in children with heavy prenatal alcohol exposure', *Journal of Studies on Alcohol*, 62: 239–46.

Schonfeld, A.M., Paley, B., Frankel, F. and O'Connor, M.J. (2006) 'Executive functioning predicts social skills following prenatal alcohol exposure', *Child Neuropsychology*, 12: 439–52.

Simmons, R.W., Levy, S.S., Riley, E.P., Madra, N.M. and Mattson, S.N. (2009) 'Central and peripheral timing variability in children with heavy prenatal alcohol exposure', *Alcoholism: Clinical and Experimental Research*, 33: 400–7.

Simmons, R.W., Nguyen, T.T., Levy, S.S., Thomas, J.D., Mattson, S.N. and Riley, E.P. (2012) 'Children with heavy prenatal alcohol exposure exhibit deficits when regulating isometric force', *Alcoholism: Clinical and Experimental Research*, 36: 302–9.

Simmons, R.W., Thomas, J.D., Levy, S.S. and Riley, E.P. (2006) 'Motor response selection in children with fetal alcohol spectrum disorders', *Neurotoxicology and Teratology*, 28: 278–85.

Simmons, R.W., Thomas, J.D., Levy, S.S. and Riley, E.P. (2010) 'Motor response programming and movement time in children with heavy prenatal alcohol exposure', *Alcohol*, 44: 371–8.

Simmons, R.W., Wass, T., Thomas, J.D. and Riley, E.P. (2002) 'Fractionated simple and choice reaction time in children with prenatal exposure to alcohol', *Alcoholism: Clinical and Experimental Research*, 26: 1412–19.

Sowell, E.R., Jernigan, T.L., Mattson, S.N., Riley, E.P., Sobel, D.F. and Jones, K.L. (1996) 'Abnormal development of the cerebellar vermis in children prenatally exposed to alcohol: size reduction in lobules I–V', *Alcoholism: Clinical and Experimental Research*, 20: 31–4.

Sowell, E.R., Johnson, A., Kan, E., Lu, L.H., Van Horn, J.D., Toga, A.W., O'Connor, M.J. and Bookheimer, S.Y. (2008a) 'Mapping white matter integrity and neurobehavioral correlates in children with fetal alcohol spectrum disorders', *Journal of Neuroscience*, 28: 1313–19.

Sowell, E.R., Lu, L.H., O'Hare, E.D., McCourt, S.T., Mattson, S.N., O'Connor, M.J. and Bookheimer, S.Y. (2007) 'Functional magnetic resonance imaging of verbal learning in children with heavy prenatal alcohol exposure', *NeuroReport*, 18: 635–9.

Sowell, E.R., Mattson, S.N., Thompson, P.M., Jernigan, T.L., Riley, E.P. and Toga, A.W. (2001a) 'Mapping callosal morphology and cognitive correlates: effects of heavy prenatal alcohol exposure', *Neurology*, 57: 235–44.

Sowell, E.R., Mattson, S.N., Kan, E., Thompson, P.M., Riley, E.P. and Toga, A.W. (2008b) 'Abnormal cortical thickness and brain-behavior correlation patterns in individuals with heavy prenatal alcohol exposure', *Cerebral Cortex*, 18: 136–44.

Sowell, E.R., Thompson, P.M., Mattson, S.N., Tessner, K.D., Jernigan, T.L., Riley, E.P. and Toga, A.W. (2001b) 'Voxel-based morphometric analyses of the brain in children and adolescents prenatally exposed to alcohol', *NeuroReport*, 12: 515–23.

Sowell, E.R., Thompson, P.M., Mattson, S.N., Tessner, K.D., Jernigan, T.L., Riley, E.P. and Toga, A.W. (2002a) 'Regional brain shape abnormalities persist into adolescence after heavy prenatal alcohol exposure', *Cerebral Cortex*, 12: 856–65.

Sowell, E.R., Thompson, P.M., Peterson, B.S., Mattson, S.N., Welcome, S.E., Henkenius, A.L., Riley, E.P., Jernigan, T.L. and Toga, A.W. (2002b) 'Mapping cortical gray matter asymmetry patterns in adolescents with heavy prenatal alcohol exposure', *Neuroimage*, 17: 1807–19.

Spadoni, A.D., Bazinet, A.D., Fryer, S.L., Tapert, S.F., Mattson, S.N. and Riley, E.P. (2009) 'BOLD response during spatial working memory in youth with heavy prenatal alcohol exposure', *Alcoholism: Clinical and Experimental Research*, 33: 2067–76.

Steinhausen, H.C., Willms, J. and Spohr, H.L. (1993) 'Long-term psychopathological and cognitive outcome of children with fetal alcohol syndrome', *Journal of the American Academy of Child and Adolescent Psychiatry*, 32: 990–4.

Streissguth, A.P., Aase, J.M., Clarren, S.K., Randels, S.P., LaDue, R.A. and Smith, D.F. (1991) 'Fetal alcohol syndrome in adolescents and adults', *Journal of the American Medical Association*, 265: 1961–7.

Streissguth, A.P., Barr, H.M., Sampson, P.D., Parrish-Johnson, J.C., Kirchner, G.L. and Martin, D.C. (1986) 'Attention, distraction and reaction time at age 7 years and prenatal alcohol exposure', *Neurobehavioral Toxicology and Teratology*, 8: 717–25.

Streissguth, A.P., Barr, H.M. and Sampson, P.D. (1990) 'Moderate prenatal alcohol exposure: effects on child IQ and learning problems at age 7½ years', *Alcoholism: Clinical and Experimental Research*, 14: 662–9.
Streissguth, A.P., Barr, H.M., Olson, H.C., Sampson, P.D., Bookstein, F.L. and Burgess, D.M. (1994a) 'Drinking during pregnancy decreases word attack and arithmetic scores on standardized tests: adolescent data from a population-based prospective study', *Alcoholism: Clinical and Experimental Research*, 18: 248–54.
Streissguth, A.P., Martin, D.C., Barr, H.M. and Sandman, B.M. (1984) 'Intrauterine alcohol and nicotine exposure: attention and reaction time in 4-year-old children', *Developmental Psychology*, 20: 533–41.
Streissguth, A.P., Sampson, P.D., Olson, H.C., Bookstein, F.L., Barr, H.M., Scott, M., Feldman, J. and Mirsky, A.F. (1994b) 'Maternal drinking during pregnancy: attention and short-term memory in 14-year-old offspring: a longitudinal prospective study', *Alcoholism: Clinical and Experimental Research*, 18: 202–18.
Stromland, K. and Pinazo-Duran, M.D. (2002) 'Ophthalmic involvement in the fetal alcohol syndrome: clinical and animal model studies', *Alcohol and Alcoholism*, 37: 2–8.
Swayze, V.W., 2nd, Johnson, V.P., Hanson, J.W., Piven, J., Sato, Y., Giedd, J.N., Mosnik, D. and Andreasen, N.C. (1997) 'Magnetic resonance imaging of brain anomalies in fetal alcohol syndrome', *Pediatrics*, 99: 232–40.
Thorne, J.C., Coggins, T.E., Olson, H.C. and Astley, S.J. (2007) 'Exploring the utility of narrative analysis in diagnostic decision making: picture-bound reference, elaboration, and fetal alcohol spectrum disorders', *Journal of Speech Language and Hearing Research*, 50: 459–74.
Timler, G.R., Olswang, L.B. and Coggins, T.E. (2005) '"Do I know what I need to do?" A social communication intervention for children with complex clinical profiles', *Language, Speech, and Hearing Services in Schools*, 36: 73–85.
Uecker, A. and Nadel, L. (1996) 'Spatial locations gone awry: object and spatial memory deficits in children with fetal alcohol syndrome', *Neuropsychologia*, 34: 209–23.
Uecker, A. and Nadel, L. (1998) 'Spatial but not object memory impairments in children with fetal alcohol syndrome', *American Journal of Mental Retardation*, 103: 12–18.
Vaurio, L., Riley, E.P. and Mattson, S.N. (2008) 'Differences in executive functioning in children with heavy prenatal alcohol exposure or attention-deficit/hyperactivity disorder', *Journal of the International Neuropsychological Society*, 14: 119–29.
Wass, T.S., Simmons, R.W., Thomas, J.D. and Riley, E.P. (2002) 'Timing accuracy and variability in children with prenatal exposure to alcohol', *Alcoholism: Clinical and Experimental Research*, 26: 1887–96.
Willford, J.A., Richardson, G.A., Leech, S.L. and Day, N.L. (2004) 'Verbal and visuospatial learning and memory function in children with moderate prenatal alcohol exposure', *Alcoholism: Clinical and Experimental Research*, 28: 497–507.
Willoughby, K.A., Sheard, E.D., Nash, K. and Rovet, J. (2008) 'Effects of prenatal alcohol exposure on hippocampal volume, verbal learning, and verbal and spatial recall in late childhood', *Journal of the International Neuropsychological Society*, 14: 1022–33.
Wisniewski, K., Dambska, M., Sher, J.H. and Qazi, Q. (1983) 'A clinical neuropathological study of the fetal alcohol syndrome', *Neuropediatrics*, 14: 197–201.
Wozniak, J.R., Mueller, B.A., Chang, P.N., Muetzel, R.L., Caros, L. and Lim, K.O. (2006) 'Diffusion tensor imaging in children with fetal alcohol spectrum disorders', *Alcoholism: Clinical and Experimental Research*, 30: 1799–806.
Wozniak, J.R., Mueller, B.A., Muetzel, R.L., Bell, C.J., Hoecker, H.L., Nelson, M.L., Chang, P.N. and Lim, K.O. (2011) 'Inter-hemispheric functional connectivity disruption in children with prenatal alcohol exposure', *Alcoholism: Clinical and Experimental Research*, 35: 849–61.
Wozniak, J.R., Muetzel, R.L., Mueller, B.A., McGee, C.L., Freerks, M.A., Ward, E.E., Nelson, M.L., Chang, P.N. and Lim, K.O. (2009) 'Microstructural corpus callosum anomalies in children with prenatal alcohol exposure: an extension of previous diffusion tensor imaging findings', *Alcoholism: Clinical and Experimental Research*, 33: 1825–35.
Yang, Y., Roussotte, F., Kan, E., Sulik, K.K., Mattson, S.N., Riley, E.P., Jones, K.L., Adnams, C.M., May, P.A., O'Connor, M.J., Narr, K.L. and Sowell, E.R. (2012) 'Abnormal cortical thickness alterations in fetal alcohol spectrum disorders and their relationships with facial dysmorphology', *Cerebral Cortex*, 22: 1170–9.

19

DEVELOPMENTAL PSYCHIATRIC DISORDERS IN CHILDREN, ADOLESCENTS AND YOUNG ADULTS WITH FETAL ALCOHOL SPECTRUM DISORDERS (FASD)

A transgenerational approach to diagnosis and management

Kieran D. O'Malley

Introduction

Fetal alcohol spectrum disorders (FASD)[1] can be understood as specific developmental psychiatric disorders. There are two conditions: dysmorphic fetal alcohol syndrome (FAS), and the far more common, non-dysmorphic alcohol-related neurodevelopmental disorder (ARND).[2] Continuing clinical and epidemiological work in different settings has consistently shown the long-term psychiatric, cognitive and functional consequences of FASD (Densmore 2011; Fast *et al.* 1999; Hagerman 1999; Moore and Green 2004; Nowick Brown *et al.* 2011; Page 2008; Streissguth and O'Malley 2000), and longitudinal studies have suggested that individuals with FASD are at high risk for psychiatric disorders and poor social life adjustment.

Although the first Irish published psychiatric/psychological academic paper on FASD appeared only in 2010 (Orakwue *et al.* 2010), the preponderance of psychiatric disorders among adult patients with FAS was first reported by Lemoine and Lemoine (1992) in a 30-year follow-up of his original child patients. Later, Streissguth and colleagues at the University of Washington (UW) in their 1996 Secondary Disabilities Study (Streissguth and Kanter 1997; Streissguth *et al.* 1996) highlighted the prevalence of mental health problems and psychiatric disorders.

Streissguth *et al.*'s study investigated the lifespan progression of ARND (Hoyme *et al.* 2005; Smith 1981). Disturbingly, they found that over 90 per cent of individuals in the study, from age six years to adulthood, had mental health problems or psychiatric disorders. The conditions were often undiagnosed, poorly understood, and had no systematic management plan. Of the 62 adults with FAS or fetal alcohol effects (FAE) (now ARND), 92 per cent had a mental health diagnosis (psychiatric disorder), 65 per cent were diagnosed with attention deficit/hyperactivity disorder (ADHD), 45 per cent with depression, and 21 per cent with panic disorder. In the current UK and Irish contexts, these findings are still very relevant.

The impact of prenatal alcohol exposure on the brain

Alcohol is a teratogenic prenatal neurotoxin that not only differentially affects the structure of the developing brain (e.g. the developing hippocampus, cerebellum and corpus callosum) throughout pregnancy, but also critically changes the balance of the developing neurotransmitters. Animal research has identified that the short allele of the serotonin transporter gene (5-hydroxytryptamine (5HT)) is affected by prenatal alcohol exposure. This gene influences the appearance of anxiety disorders through increasing hypothalamic pituitary adrenal (HPA) axis activation (Archibald et al. 2001; British Medical Association 2007; Goodlett et al. 2005; Hagerman 1999; Kraemer et al. 2008; Mukherjee et al. 2012; Nowick Brown et al. 2011; O'Malley and Mukherjee 2010; Riley et al. 1995; Sowell et al. 2008; Stratton et al. 1996). Furthermore, animal research has identified the effect of prenatal alcohol exposure on Dopamine 2 Receptors (D2R) as a key biochemical factor in the development of sensory under- or over-responsiveness (Screiber et al. 2008). Also, the effects of prenatal alcohol exposure on inhibitory gamma-aminobutyric acid (GABA) and excitatory N-methyl-D-aspartic acid (NMDA) can kindle seizures.

Infants exposed to prenatal alcohol may show immediate neurological sequelae, as shown in the 1974/1975 Seattle 500 Longitudinal Study. Streissguth and colleagues demonstrated that on neonate days one and two infants showed problems in habituation, and state regulation, decreased suck reflex and longer latency to suck (Smith 1981; Streissguth et al. 2004). The immediate temperament challenges of these brain-damaged infants and neonates may result in abnormal attachment, bonding and dyadic connections. Although this is often attributed to postpartum depression in birth mothers (Murray et al. 2011), it may be the temperamental difficulties of the infant from basic feeding, state regulation, habituation and general reactivity that drive the mother/infant dyad and not the other way around. The 'difficult to settle' or the 'slow to warm' temperaments offer clinical frames for understanding infants with FASD (Chess and Thomas 1977).

CLINICAL VIGNETTE[3]

A 22-month Irish/Lithuanian boy (GH) was assessed for possible effects of prenatal alcohol exposure. His birth mother disclosed that she drank vodka steadily for the first six months of her pregnancy, then stopped as she would become nauseous when she drank. There was no history of intellectual disability in either birth parent. GH was born at term in a local maternity hospital but at birth his weight was low for his gestational age. His temperament was 'difficult to settle' in infancy, and this temperament persists. He was removed from his birth home at three months because of concerns about neglect and the birth mother's return to alcohol addiction postnatally. GH is still with his initial foster placement.

He was monitored closely by a health visitor, and his height and weight indicated a marked failure to thrive up to 12 months. Since 12 months of age, his weight remained at the twenty-fifth percentile, but his height was just below the tenth percentile, although his birth parents are normal or above average height. The health visitor also carefully documented delays in gross and fine motor skills, early social/emotional development difficulties and language difficulties. She struggled to obtain an accurate hearing test as

GH was so restless and reactive to sound and light in the examining room. He had evidence of a right eye strabismus which needed ophthalmologist examination.

GH had little spontaneous play with few vocalizations, and was incapable of co-operative or imitative play as he was too sensory seeking and distracted by his surroundings. Formal assessment of sensory motor function showed auditory, visual, olfactory, tactile and co-ordination problems.

GH had classic FAS facial dysmorphology with microcephaly. He also had global developmental delay with early features consistent with ARND, and presented a regulatory disorder (sensory stimulation seeking/impulsive).

At this age it would be important for GH to have genetic and ophthalmology consultations, but immediate multi-modal strategies include sensory integration therapy, speech and language therapy and occupational therapy for co-ordination.

Diagnostic classification of FASD

The diagnosis and, ultimately, the treatment and management of individuals affected by prenatal alcohol exposure have been complicated for many years by the lack of appropriate neuropsychiatric diagnostic formulation. These difficulties are illustrative of the lack of understanding around environmentally induced disorders (Howlin *et al.* 2011; O'Malley 2011a). This continues to prevent any proper epidemiological research on the multitude of psychiatric and cognitive problems found in significant numbers of individuals with a clear history of prenatal alcohol exposure from an early age.

Three diagnostic classification systems are commonly used to communicate diagnostic findings:

1. *International Classification of Diseases* (ICD) (World Health Organization 2004);
2. *Diagnostic and Statistical Manual of Mental Disorders* (DSM) (American Psychiatric Association 2000);
3. *Diagnostic Classification of Mental Health and Developmental Disorders of Infancy and Early Childhood* (DC: 0–3) (Zero to Three 2005).

The ICD is used for both medical and mental health diagnoses, whereas the DSM is used solely for mental health diagnoses. Both are necessary for communicating the complex deficits and conditions associated with FASD, but currently these classification systems present problems with respect to FASD diagnosis because they do not acknowledge the more prevalent condition of ARND and they do not place FASD in a neurodevelopmental disorder frame. However, this is being considered for the most recent edition of the DSM (Pine *et al.* 2012).

The ICD lists 'Fetal Alcohol Syndrome (dysmorphic)' as a specific medical diagnosis under its congenital malformations section, and developmental psychiatric disorder can be established through a full ICD axis profile. For example:

Axis I: Described a ten-year-old Irish boy in a foster home placement who had a confirmed history of prenatal alcohol exposure and clinical features of FAS. Recent clinical assessment established there was no evidence of attachment disorder; the boy had been in the same foster home placement since 12 months of age and was well attached to his foster parents. Hyperkinetic disorder (or you could say ADHD) – Inattention/Impulsive subtype – was identified.

Axis II: Evidence of complex learning disorder with specific spelling disorder and specific disorder of arithmetic skills [assess using the Wechsler Intelligence Scale for Children (WISC-IV), the Wechsler Individual Achievement Test (WIAT-2) or another appropriate psychological test]; evidence of language disorder with problems in expressive and receptive language [assess using the Clinical Evaluation of Language Fundamentals (CELF-2) or another language pragmatics test which can identify social communication disorder with problems in social cognition and social communication (Coggins *et al.* 2008; Greenbaum *et al.* 2009)].

Axis III: 12-point difference between verbal IQ (=88) and performance IQ (=76) [assess using WISC].

Axis IV: FAS; evidence of specific developmental disorder of motor function with developmental co-ordination disorder.

Axis V: Early psychosocial stressor of separation from birth parents at one year.

Axis VI: Level of functioning 50/100 as in school.

In a similar way, the DSM allows mental health professionals to code anxiety, mood or psychotic disorder due to the general medical condition of prenatal alcohol exposure with clinical evidence of ARND. 'Cognitive disorder not otherwise specified (NOS)' is the best DSM descriptor of the learning disorder associated with FASD, along with psychiatric diagnoses such as ADHD or mood disorder, and provides the option for mental health professionals to diagnose this disorder as 'secondary to FAS or ARND'. As with the ICD, the DSM's five-axis structure supports the same diagnostic descriptive approach. For example:

Axis I: Describes an eight-year-old girl with mood disorder and intermittent explosive disorder with history of prenatal alcohol exposure and clinical evidence of ARND.

Axis II: A verbal IQ of 77 and a performance IQ of 81 identified; subtests showed reading disorder, writing disorder, mathematics disorder and working memory at first percentile [assess using WISC].

Axis III: Evidence of developmental co-ordination disorder identified; also right eye strabismus and ventricular septal defect – both recognized alcohol-related birth defects (ARBD) (Stratton *et al.* 1996; O'Malley 2008).

Axis IV: Psychosocial stressor of continual school failure with no special needs support in school identified.

Axis V: Level of functioning 40/100 as currently out of school.

Zero to Three's DC: 0–3 (2005) is an essential validated instrument which can describe the initial presentation of ARND. The three most common presentations of psychiatric disorder in infants or young children with either FAS or ARND come under the 'regulatory disorders of sensory processing' category, and capture quite accurately the range of sensory integration problems caused by the prenatal neurotoxic impact of alcohol. They are:

1. Hypersensitive (subtypes: Type A – fearful/cautious; Type B – negative/defiant)
2. Hyposensitive/underresponsive
3. Sensory stimulation seeking/impulsive.

Psychiatric diagnosis and management of FASD

Both FAS and ARND present well-recognized behavioural phenotypes including regulatory disorders, ADHD, autistic spectrum disorders (ASD) or Asperger's syndrome, intermittent explosive disorder and mood/affective instability. As a result, FASD – whether dysmorphic FAS or non-dysmorphic ARND – may be overlooked and misdiagnosed as one or more of its associated 'phenotype' disorders, even when the phenotype diagnosis does not meet the full diagnostic criteria. In childhood, ADHD or hyperkinetic disorders are the most common diagnoses that 'mask' prenatal alcohol exposure. It is only when the child does not respond to standard treatment (e.g. methylphenidate) or experiences many school academic difficulties that an organic hypothesis for FAS or ARND enters into the diagnostic and management frame.

CLINICAL VIGNETTE

A 35-year-old single Caucasian mother (AB), with a history of depression and domestic violence in a common-law relationship, delivered an infant exposed to alcohol. The infant boy (GD) had a 'difficult to settle' temperament from birth, continuing into early childhood. The birth mother struggled with basic parenting, and the young child became unmanageable with temper tantrums, explosive episodes and periods of severe anxiety or panic.

The mother saw a number of psychologists with her son between ages four and six years. GD was prescribed play therapy which did not work. He was then assessed by the local Child and Adolescent Mental Health Service team a number of times between seven and ten years of age. His behavioural profile was attributed to a range of diagnoses including ADHD, oppositional defiant disorder (ODD), ASD, possible psychotic disorder and finally inconsistent/inadequate parenting (the latter being the most destructive to the mother). A prescription of methylphenidate made his problems worse, and a subsequent switch to biphasic, Concerta, did not improve the situation.

The mother became overwhelmed, but sought a further opinion, recognizing that the alcohol in pregnancy that she took in response to severe depression and domestic violence might be related to her child's unusual behaviours. Her feelings of guilt had prevented her from disclosing this in previous assessments, but neither had professionals questioned her about the possibility of her son's prenatal alcohol exposure.

This gave rise to a hypothesis of prenatal alcohol, linked to a presentation consistent with ARND, being suggested. It fitted the child's profile, and afforded an opportunity for a more specialized multi-modal treatment programme, including sensory integration and a specialized school placement. Formal academic cognitive testing quantified the child's social communication disorder and severe problems in verbal processing of information. This led to a transdisciplinary conceptualization of a developmental psychiatric disorder – a combination of learning disorder and psychiatric disorder. An essential component of ongoing management was mother/child dyadic support.

Co-occurring psychiatric disorders in patients with FASD should always be considered in relation to the brain damage that can be caused by the prenatal alcohol exposure (Archibald et al. 2001; Bookstein et al. 2002; Mattson et al. 1996; Riley et al. 1995; Sowell et al. 2007, 2008). For example the association between brain circuits and structural brain damage has been well established in relation to such problematic conditions as antisocial personality disorder (Raine et al. 2000). The prenatal alcohol effect on the developing corpus callosum, frontal lobes, hippocampus and cerebellum all have potential effects on executive function decision making, impulsivity and memory which must be incorporated in the diagnostic understanding of the patient's clinical presentation.

Age related shifts in developmental psychiatric presentations of FASD

Presentation of FASD in childhood is commonly coupled with physical symptoms such as disruptive behavioural problems, chronic headaches, abdominal pain or unspecified pain. This somatic expression and externalization are due to the common inability of children with FASD to express their emotional distress in words. For example, in the language disability alexithymia, patients somaticize their emotional pain and present physical pain as the focus of their distress (Sifneos 1973; Sullivan 2008).

One of the confusing clinical issues in diagnosis and management of FASD is that the developmental impairments do not appear at uniform times, but present differently depending on the chronological and mental age of the patient. According to the regulatory disorders guidelines in DC: 0–3R (Zero to Three 2005), sensory integration problems are identifiable in infancy, while social cognition and communication problems are more easily identified during the toddler years; developmental executive function problems commonly surface in

TABLE 19.1 Percentages of psychiatric disorders found in children, adolescents and adults with FASD in certain research populations

	Percentage psychiatric disorders in population			
Study and cohort details	ADHD/ ADD	Depression/mood disorder	PDD/Anxiety disorder	Addictive disorder
Streissguth et al. 1996, n=417, 6–51 years old, parent/patient report	60%	20%	20%	–
O'Malley 2001, n=51, 3–33 years old, psychiatric examination	58%	44%	–	–
O'Malley 2011a★, n=59, infancy to 20 years old, psychiatric examination	60%	20%	15%	–
Famy et al. 1998, n=25, adults, Structured Clinical Interview for DSM-IV I and II	–	44%	20%	60%

★ Intermittent explosive disorder and regulatory disorder; other disorders in sample.

the school setting disguised as multiple psychiatric disorders (e.g. ADHD – commonly the inattention type coupled with impulsivity – disruptive behaviour disorder, intermittent explosive disorder, affective instability or ASD, with comorbid complex learning disabilities) that can be quantified on standard cognitive tests such as the Wechsler Preschool and Primary Scale of Intelligence (WPPSI) or WISC (Althoff 2010; Brown 2009; Mukherjee *et al.* 2008; Nanson 1992; O'Connor *et al.* 2002; O'Malley 2008; O'Malley and Nanson 2002; Vidal 2012). These developmentally distinct psychiatric disorders form the evolving and shifting behavioural phenotype of infants and children with FASD. In many ways they reflect changing brain maturation.

Developmental psychiatric presentations also vary across the age range. This is not unlike the presentation of the classic FAS dysmorphic facial features which are 'fleeting' (i.e. evident in infancy, most obvious from 6 to 12 years of age, but increasingly less identifiable in adolescence or young adulthood). Thus regulatory disorder (hypersensitive type) later becomes diagnosable as ADHD; regulatory disorder (hyposensitive type) becomes ASD or mood disorder; and regulatory disorder (sensory seeking/impulsive) can become co-occurring ADHD/ASD/pervasive developmental disorder (PDD). Recent interest in early onset bipolar disorder (EOBD) in the USA is offering clinical insights into the understanding of the initial psychiatric presentation of FAS or ARND (Althoff 2010; Carlson *et al.* 2009). In adolescence ADHD can become early alcohol addictive disorder, or mood disorder with impulsive suicide risk (O'Malley 2011a; Turk 2007).

The developmental psychiatric disorders have to be seen within the context of the comorbid complex learning disabilities, and therefore ARND, which can impair the patient's ability to communicate or understand their emotional distress (Sullivan 2008). For example:

- Conditions such as alexithymia, the inability to have words for emotions (well recognized in the field of psychosomatic disorders; Sifneos 1973) were critical constructs necessary to unravel the intermittent explosive disorder in a nine-year-old boy with ARND.
- The social communication disorder in a 12-year-old girl with ARND and ADHD presented a co-occurring pseudo 'autistic' picture which changes markedly in response to ADHD medication; the medication ameliorates the pervasive auditory and visual distractibility that impedes the processing of social information.
- Affective or mood instability can present features of 'emotional incontinence' similar to that in children with traumatic brain injury.

Effective clinical case management of FASD

Effective clinical case management of FASD requires:

1. constructing a '*scaffolding containment system*' around the patient and his/her family;
2. adopting a '*family-based systemic approach*';
3. *forming a diagnostic or working hypothesis*;
4. *ensuring multi-system involvement* (i.e. different educational, psychological, medical, nursing, social service systems, etc.) which addresses the transgenerational problem.

Always remember that alcohol is at the core of the FASD transgenerational problem; always think about multi-generational diagnoses and multi-system involvement.

> **CLINICAL VIGNETTE**
>
> A 15-year-old Irish teenager (KM) had been binge drinking weekly for two years. She reported being pregnant a year ago, but losing the pregnancy in the first few months. She did not follow-up at the maternity hospital, but became involved with child and adolescent psychiatry after a serious, self-harm overdose of paracetamol, and a short crisis hospitalization in a paediatric hospital.
>
> She was found to have been prenatally exposed to alcohol. Hospital and school records revealed a history of developmental delay, academic school failure with particular problems in mathematics and English. The school had not carried out any formal academic tests because her school attendance had been inconsistent, but she had been labelled as having ODD. The hospital school assessments showed clear evidence of dyslexia, dyscalculia and poor working memory. As KM had no dysmorphic FAS facial features, she was diagnosed with ARND.
>
> KM presented a clinical picture of a combination of affective instability with some emotional incontinence and intermittent explosive disorder that had not responded to previous individual insight-orientated psychotherapy in the community. In conversation with professionals, she described having had a craving for alcohol from as early as nine or eleven years of age, and said that she had started drinking continuously at 12 years old.
>
> She also reported a sexual assault episode three weeks before her overdose. The A&E hospital which treated her had verified sexual assault, but would not fully believe her story as she had a learning disability and could not consistently remember the details. Child protection services in the hospital were contacted by the hospital social worker working with the consultation liaison child and adolescent psychiatrist, and the community child protection services in the teenager's group home area were contacted as the perpetrator was a well-known, violent, teenage boy who was in care.
>
> KM was the subject of an interim custody agreement between social services and her birth mother, who was still alcohol dependent and may herself have had an ARND due to her own prenatal alcohol exposure.
>
> On the positive side KM responded to carbamazepine, and her mood became much more settled with no explosive episodes in over two months.
>
> With the epidemic of underage drinking in Ireland and the UK, this type of case could become a 'new norm'. How could services protect this vulnerable teenager with ARND, protect her from an unplanned, possibly alcohol-exposed pregnancy, and approach/ support her birth mother's home environment? Effective management in this case would have to begin with 'joining up' of child and adult services in obstetrics, developmental paediatrics, psychiatry, social service and addiction.

Constructing a scaffolding containment system

The first principle in effective clinical case management of FASD is the construction of a 'scaffolding containment system' around the patient and his/her family (Page 2008).

The quality and stability of the childhood home environment is a crucial factor in the ultimate outcome of those with FAS or ARND. Children, especially in early childhood, who are provided with positive, structured and nurturing environments where their challenges are met with consistent parenting, will be more likely to cope with their developmental or psychiatric disabilities. Therefore, it is essential to contain the vulnerable infant or child early in development in a suitable safe, structured, predictable nurturing environment. Social Services have an essential role in assessing the safety of the home environment and, if necessary, facilitating placement in safer environments. The impact of alcohol addiction in home environments is multi-factorial: it affects physical, emotional and cognitive development at many levels, while possibly exposing the vulnerable infant or child to risk of abuse due to lack of safe boundaries (Abudabo and Cohen 2011; Dumaret *et al.* 2009; Streissguth *et al.* 1996, 2004).

Adopting a family-based systemic approach

Clinical presentations of patients with dysmorphic FAS or non-dysmorphic ARND show a combination of developmental disorder and co-occurring psychiatric disorder. The latter may arise as a result of the environmental impact of the rearing home. All alcohol-exposed infants are subsequently reared in environments that have a modulating effect one way or another on clinical expression of the neurotoxic effects of that exposure. Clinicians need to adopt a family-based systemic approach that identifies key environmental supports and stressors in the patient's environment (Grant *et al.* 2009; Nowick Brown *et al.* 2011; O'Malley 2008, 2011a; Page 2008).

In particular, a mother who drinks during pregnancy and suffers postpartum depression creates an immediate challenge to parent/infant bonding. The rearing environment must therefore be assessed, especially if there is evidence that direct or indirect violence (i.e. abuse or witnessing domestic violence) has occurred beyond the typical impact of a chaotic home environment and/or insecure attachment disorders often seen in the children of alcoholics (COA).

When the family environment is protective and nurturing, challenging behaviours are most likely to be caused by deficient adaptive, social and executive functioning stemming from the neurotoxin central nervous system dysfunction (Nowick Brown *et al.* 2011; O'Malley 2011a). However, as well as organic brain damage from their FASD condition, children (including many of those adopted from Romanian and Russian orphanages) may suffer the effects of early emotional deprivation. Prenatal stress (e.g. due to developing *in utero* within a violent, disorganized home setting) or post-traumatic stress disorder (PTSD) in a pregnant mother also have certain neurochemical sequelae on the HPA axis function resulting in a synergistic effect on fetal brain development from combined cortisol and prenatal alcohol (Meewise *et al.* 2007). Emotional deprivation may also be due to familial mental illness where a parent is emotionally unavailable for active parenting. Sometimes this is reflective of the transgenerational cognitive legacy of alcohol, which impairs maternal and paternal organizational and emotional regulation abilities.

This can lead to challenging (but not untreatable) insecure ambivalent resistant, or ambivalent avoidant attachment patterns. As a result, among the postnatal and early childhood vulnerabilities in FASD is a tendency for infants and young children to experience multiple placements before the fifth birthday due to their difficult and un-predictable behaviours.

Forming a diagnostic or working hypothesis

The essential clinical component related to prenatal alcohol exposure is the presence of a developmental psychiatric disorder, and the aetiology being sought is either genetic or environmental. Management of psychiatric disorders in FASD begins with medical and mental health professionals 'forming a diagnostic or working hypothesis'.

An early diagnosis or neurodevelopmental working hypothesis is crucial as it avoids the impasse of a 'reactive attachment disorder' diagnosis. This diagnosis sites the infant or young child's difficulties with the parents, instead of attributing them to complex brain damage caused through prenatal alcohol exposure. In making such a diagnosis, professionals invalidate the valuable objective observations of foster or adoptive parents and immobilize many, thus, through misdiagnosis, denying the child effective parenting. However, in some birth families where parents continue to abuse alcohol and provide an adverse rearing environment, this diagnosis, although painful, may offer an opportunity to break a cycle of transgenerational addiction and subsequent transgenerational prenatally created brain damage.

Ensuring multi-system involvement

The involvement of different health, education and social service systems in the diagnosis and management of FASD is essential, and should include addiction services. Although the USA, Canada and France are many years ahead of the rest of Europe in the integrated understanding of these issues, they have still not developed consistent diagnostic or management strategies which incorporate a developmental psychiatric understanding.

Multi-system involvement begins with the transgenerational approach to alcohol. The idea that alcohol craving and subsequent abuse or dependence in prepubertal children, adolescents and young adults with FASD may have their origins in prenatal alcohol exposure has been demonstrated by animal and human researchers for many years (Baer *et al.* 2003; Barr and Streissguth 2001; Barr *et al.* 2006; Reyes *et al.* 1985). Thus effective management of transgenerational drinking has to involve general acceptance that maternal drinking may reflect a prenatally kindled biochemical craving for alcohol due to the effect of prenatal alcohol exposure on the developing brain, especially the nucleus accumbens (O'Malley 2003, 2011a).

When children or adolescents with FASD live with birth parents who have FAS or ARND themselves, this can cause diverse clinical management problems compounded by the historical pervasive disconnection between addiction services for adolescents and adults and psychiatry and/or learning disability (O'Malley 2003, 2011b). The impact of parental FASD-associated difficulties include the chronic crisis and chaos arising from problems in dependent living and employment, and also those associated with problem solving (e.g. poor judgement, poor organizational skills, coupled with impulsivity, difficulty in making decisions and inadequate interpersonal relationships (Fast *et al.* 1999; Streissguth *et al.* 1996).

At this juncture there is little formal connection between adult mental health or adult learning disability services and child/adolescent mental health or learning disability services and so there is no natural case management forum to discuss the family/parenting challenges. Transgenerational alcohol abuse and dependence management requires Health and Social Service systems collaborating across traditional age-divides (i.e. child/adolescent/ adult). Obstetricians and midwives need to become sensitive to implicit risks in the developing fetus from alcohol use in any trimester of pregnancy. One effective model is the Parent Child Assistance Program (PCAP), an advocacy programme in Seattle, which began working with substance-abusing pregnant mothers in 1991. They acknowledge the complexity of working with a parent/infant dyad if the parent has FASD (Grant *et al.* 2009; Werner *et al.* 1986).

In the UK, hospital-based services are beginning to address the critical area of perinatal psychiatry which seeks to identify mentally or developmentally vulnerable pregnant mothers and their potentially vulnerable newborn infants. The vulnerable pregnant woman may have a mixture of psychiatric disorder, addictive disorder and even developmental disorder (Henshaw *et al.* 2009).

Education-based approaches

School failure was first identified as a major problem by Streissguth and colleagues and continues to present significant management challenges. These children are often 'hidden' under diagnoses such as ADHD, ASD, ODD or bipolar disorder and the organic roots to their learning, behavioural, psychiatric and language problems are not recognized (Streissguth *et al.* 1996).

School-based assessment typically focuses not only on the child's learning disabilities, but also any classroom behaviours that may be affecting a child's learning progress. This may include history of suspension from school. However, standard school testing is often limited and can miss the multiple functional, academic, social and language impairments associated with FASD which impede the child's ability to learn in a standard classroom environment. Most frequently it is when the child displays attention problems and/or disruptive behaviours in the classroom, ADHD is considered and a referral is made, often resulting in a prescription of methylphenidate (brand name: Ritalin). However, for FASD patients, often Ritalin is not effective and so the school-based problems continue. It is at this juncture, or in the context of a suspension, that a comprehensive child psychiatric assessment of a possible neurodevelopmental disorder should be carried out, preferably by a paediatrician.

Embedded in the Streissguth *et al.*'s secondary disability study was the demonstration that over 60 per cent of children with FASD had a disrupted school experience which progressively increased during the adolescent years. Obviously school systems were not meeting the patients' needs. The early recognition of FASD is critical to school success and the avoidance of disrupted school experiences identified by Streissguth and colleagues (Streissguth *et al.* 1996), and a **neurodevelopmental assessment is the kernel of understanding FAS or ARND** developmental psychiatric presentations. There was therefore a critical need to understand the complexity of the developmental of psychiatric FASD (FAS or ARND) in terms of broader-based functional assessments including four clinical assessment areas which contribute to the overall presentation (O'Malley and Rich 2013):

1. language and social skills assessment;
2. mood dysregulation and autonomic arousal;
3. cognitive and executive dysfunctions;
4. multisensory functional and perceptual deficits.

An assessment of functional ability compared with IQ (e.g. using the Vineland Adaptive Behaviour Scales (VABS) (Elias *et al.* submitted)) within a school's evaluation of a child or adolescent has already resulted in many gains in knowledge and understanding in the USA and Canada, and informed school curriculum planning in places such as British Columbia and Alberta in Canada. Early school recognition of FASD could become the lynchpin of multi-system intervention, including a more holistic approach to vocational training, which could incorporate the many strengths of learners with FASD – music, drama, sport, beauty care, mechanics, woodwork, home cooking, to name but a few.

The child protection system

There are situations when a referral to child protection services during pregnancy would be a safety and prophylactic measure for both mother and infant. There is a need for more parent/family support services for alcohol-abusing pregnant women who are often exposed to domestic violence.

Psychological management

Although few evidence-based psychological treatments have been shown to work consistently in FAS or ARND populations, and few have scientific validity (Kodituwakku and Kodituwakku 2011), some psychological management approaches have proven value (O'Malley 2008, 2011a; Mattson et al. 2011). Unfortunately standard outpatient Child and Adolescent Mental Health Service (CAMHS) practice in the UK and Ireland generally does not incorporate developmental psychiatric patients. When this is the case, children with FASD become further disadvantaged by being effectively excluded from mainstream psychological or even psychiatric systems. A psychological management approach may include any of the following, but remember that these therapies work best in a multi-modal context; that is, with concurrent speech and language therapy, occupational therapy for sensory integration, or medication therapy (O'Malley 2008):

1. *individual play therapy*, especially if child has also experienced abuse or domestic violence;
2. *reality-based therapy* to help child or adolescent navigate life stages and family transitions;
3. *trauma-based therapy* for severely vulnerable child with features of developmental trauma disorder as well as FAS or ARND;
4. *dyadic therapy* for child and parent (usually the mother) at different stages (e.g. early childhood, later in adolescence, etc.); this may include work on identity, conflict and antipathy towards birth parent;
5. *family therapy* related to family education and family instrumental work on daily living organization, or family stress resulting from the burden of caring for someone with chronic neurodevelopmental disorder;
6. *group therapy* has been used sporadically but has real potential in the realm of socialization skills training in adolescents and young adults;
7. *parallel therapy* between adult psychiatric and addiction providers and child psychiatric/ psychological providers to address the transgenerational issues (O'Malley 2003; Nowick Brown et al. 2011; Turk 2007);
8. *intergenerational psychotherapy and support* is needed, especially in countries with transgenerational FASD such as Ireland and the UK; here there needs to be integration

of services between adult psychiatric and addiction providers and child psychiatric and psychological providers (O'Malley 2003; Turk 2007);
9. *addiction counselling* is an important approach for birth mothers, but this type of therapy may not be suitable for birth parents who have FASD themselves and therefore have differing levels of cognitive processing impairment;
10. *parent support* with respite care utilizing the concept of an 'auxiliary brain' for the patient to help them navigate life's tasks and stages (Bertrand 2009).

Animal research is now involved in exploring models of experience-based interventions to decrease or manage the behavioural deficits caused by prenatal alcohol exposure (Hannigan *et al.* 2007). A recent review by Bertrand in 2009 delineated a number of interventions that had positive results.

Medical medication management

There is continuing research on new medications that may modulate or decrease the neurotoxic alcohol damage (Savage *et al.* 2010). Medication may also improve the participation of FASD patients in other important treatment modalities such as non-verbal play therapy, speech and language therapy or sensory integration therapy (O'Malley 2008). However, medication management must always be part of a multi-modal array of services for both the child and his/her family (O'Malley 2008) including family therapy and support, which are essential.

Combined pharmacotherapy inevitably involves more risks in this unpredictable brain-damaged population due to potential ARBD-associated cardiac, renal or even liver dysfunction. There have been few studies of single medications in FASD, let alone combinations of medications (Wilens 2009). Although medication, and especially polydrug therapy, is used extensively in co-occurring psychiatric disorders associated with FASD, this is done without approval from the Food and Drug Administration (FDA) of the United States or from the National Institute of Clinical Excellence (NICE) in the United Kingdom. In fact, despite co-occurring mood disorders presenting in almost all children and adults with FASD, there are no medium- or large-scale scientific drug industry or government-sponsored randomized clinical studies in any age group of this patient population (Kodituwakku and Kodituwakku 2011; Nowick Brown *et al.* 2011; O'Malley 2011a).

The following paragraphs set out possible medication management related to certain clinical presentations of FAS or ARND in which medication has a proven role:

ADHD symptoms

The complexity of ADHD comorbidities has been long recognized (Brown 2009). The co-occurrence of ADHD appears to be the commonest psychiatric condition in FASD, most often presenting inattention and impulsivity, without physical hyperactivity, in both children and adults (O'Malley 2010; O'Malley and Nanson 2002; O'Malley and Storoz 2003; Streissguth *et al.* 1996). Medications such as psychostimulants do have an ameliorating role, and some initial small clinical studies have shown that Dextroamphetamine seems more efficacious than methylphenidate (O'Malley 2008). Long-acting biphasic or bimodal (in USA) agents such as Concerta (USA), Equasym, and Medikinet (UK) may be helpful and can increase medication compliance. However, proper double-blind placebo studies have yet to be performed in patients with FASD.

In addition, prenatal nicotine also has been identified as a synergistic biochemical agent that kindles ADHD (Altink *et al.* 2009; Mick *et al.* 2002; Milberger *et al.* 1996) Long-acting guanfacine (which is not available in the UK) may be useful in such cases, as is the short-acting version, but this needs to be studied in this patient population (Salee *et al.* 2009). There is a proposal for a study of this medication versus atomoxetine in ADHD being carried out in Ireland (McNicholas 2011, pers. comm.).

Mood disorders

In FASD, mood disorders are really emotional dysregulations caused by the effects of prenatal exposure on developing neurotransmitters. These can range from deep-rooted depressive feelings to uncontrollable mood instability which mimics a rapid cycling bipolar disorder. Early childhood regulatory disorders are often a combination of a disturbance of autonomic arousal, attention, behaviour and mood. Recent interest in EOBD in the USA is beginning to offer clinical insights into the understanding of the initial psychiatric presentation of FASD (Carlson *et al.* 2009; Geller *et al.* 2002). Patients with co-occurring mood disorders may present with what is called 'emotional incontinence', or unprovoked cascades of crying or laughing. Carbamazepine, valproic acid or even GABA agents such as gabapentin or progablin can be effective in treating these symptoms (Wozniak and Biederman 1996).[4]

Mood disorder medications that have shown to be useful include fluoxetine (in liquid or tablet form), sertraline and citalopram. It is best to start with low dosage fluoxetine and build slowly, being especially aware of an activation effect in the first week which may bring forth increased agitation or even increased suicidal tendencies.

Tricyclic antidepressants are contraindicated as they can increase the risk of cardio-toxicity in a patient population known to have potential cardiac problems (ARBD effect) from their prenatal alcohol exposure (Byrne 2008; Hagerman 1999; O'Malley 2008). Therefore, a pre-treatment electrocardiograph (ECG) is essential before prescribing.

If the antidepressants, serotonin-specific reuptake inhibitors (SSRIs) are used, and the patient becomes pregnant, dosage needs to be carefully monitored as neonatal neurobehavioral effects have been described as a result of prenatal exposure (Oberlander *et al.* 2009). SSRIs may be teratogenic to heart in pregnancy.

Mood disorders also must always be assessed in the context of the family, as environmental factors (e.g. abuse, recent losses or separations, change in family constellation such as arrival of a new sibling, or illness in a parent) may have a profound kindling, or synergistic effect, on the appearance or severity of the mood disorder (O'Malley 2008, 2010).

Conduct disorders

Frequent problems with conduct are seen in children who come from family environments where there is a transgenerational history of disorganized or even absent parenting. FASD tends to run through multiple generations in a family, and recent clinical work in the UK and Ireland has focused on the risk of conduct disorders when FASD affects several generations within a family. Conduct disorders frequently include aggressive/explosive episodes and may progress to fire setting or even cruelty to animals. A sleep-deprived electroencephalogram (EEG) may rule out a complex partial seizure disorder, and a supplementary examination may uncover sexual or physical abuse.

Medications such as carbamazepine and valproic acid are useful, especially if intermittent explosive disorder is present with the conduct disorder. Also, fluoxetine – in liquid form for young children and tablet form for adolescents (20 mg tablet only available in UK) – may help if there has been a traumatic history, and clinical signs of PTSD with the conduct disorder, as it has an antidepressant quality.

Chronic anxiety

Chronic anxiety occurs in children and adults with FASD, partly because of an inability to self-soothe. A combination of psychostimulant and guanfacine or clonidine has been effective in the treatment of such symptoms, if they are present in the context of ADHD with co-occurring anxiety disorder. It is important to check blood pressure and pulse and do an ECG prior to prescribing these medications due to their possible cardio-toxicity when used in combination.

If the anxiety disorder is the primary psychiatric presentation, it also is essential to unravel the environmental stressors in the history as individual non-verbal play therapy may be better than medication as the first option in young children. If medication is indicated, then Buspirone or lorazepam may be helpful.

Patients with acute anxiety may respond to clonidine, guanfacine or even propranolol, especially if there is a 'panic' component. Pervasive social anxiety has responded to Buspirone.

Psychotic symptoms

These may be quite difficult to unravel as patients with FASD with average or higher IQs may make up (confabulate) exaggerated stories that are not delusional but rather the individual's way of 'filling in the blanks' due to severe deficits in working memory, social cognition and communication. Newer atypical antipsychotic agents may have a role in management (i.e. Risperidone), but it can precipitate a manic switch due to its differential effect on the 5HT receptor. Clinically, Olanzapine seems to be most effective if the patient is displaying features of acute mania, but here the weight gain can be a significant problem.

Symptoms of ASD or Asperger's syndrome

These can be seen in FASD, with the coupling of developmental impairments in executive function, theory of mind reasoning and sensory integration. The developmental impairments in social cognition and communication appear to be related to psychiatric problems such as anxiety disorders or sometimes even psychotic disorders. Psychostimulants must be used with caution as they can precipitate a schizoid personality change, sometimes described as 'zombie' type states in the USA, or increase perseveration due to enhanced focus. However, for the FAS or ARND patient with ADHD and co-occurring symptoms of ASD, the psychostimulant can have a positive effect on visual or auditory focus. This increases the child's social awareness and connection. Atomoxetine seems to be a good fit in older teenage patients.

Alcohol dependency

Ireland and the UK have the highest underage and binge-drinking patterns in the world. Animal researchers for over 40 years have established links between teratogenic prenatal alcohol exposure and alcohol craving. This concept and its potential impact for the developmentally delayed, alcohol-craving children of the Irish and UK binge-drinking generation has still not been fully realized in the adult mental health or adult addiction field (Baer et al. 2003; O'Malley 2011a; Orakwue et al. 2010; Reyes et al. 1985).

Lack of understanding of children's difficulties by the school authorities can precipitate disconnection from school, leading to school expulsion, leading in turn to aimless behaviour, excessive alcohol consumption, impulsive early sexual intercourse and pregnancy, giving rise to the next generation of children with FASD.

Where addiction counselling is ineffective, the use of psychopharmacology (borrowing from work in cocaine addiction) has been used successfully in blocking the central nervous system craving (Sinha and O'Malley 1999). Agents such as Naltrexone or Acamprosate have been used successfully in patients with FASD but still require rigorous scientific testing, especially if considered as a strategy in pregnancy with the alcohol addicted patient (Handley and Chassin 2009). Treatment strategies can be borrowed from studies on narcotic dependent mothers and the mother/infant dyad (Velez and Jansson 2008).

Conclusion

The medical community continues to fail to acknowledge FAS (dysmorphic) and ARND (non-dysmorphic) as developmental psychiatric disorders in their own right. It is becoming increasingly self-evident that a transgenerational management perspective with alcohol abuse at the core of understanding is the only effective way to approach FASD. A family-centred, transgenerational approach spans all age groups and is, by its nature, multi-modal and multi-systemic as it encompasses every discipline involved in FASD assessment and management: medicine, education, social welfare, psychology, occupational, language therapy and legal advocacy.

The beginning of the therapeutic process begins with the honest acknowledgement of the prevalence and extent of the transgenerational alcohol-related problem. After that it is no mean step to start to construct a 'scaffolding containment of the patient and family'. Judicious use of medicine for parent and child is a key component, but science needs to step in and test these types of unique but essential interventions. Already the animal researchers in alcohol teratology have shown the way (Hannigan et al. 2007; Kodituwakku and Kodituwakku 2011). It is up to society (us) to take this proverbial ball and run with it!

Notes

1. The term fetal alcohol spectrum disorders (FASD) was initially coined and published in the USA by Streissguth and O'Malley (2000). It is an umbrella term capturing the range of disorders caused by prenatal alcohol exposure.
2. Countries such as Australia, Canada and the UK use 'fetal alcohol spectrum disorder' (singular), as a diagnostic category, but this is a misnomer and not the intended usage for this umbrella term. Hopefully international clinicians will begin to understand that non-dysmorphic ARND is really what has been called FASD singular.

3   The names, ages and ethnic groups of all clinical cases cited have been changed to protect their identities.
4   If these types of agents are used, there must be awareness of potential teratogenic problems if the patient with FAS or ARND becomes pregnant. Fetal valproate syndrome, for example, has many of the physical and some of the central nervous system dysfunctions seen in FASD.

References

Abudabo, S. and Cohen, D. (2011) *Prenatal Alcohol Use and Fetal Alcohol Spectrum Disorders: Diagnosis, assessment and new directions in research and multimodal treatment*, Oak Park, IL: Bentham On Line Publishing.

Althoff, R.R. (2010) 'Dysregulated children reconsidered', *Journal of the American Academy of Child and Adolescent Psychiatry*, 49: 302–4.

Altink, M.E., Slaate-Willense, D.I.E., Ronnelse, N.N.J., Buschgens, C.J.M., Fliers, E.A., Arias-Vasquez, A., Xi, X., Franke, B., Sergeant, J.A., Farone, S.V. and Buitelaar, J.K. (2009) 'Effects of maternal and paternal smoking on attentional control in children with and without ADHD', *European Child and Adolescent Psychiatry*, 18: 465–75.

American Psychiatric Association (2000) *Diagnostic and Statistical Manual of Mental Disorders (4th edn) (DSM-IV)*, Arlington, VA: APA.

Archibald, S.L., Fennema-Notestine, C., Ganst, A., Riley, E.P., Mattson, S.N. and Jernigan, T.L. (2001) 'Brain dysmorphology in individuals with severe prenatal alcohol exposure', *Developmental Medicine and Child Neurology*, 43: 148–54.

Baer, J.S., Sampson, P.D., Barr, H.M., Connor, P.D. and Streissguth, A.P. (2003) 'A 21-year longitudinal analyses of the effects of prenatal alcohol exposure on young adult drinking', *Archives of General Psychiatry*, 60: 377–85.

Barr, H.M. and Streissguth, A.P. (2001) 'Identifying maternal self-reported alcohol use associated with fetal alcohol spectrum disorders', *Alcoholism: Clinical and Experimental Research*, 25: 283–7.

Barr, H.M., Bookstein, F.L., O'Malley, K.D., Connor, P.D., Huggins, J. and Streissguth, A.P. (2006) 'Binge drinking during pregnancy as a predictor of psychiatric disorders on the Structured Clinical Interview for DSM-IV in young adult offspring', *American Journal of Psychiatry*, 163: 1061–5.

Bertrand, J. (2009) 'Interventions for children with fetal alcohol spectrum disorders (FASD): overview of findings for five innovative research projects', *Research in Developmental Disabilities*, 30: 986–1006.

Bookstein, F.L., Sampson, P.D., Connor, P.D. and Streissguth, A.P. (2002) 'Midline corpus callosum is a neuroanatomical focus of fetal alcohol damage', *The Anatomical Record*, 269: 162–74.

British Medical Association (2007) *Fetal Alcohol Spectrum Disorders: A guide for professionals*, London: BMA Science and Education Department and the Board of Science.

Brown, T.E. (ed.) (2009) *ADHD Comorbidities: Handbook for ADHD complications in children and adults*, Arlington, VA: American Psychiatric Press.

Byrne, C. (2008) 'Psychopharmacology basics for FASD', workshop presentation, 3rd National Biennial Conference on Adolescents and Adults with Fetal Alcohol Spectrum Disorder, 9–12 April, Vancouver, British Columbia.

Carlson, G.A., Findling, R.L., Post, R.M., Birmaher, B., Blumberg, H.P., Correll, C., Delbello, M.P., Fristad, M., Frazier, J., Hammen, C., Hinshaw, S.P., Kowatch, R., Leibenluft, E., Mayer, S.E., Pavulrui, M.N., Dineen Wagner, K. and Tohen, M. (2009) 'Advancing research in early-onset bipolar disorder: barriers and suggestions', *Journal of Child and Adolescent Psychopharmacology*, 19: 3–12.

Chess, S. and Thomas, A. (1977) *Temperament and Development*, New York, NY: Brunner/Mazel.

Coggins, T.E., Timler, G.R. and Olswang, L.B. (2008) 'Identifying and treating social communication deficits in school-age children with fetal alcohol spectrum disorders', in K.D. O'Malley (ed.) *ADHD and Fetal Alcohol Spectrum Disorders* (FASD), New York, NY: Nova Science.

Densmore, R. (2011) *FASD Relationships: What I have learned about fetal alcohol spectrum disorder*, Altoma, MB: Freisen Corporation.

Dumaret, A.-C., Cousin, M. and Titran, M. (2009) 'Two generations of maternal alcohol abuse: impact on cognitive levels in mothers and their children', *Early Childhood Development and Care*, 9: 1–11.

Elias, S., Coughlan, B. and O'Malley, K.D. (submitted) 'Fetal alcohol spectrum disorders, children, parents and carers living with the disorder: a mixed methods approach'.

Famy, C., Streissguth, A.P. and Unis, A.S. (1998) 'Mental illness in adults with FAS', *American Journal of Psychiatry*, 155: 552–4.

Fast, D.K., Conry, J. and Loock, C.A. (1999) 'Identifying fetal alcohol syndrome among youth in the criminal justice system', *Journal of Developmental and Behavioral Pediatrics*, 20: 370–2.

Geller, B., Zimerman, B., Williams, M., Delbello, M.P., Frazier, J. and Beringer, L. (2002) 'Phenomenology of prepubertal and early onset adolescent bipolar disorder: examples of elated mood, grandiose behaviours, decreased need for sleep, racing thoughts, hypersexuality', *Journal of Child and Adolescent Psychopharmacology*: 12: 3–9.

Goodlett, C.R., Horn, K.H. and Zhou, F.C. (2005) 'Alcohol teratogenesis: mechanisms of damage and strategies for intervention', *Experimental Biology and Medicine*, 230: 394–406.

Grant, T.M., Huggins, J.E., Sampson, P.D., Ernst, C.C., Barr, H.M. and Streissguth, A.P. (2009) 'Alcohol use before and during pregnancy in western Washington, 1989–2004: implications for the prevention of fetal alcohol spectrum disorders', *American Journal of Obstetrics and Gynecology*, 200: 278.e1–8.

Greenbaum, R.L., Stevens, S.A., Nash, K., Koren, G. and Rovet, J. (2009) 'Social cognitive and emotion processing abilities of children with fetal alcohol spectrum disorders: a comparison with attention deficit hyperactivity disorder', *Alcoholism: Clinical and Experimental Research*, 33: 1656–70.

Hagerman, R.J. (1999) *Neurodevelopmental Disorders: Diagnosis and treatment*, Oxford: Oxford University Press.

Hannigan, J.H., O'Leary-Moore, S.K. and Berman, R.F. (2007) 'Postnatal environmental or experimental amelioration of neurobehavioural effects of prenatal alcohol exposure in rats', *Neuroscience and Behavioural Review*, 31: 202–11.

Handley, E. and Chassin, L. (2009) 'Intergenerational transmission of alcohol expectancies in a high-risk sample', *Journal of Studies on Alcohol and Drugs*, 70: 675–82.

Henshaw, C., Cox, J. and Barton, J. (2009) *Modern Management of Perinatal Psychiatric Disorders*, London: Royal College of Psychiatrists.

Howlin, P., Charman, T. and Ghazziuddin, M. (eds) (2011) *The Sage Handbook of Developmental Disorders*, London: Sage.

Hoyme, H.E., May, P.A., Kalberg, M.A., Kodituwakku, P., Gossage, J.P., Truijillo, P.M., Buckley, D.G., Miller, J.H., Aragon, A.S., Khaole, N., Viljoen, D.L., Jones, K.L. and Robinson, L.K. (2005) 'A practical clinical approach to diagnosis of fetal alcohol spectrum disorders: clarification of the 1996 Institute of Medicine criteria', *Pediatrics*, 115: 39–47.

Kodituwakku, P.W. and Kodituwakku, E.L. (2011) 'From research to practice: an integrative framework for the development of interventions for children with fetal alcohol spectrum disorders', *Neuropsychology Review*, 21; 204–23.

Kraemer, G.W., Moore, C.F., Newman, T.K., Barr, C.S. and Schneider, M.L. (2008) 'Moderate fetal alcohol exposure and serotonin transporter gene promoter polymorphism effect neonatal temperament and limbic-hypothalamic-pituitary-adrenal axis regulation in monkeys', *Biological Psychiatry*, 63: 317–24.

Lemoine, P. and Lemoine, P.H. (1992) 'Avenir des enfants de mères alcooliques (Étude de 105 cas retrouvés à l'âge adulte) et quelques constatations d'intérêt prophylactique' [Outcome in the offspring of alcoholic mothers (study of 105 adults) and considerations with a view to prophylaxis], *Annales depédiatrie, Paris*, 39: 226–35.

Mattson, S.N., Riley, E.P., Sowell, E.R., Jernigan, T.L., Sobel, D.F. and Jones, K.L. (1996) 'A decrease in the size of the basal ganglia in children with FAS', *Alcoholism: Clinical and Experimental Research*, 20: 1088–93.

Mattson, S.N., Crocker, N. and Nyguen, T.T. (2011) 'Fetal alcohol spectrum disorders: neuropsychological and behavioural features', *Neuropsychology Review*, 2: 84–101.

Meewise, M.L., Reitsma, J.B., De Vries, G.J., Gersons, B.P.R. and Olff, M. (2007) 'Cortisol and post-traumatic stress disorder in adults: systematic review and meta-analysis', *British Journal of Psychiatry*, 191: 387–92.

Mick, E., Biederman, J., Farone, S., Sayer, J. and Kleinman, S. (2002) 'Case-control study of ADHD and maternal smoking, alcohol use and drug use during pregnancy', *Journal of the American Academy of Child and Adolescent Psychiatry*, 41: 378–85.

Milberger, S., Biederman, J., Farone, S.V., Chen, L. and Jones, J. (1996) 'Is maternal smoking during pregnancy a risk factor for attention deficit hyperactivity disorder in children?' *American Journal of Psychiatry*, 153: 1138–42.

Moore, T.E. and Green, M. (2004) 'Fetal alcohol spectrum disorder: a need for closer examination by the criminal justice system', *Criminal Reports*, 19: 99–108.

Mukherjee, R.A.S., Hollins, S. and Turk, J. (2008) 'Fetal alcohol spectrum disorder', *Journal of the Royal Society of Medicine*, 99: 298–302.

Mukherjee, R.A., Hollins, S. and Curfs, L. (2012) 'Fetal alcohol spectrum disorders: is it something we should be more aware of?' *Journal of the Royal College of Physicians of Edinburgh*, 42: 143–50.

Murray, L., Arteche, A., Fearon, P., Halligan, S., Goodyer, I. and Cooper, P. (2011) 'Maternal postnatal depression and the development of depression in offspring up to 16 years of age', *Journal of the American Academy of Child and Adolescent Psychiatry*, 50: 460–70.

Nanson, J. (1992) 'Autism in fetal alcohol syndrome: a report of 6 cases', *Alcoholism: Clinical and Experimental Research*, 16: 558–65.

Nowick Brown, N., O'Malley, K.D. and Streissguth, A.P. (2011) 'FASD: diagnostic dilemmas and challenges for a modern transgenerational approach', in S.A. Abudato and S. Cohen (eds) *Prenatal Alcohol Use and Fetal Alcohol spectrum Disorders: Diagnosis, assessment, and new directions in research and multimodal treatment*, Oak Park, IL: Bentham On Line Publishing.

Oberlander, T.F., Gingrich, J.A. and Ansorge, M.S. (2009) 'Sustained neurobehavioral effects of exposure to SSRI antidepressants during development: molecular to clinical evidence', *Clinical Pharmacology and Therapeutics*, 86: 672–7.

O'Connor, M.J., Shah, B., Whaley, S., Cronin, P., Gunderson, B. and Graham, J. (2002) 'Psychiatric illness in a clinical sample of children with prenatal alcohol exposure', *American Journal of Drug and Alcohol Abuse*, 28: 743–54.

O'Malley, K.D. (2001) 'Medication in FASD: uses in primary, secondary and tertiary prevention', presentation to the National FAS Conference, Centers for Disease Control and Prevention, 27–28 April, Atlanta, USA.

O'Malley, K.D. (2003) 'Youth with comorbid disorders', in A.J. Pumariega and N.C. Winters (eds) *The Handbook of Child and Adolescent Systems of Care: The new community psychiatry*, Hoboken, NJ: Jossey-Bass.

O'Malley, K.D. (2008) 'Multimodal management strategies through the lifespan', in K.D. O'Malley (ed.) *ADHD and Fetal Alcohol Spectrum Disorders (FASD)*, New York, NY: Nova Science.

O'Malley, K.D. (2010) 'FASD', in I.P. Stolerman (ed.) *Encyclopedia of Psychopharmacology*. Berlin: Springer Verlag.

O'Malley, K.D. (2011a) 'Fetal alcohol spectrum disorders', in P. Howlin, T. Charman and M. Ghazziuddin (eds) *The Sage Handbook of Developmental Disorders*, London: Sage.

O'Malley, K.D. (2011b) 'Psychiatric review of 95 to 100 transgenerational patients with FASD, Ireland 2006–2011', plenary talk to the 4th International Conference on FASD, 3–6 March, Vancouver.

O'Malley, K.D. and Mukherjee, R. (2010) 'Fetal alcohol syndrome/alcohol related neurodevelopmental disorder' (Syndrome sheet), Bourne End, Buckinghamshire: Society for Study of Behavioural Phenotypes [online at: www.ssbp.org.uk/site/images/stories/ssbp/downloads/Foetal_alcohol.pdf; accessed: 21 January 2013].

O'Malley, K.D. and Nanson, J. (2002) 'Clinical implications of a link between fetal alcohol spectrum disorder and attention-deficit hyperactivity disorder', *Canadian Journal of Psychiatry*, 4: 349–54.

O'Malley, K.D. and Rich, S. (2013) 'Clinical implications of a link between fetal alcohol spectrum disorders (FASD) and autism or Asperger's disorder: a neurodevelopmental frame for helping understanding and management', in M. Fitzgerald (ed.) *Recent Advances in Autism Spectrum Disorders (Volume 1)*, Rijeka, Croatia: INTECH [online at: www.intechopen.com/books/recent-advances-in-autism-spectrum-disorders-volume-i; accessed: 17 June 2013].

O'Malley, K.D. and Storoz, L. (2003) 'Fetal alcohol spectrum disorder and ADHD: diagnostic implications and therapeutic consequences', *Expert Review of Neurotherapeutics*, 3: 477–89.

Orakwue, N., McNicholas, F. and O'Malley, K.D. (2010) 'Fetal alcohol spectrum disorders: the Irish perspective', *Irish Journal Psychological Medicine*, 27: 223–7.

Page, K. (2008) 'Adult neuropysychology of fetal alcohol spectrum disorders', in K.D. O'Malley (ed.) *ADHD and FASD*, New York, NY: Nova Science.

Pine, D., Regier, D.A., Chmura Kraemer, H., Fisher, P. and Shaffer, D. (2012) 'Symposium 21: the making of DSM 5 (Part 1)', presentation to the American Academy of Child and Adolescent Psychiatry 59th Annual Meeting, San Francisco, 25 October.

Raine, A., Lencz, T., Bihrie, S., Lacasse, C. and Colletti, P. (2000) 'Reduced prefrontal gray matter volume and reduced autonomic activity in antisocial personality disorder', *Archives of General Psychiatry*, 57: 119–27.

Reyes, E., Garcia, K.D. and Jones, B.C. (1985) 'Effects of maternal consumption of alcohol on alcohol selection in rats', *Alcohol*, 2: 323–6.

Riley, E.P., Mattson, S.N., Sowell, E.R., Jernigan, T.L., Sobel, D.F. and Jones, K.L. (1995) 'Abnormalities of the corpus callosum in children prenatally exposed to alcohol', *Alcoholism: Clinical and Experimental Research*, 19: 1198–202.

Salee, F.R., Lyne, A., Wigal, T. and McGough, J.J. (2009) 'Long term safety and efficacy of guanfacine extended release in children and adolescents with attention-deficit/hyperactivity disorder', *Journal of Child and Adolescent Psychopharmacology*, 19: 215–26.

Savage, D.D., Rosenberg, M.J., Wolff, C.R., Akers, K.G., El-Emawy, A., Staples, M.C., Varaschin, R.K., Wright, C.A., Seidel, J.L., Caldwell, K.K. and Hamilton, D.A. (2010) 'Effects of a novel cognition-enhancing agent on fetal ethanol induced learning deficits', *Alcoholism: Clinical and Experimental Research*, 34: 1793–802.

Screiber, M.L., Moore, C.F., Gajewski, L.L., Larson, J.A., Roberts, A.D., Converse, A.K. and De Jesus, O.T. (2008) 'Sensory processing disorder in primate models: evidence from a longitudinal study of prenatal alcohol and prenatal stress effects', *Child Development*, 79: 100–13.

Sifneos, P. (1973) 'The prevalence of "alexithymic" characteristics in psychosomatic patients', *Psychotherapy and Psychosomatics*, 22: 225–62.

Sinha, R. and O'Malley, S.S. (1999) 'Craving for alcohol: findings from the clinic and the laboratory', *Alcohol and Alcoholism*, 34: 223–30.

Smith, D.W. (1981) 'Fetal alcohol syndrome and fetal alcohol effects', *Neurobehavioral Toxicology and Teratology*, 3: 127.

Sowell, E.R., Lu, L.H., O'Hare, E.D., McCourt, S.T., Mattson, S.N., O'Connor, M.J. and Bookheimer, S.Y. (2007) 'Functional magnetic resonance imaging of verbal learning in children with heavy prenatal alcohol exposure', *Neuroreport*, 18: 636–9.

Sowell, E., Johnson, A., Kan, E., Lu, L.H., Van Horn, J.D., Toga, A.W., O'Connor, M.J. and Bookheimer, S.Y. (2008) 'Mapping white matter integrity and neurobehavioral correlates in children with fetal alcohol spectrum disorders', *Journal of Neuroscience*, 28: 1313–19.

Stratton, K., Howe, C. and Battaglia, F. (eds) (1996) *Fetal Alcohol Syndrome: Diagnosis, epidemiology, prevention, and treatment*, Washington, DC: National Academy Press.

Streissguth, A.P. (1997) *Fetal Alcohol Syndrome: A guide for families and communities*, Baltimore, MD: Brooks.

Streissguth, A.P. and Kanter, J. (1997) *The Challenges of Fetal Alcohol Syndrome: Overcoming secondary disabilities*, Seattle, WA: University of Washington Press.

Streissguth, A.P. and O'Malley, K.D. (2000) 'Neuropsychiatric implications and long-term consequences of fetal alcohol spectrum disorders', *Seminars in Clinical Neuropsychiatry*, 5: 177–90.

Streissguth, A.P., Barr, H.M., Kogan, J. and Bookstein, F.L. (1996) *Understanding the Occurrence of Secondary Disabilities in Clients with Fetal Alcohol Syndrome (FAS) and Fetal Alcohol Effects (FAE): Final report to the Centers for Disease Control and Prevention (CDC)*, Seattle, WA: University of Washington.

Streissguth A.P., Bookstein, F.L., Barr, H.M., Sampson, P.D., O'Malley, K. and Kogan Young, J. (2004) 'Risk factors for adverse life outcomes in fetal alcohol syndrome and fetal alcohol effects', *Journal of Developmental and Behavioral Pediatrics*, 25: 228–38.

Sullivan, A. (2008) 'Fetal alcohol spectrum disorders in the adult: vulnerability, disability or diagnosis – a psychodynamic perspective', in K.D. O'Malley (ed.) *ADHD and Fetal Alcohol Spectrum Disorders (FASD)*, New York, NY: Nova Science.

Turk, J. (2007) 'Behavioural phenotypes: their applicability to children and young people who have learning disabilities', *Advances in Mental Health and Learning Disabilities*, 1: 4–13.

Velez, M. and Jansson, L.M. (2008) 'The opoid dependent mother and newborn dyad: non pharmacological care', *Journal of Addiction Medicine*, 2: 113–20.

Vidal, B.V. (2012) 'Sensory processing in children with fetal alcohol spectrum disorders' (session 52), presentation to the Second European Conference on FASD, Barcelona, 21–24 October.

Werner, E.E. (1986) 'Resilient offspring of alcoholics: a longitudinal study from birth to age 18', *Journal of Studies on Alcohol*, 47: 34–40.

Wilens, T.E. (2009) 'Combined pharmacotherapy in pediatric psychopharmacology: friend or foe?' *Journal of Child and Adolescent Psychopharmacology*, 19: 483–4.

Wozniak, J. and Biederman, J. (1996) 'A pharmacological approach to the quagmire of comorbidity in juvenile mania', *Journal of the American Academy of Child and Adolescent Psychiatry*, 35: 826–8.

World Health Organization (2004) *International Statistical Classification of Diseases and Related Health Problems 10th Revision (ICD-10)*, Geneva: WHO.

Zero to Three (2005) *Diagnostic Classification of Mental Health and Developmental Disorders of Infancy and Early Childhood (revised edition)*, Washington, DC: Zero to Three.

PART V
International perspectives

20

NORTH AMERICAN PERSPECTIVES ON FETAL ALCOHOL SPECTRUM DISORDERS

Therese M. Grant and Sterling K. Clarren

Introduction

Alcohol is legal, widely available, heavily advertised and popular among women in the United States (US) and Canada. World Health Organization (WHO 2004) data indicate that approximately 62 per cent of adult women in the US drink alcohol and 15.1 per cent report binge drinking (five or more drinks) at least once in the past 30 days. Among Canadian women, 73.9 per cent drink alcohol and 11.2 per cent report binge drinking 12 or more times in the past year (WHO 2004).

Alcohol is also a known teratogen, that is, depending on dose, timing, frequency and genetic susceptibility, a woman's use of alcohol during pregnancy can result in a range of damaging and irreversible neurodevelopmental effects to the fetus, known as fetal alcohol spectrum disorders (FASDs) and among those conditions, fetal alcohol syndrome (FAS) itself.

Over the 40 years since FAS was first named by Drs David Smith and Kenneth Lyon Jones (Jones and Smith 1973; Jones *et al*. 1973), a great deal of publicly funded research has been conducted worldwide examining scientific questions associated with alcohol teratogenicity (e.g. animal models, brain imaging, mechanisms of action), developing diagnostic and screening methods, and testing strategies for intervention and prevention. Since 1973 nearly 3,900 articles have been published on aspects of fetal alcohol exposure, with nearly 40 per cent of these appearing since 2000 (Goodlett 2010).

The US and Canada share similar perspectives on FAS and FASDs. Both countries recognize that maternal alcohol use during pregnancy is a serious problem, and have invested considerable efforts in understanding this disability and how to respond with effective practices and policies. Their history is one of sharing information and collaborating to address the goals of reducing the incidence of this preventable birth defect and ameliorating the suffering of affected individuals and families.

In this chapter we will describe the evolution of current North American policies and practices regarding FASDs and maternal alcohol use during pregnancy, and provide an overview of diagnostic guidelines, screening recommendations, public health messaging and prevention and intervention efforts.

Public policy development

Alcohol was first identified as a teratogen in 1973, and by the mid-1970s epidemiologic and animal studies were beginning to demonstrate adverse effects among offspring exposed prenatally to alcohol (Ellis and Pick 1980; Harlap and Shiono 1980; Little 1977; Sulik *et al.* 1981). By 1978 two of the first FAS prevention programmes had been funded in the US by the National Institute of Alcohol Abuse and Alcoholism, including a community-wide programme to directly address the problem of female alcohol abuse during pregnancy (Little *et al.* 1980).

Broader policy responses did not evolve without some controversy. Following publication of a summary paper reviewing the available scientific evidence on FAS at the time (Eckardt *et al.* 1981), the US Surgeon General issued an advisory at the federal policy level recommending that women who are, or plan to become, pregnant abstain from alcohol; health professionals who care for them are urged to ask routinely about alcohol consumption and enter this information into the medical record (Public Health Service 1981). In the early 1980s there was a failed attempt by the US Congress to mandate warning labels on all alcohol beverage containers. This act eventually passed in 1988, and in late 1990 the Alcohol Beverage Labeling Act of 1988 went into effect, requiring that all alcoholic beverage containers in the US be labelled with a specific health warning (Myers 2002). Cities and states in the US began to post warning signs about not drinking during pregnancy, beginning with New York City in 1988. By 1988 there were numerous programmes involving public education, professional training and services to educate women about the risks associated with drinking during pregnancy, all centring around the common theme of abstinence during pregnancy: 'No alcohol for our baby', 'For baby's sake, don't drink', 'A pregnant woman never drinks alone' (Robinson and Armstrong 1988). In 1993, Washington State adopted a state ordinance: three warning signs were approved and every venue selling alcohol by container or by the glass was required by law to post two of these signs. Many other states and cities have followed (Streissguth and Grant 2011).

In 1996 the Institute of Medicine (Stratton *et al.* 1996) published a public health prevention approach to FASDs that was (and continues to be) widely accepted in the US and Canada. This approach outlines three levels of prevention activities:

- *universal*: promoting general knowledge about pregnancy alcohol use and healthy practices (e.g. warning signs, public health messages, bottle labels, newspaper articles);
- *selective*: involving screening women for alcohol use, training health care professionals, working with family members of pregnant women who abuse alcohol, developing biomarkers, brief interventions and referrals;
- *indicated*: focusing directly on individuals at highest risk for adverse outcomes.

At a federal level, in 2000 the US Congress recognized FASDs as an important public health problem and developed landmark legislation, including six mandates addressing FASDs in the Children's Health Act of 2000. This Act created the Fetal Alcohol Spectrum Disorders Center for Excellence, an agency which has been instrumental in convening leadership and community partners from across the US to address the prevention and treatment of FASDs.

The US Surgeon General's advisory was reissued in 2005, urging women who are pregnant or who are considering becoming pregnant to abstain from alcohol consumption to eliminate the risk of alcohol-related birth defects (CDC 2005). Policies in the US and Canada have consistently endorsed this public health message, and medical professional organizations in North America have continued to support and endorse pregnancy alcohol abstinence as the safest course for pregnant women. For example, the American Medical Association (1999) has endorsed universal alcohol screening for all patients over the age of 14 years, and the American College of Obstetricians and Gynecologists (2008) outlined the ethical rational for using a consolidated alcohol protocol including universal screening, brief intervention and referral to treatment. The American Academy of Pediatrics (2000) endorsed the Surgeon General's recommendation for abstinence during pregnancy and additionally recommended federal legislation requiring the inclusion of health and safety messages in all print and broadcast alcohol advertisements as well as providing information about FAS and not drinking during pregnancy in marriage licences.

In August 2010 the Canadian Bar Association, noting that approximately 60 per cent of people who have FASDs become involved in the criminal justice system at some time during their lives (Streissguth et al. 2004), broke new ground in the field by recognizing the impact of this brain-based disorder on the justice system. A three-part resolution was passed recommending that the Bar Association:

> (1) support the initiative of Ministers responsible for Justice with respect to access to justice for people with FASDs and urge all levels of government to allocate additional resources for alternatives to the current practice of criminalizing individuals with FASDs; (2) urge the federal, territorial and provincial governments to develop policies designed to assist and enhance the lives of those with FASDs and to prevent persistent over-representation of FASD affected individuals in the criminal justice system; and (3) urge the federal government to amend criminal sentencing laws to accommodate the disability of those with FASDs.
>
> *(Canadian Bar Association 2010)*

In August 2012 the American Bar Association followed suit in a resolution (1) urging the justice system to help identify and respond effectively to FASDs through training to enhance awareness of FASDs and their impact, and the value of collaboration with medical, mental health and disability experts; and (2) urging the passage of laws and adoption of policies that acknowledge and treat the effects of prenatal alcohol exposure (American Bar Association 2012: 1).

Diagnosis

Because alcohol teratogenesis causes a variety of abnormal outcomes rather than only a discrete and specific syndrome, attempts have been made since 1978 to codify the disorder and bring consistency to the diagnosis (Hoyme et al. 2005; Sokol and Clarren 1989; Stratton et al. 1996). In 2002 under direction from the US Congress, the CDC (Centers for Disease Control and Prevention) collaborated with federal and non-federal partners to establish uniform diagnostic criteria for FAS and other conditions related to prenatal alcohol exposure (Floyd et al. 2005). These guidelines were published in 2004 (CDC 2004a), and in the following year Canada published their guidelines for the diagnosis of FASDs (Chudley et al. 2005). The diagnostic standards are similar in both countries, and stress the fact that the diffuse brain damage caused by alcohol is best assessed at this time through a broad battery of tests of cognition and performance. This battery both establishes the role of brain performance rather than external environment factors as a major cause of the patient's persistent maladaptation in school, society and at home and offers a road map to treatment and intervention. This means that the patient is disabled rather than disobedient and that the disability while manageable or improvable is not curable. This evaluation requires an interdisciplinary team with a minimum staff of physician, psychologist, speech and language pathologist, occupational therapist and a coordinator. This team needs to actively share their results since the information from one source informs the opinions from other sources and together the team reaches the best treatment decisions. From the patient's perspective, understanding the breadth and depth of the functional disabilities is generally far more important than the etiologic explanation. From a prevention standpoint, understanding the role of gestational alcohol exposure is a key to all forms of prevention efforts.

These guidelines have been widely accepted in North America and are endorsed by professional groups including the American College of Obstetricians and Gynecologists, the American Academy of Pediatrics and the Canadian Medical Association. Yet there is little evidence that this support has led to the funding and leadership needed to increase the diagnostic capacity that is urgently needed across most areas of both countries.

Prevalence of FAS/FASDs

Given that most communities in the US and Canada have little capacity to diagnose FAS, prevalence figures are only estimates and cannot be generalized to national populations. Depending on ascertainment methods, the prevalence of FAS in the US has been reported as 0.2 to 3.0 cases per 1,000 live births, and the rate of FASDs as 9.1 per 1,000 live births (CDC 2004b; Sampson et al. 1997).

There are no national statistics on the rates of FASDs in Canada (Albert et al. 2005), although studies have estimated its prevalence in small populations from approximately seven per 1,000 live births in north-eastern Manitoba (Williams et al. 1999) to 190 per 1,000 live births in an isolated Aboriginal community in British Columbia (Robinson et al. 1987).

There is no specific study that has been done which explains the gulf between the number of diagnostic appointments available for FASDs and the presumptive need for these evaluations based on the prevalence estimates. Capacity is driven in part by demand. Many clinics in developmental medicine will tolerate wait periods of several months, some even longer. Most programmes do report families on their waiting lists for FASD evaluation that extend into their long-term waiting period, but not beyond them. Thus the diagnostic programmes are full or over-subscribed to some extent, but not overwhelmed as one might have guessed. This could be due to (1) a lack of public interest in an FASD diagnosis, since the available treatments are not themselves widely available, affordable or truly effective (i.e. curative); (2) a lack of recommended referrals by primary care providers for the same reasons; (3) family resistance to considering an alcohol related diagnosis.

A final explanation could be related to the often standalone nature of the FASD evaluation programme. FASD diagnostic programmes are rarely incorporated into general mental health or general neurodevelopmental diagnostic centres that might more readily refer patients internally for an FASD evaluation. Most patients who seek an FASD diagnosis have been previously evaluated in these kinds of programmes, yet are often not referred for an FASD condition through them. In the end, people do not seek a 'diagnosis', they seek a solution to their problem. As treatment for FASDs improves and as supports in the community expand and demonstrate success, it is likely that demand for diagnosis will rapidly increase.

Screening and prevention

FASDs are birth defect conditions that have adverse and long-term implications not only for the health and well-being of affected individuals, but for the societies in which they live. FASDs are also preventable conditions and as such are a compelling social and public health issue (a fetus that is not exposed to alcohol during pregnancy cannot have an FASD). For communities and countries at large, there is little question that FASD prevention can mean healthier, more productive (and dare we say happier?) individuals who have a better capacity to reach their full potential.

Although the terms 'universal' and 'selective' prevention were not coined until 1996, programmes for increasing community and individual awareness about the risks of alcohol use during pregnancy have been implemented for four decades. Most US and Canadian FASD campaigns have recommended complete cessation (Clarren and Salmon 2010). For example, in one of the earliest prevention programmes, Seattle's Pregnancy and Health Program (Little *et al.* 1980) alerted the community to the message 'When you're pregnant, the best drink is no drink at all' via posters, radio and television public service announcements, signs in all Seattle buses, and fliers inserted into all purchases of alcoholic beverages at state liquor stores. In Canada, more than 350 such direct messaging campaigns have been used since 2000 (Clarren and Salmon 2010).

There is scant published research indicating that general public health campaigns about the potential risks of maternal drinking during pregnancy have been effective. In a study comparing US and Canadian respondents, Greenfield and colleagues (1999) found that in the first four years after the Alcohol Beverage Labeling Act of 1988 went into effect there was an awareness of the label in the US (which then tapered off). In terms of influencing the actual use of alcohol, several studies have found that bottle-labelling has not had a significant impact (Hankin *et al.* 1996; MacKinnon *et al.* 2000). In terms of FASD prevention, Floyd and colleagues (2009) report that universal prevention efforts have not reduced the incidence of FASDs.

There is, nevertheless, evidence from US population-based surveys suggesting that the proportion of women who drink during pregnancy has decreased over time. Nationally, any alcohol use among *non-pregnant* women ranged from 53.2 per cent in 1995 to 54.9 per cent in 2002 (CDC 2002, 2004b) while rates of any alcohol use *during pregnancy* were 12.8 per cent in 1999 (Chasnoff *et al.* 2001) and dropped to 10.1 per cent in 2002 (Tsai and Floyd 2004). Grant and colleagues (2009) similarly found that among over 12,000 mothers who were screened postpartum in western Washington between 1989 and 2004, while rates of any alcohol use in the month or so *before* pregnancy remained stable over these years (slightly > 40 per cent), rates of any alcohol use *during* pregnancy decreased significantly from 30 per cent in 1989–1991 to 12 per cent in 2002–2004.

Binge drinking in regular higher volume events seems to be a particularly dangerous pattern of embryonic exposure (Stratton *et al.* 1996). US national binge drinking rates among *non-pregnant* women have been relatively stable at about 11 per cent to 12 per cent from 1995 through 2002 (CDC 2002, 2004b); binge drinking rates *during pregnancy* went from 2.9 per cent in 1995 (CDC 1997) to 1.9 per cent in 2002 (CDC 2004b). A similar pattern emerged in the western Washington data: *non-pregnant* binge alcohol use rates were 9 per cent to 14 per cent (1989 to 2004), and *during pregnancy* rates were 3 per cent (1989–1991) to 1 per cent (2002–2004) (Grant et al. 2009). We note that concomitant to Grant et al.'s finding of reduced alcohol use during pregnancy, Astley (2004) reported a decrease in the prevalence of FAS among 264 foster children born in western Washington (King County) between 1993 and 1998. In Astley's study, five offspring were diagnosed with FAS, representing a significant decline in FAS prevalence across each birth cohort from 1993–1998 (1993, 6.67 per cent; 1994, 4.76 per cent; 1995, 0.00 per cent; 1996, 0.00 per cent; 1997, 2.17 per cent; 1998, 0.00 per cent; $p<0.03$).

These data suggest that public health messages have been effective to some extent: most women do not drink alcohol when they recognize that they are pregnant. The problem is that most women are not aware that they are pregnant for several weeks after conception, and during that early gestational period a woman may unintentionally introduce risk to the embryo by drinking (Floyd et al. 1999). Medical care providers are in an ideal position to convey a critical message: although a woman may not know that she is pregnant, heavy drinking very early in pregnancy (during the period of organogenesis) can cause injury to the particular fetal cells, organs, and limbs that are developing at the time of her alcohol use (Wilson 1973) and may be sufficient to cause permanent changes in brain development (Streissguth et al. 1989; Clarren et al. 1992).

Further complicating the public health problem is that approximately half of all pregnancies in the US are unintended (Mohllajee et al. 2007), and these rates are higher among younger women, who are also more likely to be binge drinkers. Women who are not planning to have a baby have no pregnancy-related reason to limit their alcohol intake, and women who are heavy drinkers may have unexpected, unwanted, and/or unprotected sexual encounters.

Health care and family planning providers can play a critical role in preventing FASDs by routinely screening *every* woman of child-bearing age for information about their alcohol use and their risk for pregnancy *before* they become pregnant. This concept of preconceptional health care (that is, aimed at women who have never been pregnant or are between pregnancies) has gained momentum in the US and Canada, and may be particularly powerful in preventing FASDs given the high rate of unintended pregnancy (Moos 2004). Women who are not pregnant and who report alcohol use should be counselled about contraceptive options, and educated about the potential risks of drinking at the time of conception and throughout pregnancy. Women who are pregnant and report alcohol use should be counselled to stop drinking; those who find it difficult to stop drinking should be referred for substance abuse treatment.

Advice to abstain from alcohol may run counter to messages women hear in the popular press. For example, *People Magazine* has stated, 'some doctors feel limited drinking – no more than a pint a day – after the first trimester is okay' (*People Magazine* 2006: 107). As another example, widespread media reports of research published by Kelly and colleagues (2009, 2012) in the United Kingdom misinterpreted study findings, and suggested to the public that light drinking during pregnancy may be beneficial for an unborn child (this was not what study authors reported). Messages like this can be easily misinterpreted. While a woman who drinks is likely to acknowledge some alcohol use, on further probing a clinician may find that, based on the type of alcohol or the size of the glass the woman uses, her report of 'one glass per day' actually constitutes three drinks.

If clinicians screened women for alcohol use and provided information about risks at all initial, routine and follow-up visits, large numbers of women could be identified and educated early enough to avoid alcohol-related pregnancy complications. Unfortunately, many health care providers are reluctant to ask about alcohol use because they are not trained in addictions or assessment strategies, they do not believe they have time, they assume that their patients are not problem drinkers, they lack accurate information about referral options and they question the effectiveness of treatment intervention programmes (Chasnoff *et al.* 2001; Mengel *et al.* 2006). Nevertheless, a first step for clinicians is to simply ask a woman about her use of any alcohol and binge alcohol. If warranted, brief alcohol screening instruments are available to help providers in clinical settings identify problem drinkers (e.g. CAGE, TWEAK, Audit and T-ACE instruments) (Ewing 1984; Russell 1994; Saunders *et al.* 1993; Sokol *et al.* 1989). New codes that have been established by the American Medical Association now allow physicians to screen patients for alcohol problems, deliver behavioural interventions and report these activities to health insurance programmes.

Screening for binge alcohol use in the non-pregnant population may also identify women who are under-using contraception and who may benefit from more aggressive counselling regarding risks for pregnancy and methods that do not require daily use. They may also benefit from having plan B (emergency contraceptive backup method) supplies available.

In their review of beliefs about risks related to women's alcohol use during pregnancy in six countries, Drabble and colleagues (2011) note that in Canada FASDs were initially framed primarily as a child health issue. More recently, researchers and clinicians have brought attention to FASD prevention as a women's health concern. In 2010 the Society of Obstetricians and Gynaecologists of Canada and the Public Health Agency of Canada established national standards for alcohol screening and counselling on alcohol use for women of child-bearing age and pregnant women (Carson *et al.* 2010). Based on a careful review of recently published studies that used rigorous research designs, these standards first summarize the scientific evidence on prenatal alcohol exposure, stating that there is not enough evidence to define a threshold for low-level drinking in pregnancy, and abstinence is the wisest choice for a woman who is or might become pregnant.

These national Canadian clinical guidelines are remarkable for the compassionate philosophy they reflect: one that aims to create an environment for women in which they can safely talk about their alcohol use and options for care, without being stigmatized. Advising pregnant patients who are problem drinkers to simply stop drinking is not a realistic therapeutic approach, and shaming or blaming them will simply discourage them from seeking prenatal care and help for their substance abuse disorder. The Canadian guidelines include the following recommendations:

- Universal screening for alcohol consumption should be done periodically for all pregnant women and women of child-bearing age. Ideally, at-risk drinking could be identified before pregnancy. (See recommendations later in this chapter.)
- Health care providers should create a safe environment for women to report alcohol consumption.
- The public should be informed that alcohol screening and support for women at risk is part of routine women's health care.
- Health care providers should be aware of the risk factors associated with alcohol use in women of reproductive age.

- Brief interventions are effective and should be provided by health care providers for women with at-risk drinking.
- If a woman continues to use alcohol during pregnancy, harm reduction/treatment strategies should be encouraged.
- Pregnant women should be given priority access to withdrawal management and treatment. Health care providers should advise women that low-level consumption of alcohol in early pregnancy is not an indication for termination of pregnancy.

Intervention with high-risk women

'Indicated (or targeted) prevention' activities are designed for individuals who are at highest risk for adverse outcomes. In the case of FASDs this means women who have an alcohol abuse problem, or those who have already given birth to a child with FASDs. The Parent–Child Assistance Program (PCAP), first developed in the US in 1991 and widely replicated in Canada since 1998, is an example of an indicated prevention model. PCAP began as a federally funded research demonstration project that tested the efficacy of an intensive, three-year home visitation/case management model with high-risk mothers and their children. The primary aim of the model was to prevent subsequent alcohol and drug exposed births among birth mothers who abused alcohol and/or drugs during an index pregnancy. Based on positive research findings (Ernst et al. 1999; Grant et al. 2003, 2005), the Washington State Legislature subsequently funded PCAP sites in nine counties, with a capacity to serve nearly 700 families.

The PCAP model is based on relational theory and self-efficacy constructs and emphasizes the importance of case managers building trusting, empathic relationships with their clients in order to better understand their frames of reference, and helping them develop service delivery plans that are meaningful, relevant and achievable (Grant et al. 1999). PCAP case managers are paraprofessionals who use explicit methods to help their clients identify personal goals and work with them to take incremental steps toward achieving those goals (Grant et al. 1997). They each work with a caseload of 16 families, conduct home visits approximately twice per month, connect women and their families with community services, and coordinate services among the service provider network. Case managers are highly trained and closely supervised by experienced clinicians credentialed in the mental health, social work and/or chemical dependency fields.

The first Canadian replication of the PCAP model was the Stop FAS initiative (Umlah and Grant 2003), developed at several sites in Manitoba in 1998 as part of a government strategy to address growing concern about maternal alcohol use during pregnancy, and the increasing number of children being formally diagnosed with FAS. Funded by the provincial government through Healthy Child Manitoba with collaboration from the Addictions Foundation of Manitoba, Stop FAS preliminary outcome data demonstrated programme effectiveness in helping women enter treatment, achieve sobriety and use family planning methods. The programme has expanded to sites in northern Manitoba that serve Aboriginal women by offering both contemporary and traditional approaches of support based on the medicine wheel and the seven sacred teachings.

In October 2009, the Institute of Health Economics in Alberta, Canada issued a consensus statement on 'FASD Across the Lifespan' (Institute of Health Economics and the Alberta Government 2009: 11, jury recommendation 5) that recommended a number of FASD prevention measures, including:

A high priority on ensuring that prevention services are provided to women and families at highest risk of having a child with FASD. The Parent–Child Assistance Program (PCAP) has shown great success. Canadian programs based on the PCAP model should be encouraged.

In western Canada there are currently more than 30 programmes based on the PCAP model.

Conclusion

Countries contemplating the broad problem of reducing alcohol-exposed pregnancies would do well to consider steps that we have found useful in the US and in Canada, involving a variety of public health actions. Warranted by the compelling animal and human research published in the past 40 years, government warnings regarding 'no safe level of alcohol use during pregnancy' (including bottle-labelling of all alcoholic beverages and point-of-purchase warning signs) can be an important first step. Commissioning national funds for research, women's substance abuse treatment, and development of guidelines for routine screening for women's alcohol use and abuse are all vital. Coordinating efforts with national advocacy organizations can be very effective in raising public awareness, and in providing hope and help to families of people with FASDs. Finally, incorporating successful evidence-based strategies into the ongoing public health programming of the country is an essential component of FASD prevention and intervention (Streissguth and Grant 2011). Comprehensive and effective prevention efforts will be more cost-effective for countries than managing the social and economic costs of future generations of alcohol-affected individuals.

Bibliography

Albert, E., Chudley, J., Conry, J.L., Cook, C.L., Rosales, T. and LeBlanc, L. (2005) 'Fetal alcohol spectrum disorder: Canadian guidelines for diagnosis', *Canadian Medical Association Journal*, 172(5): S1–21.

American Academy of Pediatrics (2000) 'Committee on Substance Abuse and Committee on Children with Disabilities: fetal alcohol syndrome and alcohol-related neurodevelopmental disorders', *Pediatrics*, 106(2): 358–61.

American Bar Association (2012) 'Resolution 112B ', adopted by the American Bar Association House Of Delegates Annual Meeting, Chicago, Illinois, 6–7 August [online at: www.americanbar.org/content/dam/aba/administrative/house_of_delegates/resolutions/2012_hod_annual_meeting_112b.authcheckdam.doc; accessed: 17 June 2013].

American College of Obstetricians and Gynecologists (2008) Committee on Ethics Committee Opinion #422: 'At-risk drinking and illicit drug use: ethical issues in obstetric and gynecologic practice', *Obstetrics and Gynecology*, 112(6): 1449–60.

American Medical Association (1999) *Summaries and Recommendations of Council on Scientific Affairs Reports, Interim Meeting of the AMA: 'Screening and Brief Interventions for Alcohol Problems (CSA Rep. 14, I-99)'* [online at: www.ama-assn.org/resources/doc/csaph/csai-99.pdf; accessed: 1 September 2011].

Astley, S.J. (2004) 'Fetal alcohol syndrome prevention in Washington State: evidence of success', *Paediatric and Perinatal Epidemiology*, 18(5): 344–51.

Canadian Bar Association (2010) 'Fetal alcohol spectrum disorder in the criminal justice system, certified true copy of a resolution carried by the Council of the Canadian Bar Association at the Annual Meeting held in Niagara, Ontario 14–15 August 2010' [online at: www.cba.org/CBA/resolutions/pdf/10-02-A.pdf; accessed: 2 September 2011].

Carson, G., Cox, L.V., Crane, J., Croteau, P., Graves, L., Kluka, S., Koren, G., Martel, M.J., Midmer, D., Nulman, I., Poole, N., Senikas, V., Wood. R. and Society of Obstetricians and Gynaecologists of Canada (2010) 'Alcohol use and pregnancy consensus clinical guidelines', *Journal of Obstetrics and Gynaecology Canada*, 32(8 Suppl 3): S1–31.

CDC (Centers for Disease Control and Prevention) (1997) 'Alcohol consumption among pregnant and childbearing-aged women – United States, 1991–1995', *Morbidity and Mortality Weekly Report*, 46: 346–50.

CDC (Centers for Disease Control and Prevention) (2002) 'Alcohol use among women of childbearing age – United States 1991–99', *Morbidity and Mortality Weekly Report*, 51: 273–6.

CDC (Centers for Disease Control and Prevention) (2004a) *Fetal Alcohol Syndrome: Guidelines for referral and diagnosis*, Atlanta, GA: National Center on Birth Defects and Developmental Disabilities, National Task Force on Fetal Alcohol Syndrome and Fetal Alcohol Effect.

CDC (Centers for Disease Control and Prevention) (2004b) 'Alcohol consumption among women who are pregnant or who might become pregnant – United States 2002', *Morbidity and Mortality Weekly Report*, 53: 1178–81.

CDC (Centers for Disease Control and Prevention) (2005) 'Notice to readers: Surgeon General's advisory on alcohol use in pregnancy', *Morbidity and Mortality Weekly Report*, 54: 229.

Chasnoff, I.J., Neuman, K., Thornton, C. and Callaghan, M.A. (2001) 'Screening for substance use in pregnancy: a practical approach for the primary care physician', *American Journal of Obstetrics and Gynecology*, 184(4): 752–8.

Chudley, A.E., Conry, J., Cook, J., Loock, C., Rosales, T. and LeBlanc, N. (2005) 'Fetal alcohol spectrum disorder: Canadian guidelines for diagnosis', *Canadian Medical Association Journal*, 172(5 suppl.): S1–21.

Clarren, S.K. and Salmon, A. (2010), 'Prevention of fetal alcohol spectrum disorder: proposal for a comprehensive approach', *Obstetrics and Gynecology*, 5(1): 23–30.

Clarren, S.K., Astley, S.J., Gunderson, V.M. and Spellman, D. (1992) 'Cognitive and behavioral deficits in nonhuman primates associated with very early embryonic binge exposures and ethanol', *Journal of Pediatrics*, 121(5 part 1): 789–96.Drabble, L.A., Poole, N., Magri, R., Tumwesigye, N.M., Li, Q. and Plant, M. (2011) 'Conceiving risk, divergent responses: perspectives on the construction of risk of FASD in six countries', *Substance Use and Misuse*, 46(8): 943–58.

Ebrahim, S.H., Luman, E.T., Floyd, R.L., Murphy, C.C., Bennett, E.M. and Boyle, C.A. (1998) 'Alcohol consumption by pregnant women in the United States during 1988–1995', *Obstetrics and Gynecology*, 92(2): 187–92.

Eckardt, M.J., Harford, T.C., Kaelber, C.T., Parker, E.S., Rosenthal, L.S., Ryback, R.S., Salmoiraghi, G.C., Vanderveen, E. and Warren, K.R. (1981) 'Health hazards associated with alcohol consumption', *Journal of the American Medical Association*, 246(6): 648–66.

Ellis, F.W. and Pick, J.R. (1980) 'An animal model of the fetal alcohol syndrome in beagles' *Alcoholism: Clinical and Experimental Research*, 4(2): 123–34.

Ernst, C.C., Grant, T.M., Streissguth, A.P. and Sampson, P.D. (1999) 'Intervention with high-risk alcohol and drug-abusing mothers: II. 3-year findings from the Seattle model of paraprofessional advocacy', *Journal of Community Psychology*, 27(1): 19–38.

Ewing, J.A. (1984) 'Detecting alcoholism: the CAGE questionnaire', *Journal of the American Medical Association*, 252(14): 1905–7.

Floyd, R.L., Decoufle, P. and Hungerford, D.W. (1999) 'Alcohol use prior to pregnancy recognition', *American Journal of Preventive Medicine*, 17(2): 101–7.

Floyd, R.L., O'Connor, M.J., Sokol, R.J., Bertrand, J. and Codero, J.F. (2005) 'Recognition and prevention of fetal alcohol syndrome', *Obstetrics and Gynecology*, 106(5 part 1): 1058–64.

Floyd, R.L., Weber, M.K., Denny, C. and O'Connor, M.J. (2009) 'Prevention of fetal alcohol spectrum disorders', *Developmental Disabilities Research Review*, 15(3): 193–9.

Goodlett, C.R. (2010) 'Fetal alcohol spectrum disorders: new perspectives on diagnosis and intervention', *Alcohol*, 44(7/8): 579–82.

Grant, T.M., Ernst, C.C., McAuliff, S. and Streissguth, A.P. (1997) 'The difference game: facilitating change in high-risk clients', *Families in Society: The Journal of Contemporary Human Services*, 78(4): 429–32.

Grant, T.M., Ernst, C.C. and Streissguth, A.P. (1999) 'Intervention with high-risk alcohol and drug-abusing mothers: I. administrative strategies of the Seattle model of paraprofessional advocacy', *Journal of Community Psychology*, 27(1): 1–18.

Grant, T., Ernst, C.C., Pagalilauan G. and Streissguth, A.P. (2003) 'Post-program follow-up effects of paraprofessional intervention with high-risk women who abused alcohol and drugs during pregnancy', *Journal of Community Psychology*, 31(3): 211–22.

Grant, T., Ernst, C., Streissguth, A. and Stark, K. (2005) 'Preventing alcohol and drug exposed births in Washington State: intervention findings from three Parent–Child Assistance Program sites', *American Journal of Drug and Alcohol Abuse*, 31(3): 471–90.

Grant, T.M., Huggins, J.E., Sampson, P.D., Ernst, C.C., Barr, H.M. and Streissguth, A.P. (2009) 'Alcohol use before and during pregnancy in Western Washington, 1989–2004: implications for the prevention of fetal alcohol spectrum disorders', *American Journal of Obstetrics and Gynecology*, 200(3): 278e1–8.

Greenfield, T.K., Graves, K.L. and Kaskutas, L.A. (1999) 'Long-term effects of alcohol warning labels: findings from a comparison of the United States and Ontario, Canada', *Psychology and Marketing*, 16(3): 261–82.

Hankin, J.R., Firestone, I.J., Sloan, J.J., Ager, J.W., Sokol, R.J. and Martier, S.S. (1996) 'Heeding the alcoholic beverage warning label during pregnancy: multiparae versus nulliparae', *Journal of Studies on Alcohol and Drugs*, 57(2): 171–7.

Harlap, S. and Shiono, P.H. (1980) 'Alcohol, smoking, and incidence of spontaneous abortions in the first and second trimester', Lancet, 2(8187): 173–6.

Hoyme, H.E., May, P.A., Kalberg, W.O., Kodituwakku, P., Gossage, P., Trujillo, P.M., Buckley, D.G., Miller, J.H., Aragon, A.S., Khaole, N., Viljoen, D.L., Jones, K.L. and Robinson, L.K. (2005) 'A practical clinical approach to diagnosis of fetal alcohol spectrum disorders: clarification of the 1996 Institute of Medicine criteria', *Pediatrics*, 115(1): 39–47.

Institute of Health Economics and the Alberta Government (2009) 'Consensus statement on fetal alcohol spectrum disorder (FASD) – across the lifespan' [online at: www.ihe.ca/publications/library/2009/; accessed: 1 September 2011].

Jones, K.L. and Smith, D.W. (1973) 'Recognition of the fetal alcohol syndrome in early infancy', *Lancet*, 302(7836): 999–1001.

Jones, K.L., Smith, D.W., Ulleland, C.N. and Streissguth, P. (1973) 'Pattern of malformation in offspring of chronic alcoholic mothers', *Lancet*, 1(7815): 1267–71.

Kelly, Y., Sacker, A., Gray, R., Kelly, J., Wolke, D. and Quigley, M.A. (2009) 'Light drinking in pregnancy, a risk for behavioural problems and cognitive deficits at 3 years of age?', *International Journal of Epidemiology*, 38(1): 129–40.

Kelly, Y.J., Sacker, A., Gray, R., Kelly, J., Wolke, D., Head, J. and Quigley, M.A. (2012) 'Light drinking during pregnancy: still no increased risk for socioemotional difficulties or cognitive deficits at 5 years of age?', *Journal of Epidemiology and Community Health*, 66(1): 41–8.

Little, R.E. (1977) 'Moderate alcohol use during pregnancy and decreased infant birth weight', American Journal of Public Health, 67(12): 1154–6.

Little, R.E., Streissguth, A.P., Barr, H.M. and Herman, C.S. (1980) 'Decreased birth weight in infants of alcoholic women who abstained during pregnancy', *Journal of* Pediatrics, 96(6): 974–7.

MacKinnon, D.P., Nohre, L., Pentz, M.A. and Stacy, A.W. (2000) 'The alcohol warning and adolescents: 5-year effects', *American Journal of Public Health*, 90(10): 1589–94.

Mengel, M.B., Searight, R. and Cook, K. (2006) 'Preventing alcohol-exposed pregnancies', *The Journal of the American Board of Family Medicine*, 19(5): 494–504.

Mohllajee, A.P., Curtis, K.M., Morrow, B. and Marchbanks, P.A. (2007) 'Pregnancy intention and its relationship to birth and maternal outcomes', *Obstetrics and Gynecology*, 109(3): 678–86.

Moos, M.K. (2004) 'Preconceptional health promotion: progress in changing a prevention paradigm', *Journal of Perinatal and Neonatal Nursing*, 18(1): 2–13.

Myers, J. (2002) 'Fomentation about fermentation: a study on ingredient labeling on alcoholic beverages', Legal Electronic Document Archive (LEDA) at Harvard Law School [online at: http://leda.law.harvard.edu/leda/data/513/Myers.pdf; accessed: 3 August 2011].

People Magazine (2006) 'Nesting Hollywood style', April 17.

Public Health Service (1981) 'Surgeon General's advisory on alcohol and pregnancy', *Food and Drug Administration Drug Bulletin*, 11(2): 9–10.

Robinson, G.C. and Armstrong, R.W. (eds) (1988) *Alcohol and Child/Family Health*, Vancouver, BC: University of British Columbia.

Robinson, G.C., Conry, J.L. and Conry, R.F. (1987) 'Clinical profile and prevalence of fetal alcohol syndrome in an isolated community in British Columbia', *Canadian Medical Association Journal*, 137(3): 203–7.
Russell, M. (1994) 'New assessment tools for drinking in pregnancy: T-ACE, TWEAK, and others', *Alcohol, Health and Research World*, 18(1): 55–61.
Sampson, P.D., Streissguth, A.P., Bookstein, F.L., Little, R.E., Clarren, S.K., Dehaene, P., Hanson, J.W. and Graham, J.M. Jr (1997) 'Incidence of fetal alcohol syndrome and prevalence of alcohol-related neurodevelopmental disorder', *Teratology*, 56(5): 317–26.
Saunders, J.B., Aasland, O.G., Babor, T.F., de la Fuente, J.R. and Grant, M. (1993) 'Development of the Alcohol Use Disorders Identification Test (AUDIT): WHO collaborative project on early detection of persons with harmful alcohol consumption: II', *Addiction*, 88(6): 791–804.
Sokol, R.J. and Clarren, S.K. (1989) 'Guidelines for use of terminology describing the impact of prenatal alcohol on the offspring', *Alcoholism: Clinical and Experimental Research*, 13(4): 597–8.
Sokol, R.J., Martier, S.S. and Ager, J.W. (1989) 'The T-ACE questions: practical prenatal detection of risk drinking', *American Journal of Obstetrics and Gynecology*, 160(4): 863–8.
Stratton, K., Howe, C. and Battaglia F. (eds) (1996) *Fetal Alcohol Syndrome: Diagnosis, epidemiology, prevention, and treatment*, Washington, DC: Institute of Medicine, National Academy Press.
Streissguth, A.P. and Grant, T.M. (2011) 'Prenatal and postnatal intervention strategies for alcohol-abusing mothers in pregnancy', in D. Preece and E. Riley (eds) *Alcohol, Drugs and Medication in Pregnancy: The long term outcome for the child*, London: MacKeith Press.
Streissguth, A.P., Bookstein, F.L., Sampson, P.D. and Barr, H.M. (1989) 'Neurobehavioral effects of prenatal alcohol: Part III. PLS analyses of neuropsychologic tests', *Neurotoxicology and Teratology*, 11(5): 493–507.
Streissguth, A.P., Bookstein, F.L., Barr, H.M., Sampson, P.D., O'Malley, K. and Young, J.K. (2004) 'Risk factors for adverse life outcomes in fetal alcohol syndrome and fetal alcohol effects', *Journal of Developmental and Behavioral Pediatrics*, 25(4): 228–38.
Sulik, K.K., Johnston, M.C. and Webb, M.A. (1981) 'Fetal Alcohol Syndrome: embryogenesis in a mouse model', *Science*, 214(4523): 936–8.
Umlah, C. and Grant, T. (2003) 'Intervening to prevent prenatal alcohol and drug exposure: the Manitoba experience in replicating a paraprofessional model', *Manitoba Journal of Child Welfare*, 2(1): 1–12.
Tsai, J. and Floyd, R.L. (2004) 'Alcohol consumption among women who are pregnant or who might become pregnant', *Morbidity and Mortality Weekly Report*, 53(50): 1178–81.
WHO (World Health Organization) (2004) *Global Status Report on Alcohol 2004*, Geneva: WHO, Department of Mental Health and Substance Abuse.
Williams, R.J., Odaibo, F.S and McGee, J.M. (1999) 'Incidence of fetal alcohol syndrome in northeastern Manitoba', *Canadian Journal of Public Health*, 90(3): 192–4.
Wilson, J.G. (1973) *Environment and Birth Defects*, New York: Academic Press.

21

FETAL ALCOHOL SPECTRUM DISORDERS

European perspectives

Diane Black

Introduction

Over the past centuries, many European scientists and physicians have noted negative effects of prenatal exposure to alcohol. In the early seventeenth century, Francis Bacon noted that 'the diet of women with child doth work much upon the infant; … if the mother … drink wine or strong drink immoderately … it endangereth the child to become lunatic, or of imperfect memory' (Bacon 1627: para. 977). In 1876, the British Medical Journal published an article by Dr John Haddon, describing the effects of 'intemperance in women'. He noted that:

> Children born at the full time are generally weak and puny, and likely to fall at an early age victims to disease … [I]t is possible that a large proportion of our excessive infant mortality may be due to the malnutrition of the embryo, caused by the use of alcohol.
> *(Haddon 1876: 748)*

It was only in 1968, however, that a systematic description of the characteristics of children of alcoholic mothers appeared. This seminal study, by Dr Paul Lemoine of Nantes (Lemoine *et al.* 1968), was published in a local French medical journal, and unfortunately did not receive the attention it deserved at the time. Only later, after the publication by Jones and Smith (Jones and Smith 1973: 999) in the *Lancet* of an article describing and naming 'the fetal alcohol syndrome' (FAS), did researchers become aware of the earlier French publication.

In the following years, European researchers carried out some exemplary studies (which will be mentioned in the following pages) on what we now call fetal alcohol spectrum disorders (FASDs). Unfortunately this early research did not lead to widespread awareness of the dangers of drinking during pregnancy. Why not? Certainly there are many reasons, including the fragmentation of efforts in various countries, coupled with the lack of a forum for communication and sharing of ideas or experiences. Furthermore, cultural differences (e.g. drinking patterns, beliefs of supposed health benefits of alcohol) affect drinking during pregnancy as well as what sort of messages can modify this behaviour. However, currently there is an explosion of activity in this area. Various countries and cultures have given rise to projects ranging from research to prevention to management of FAS.

This short contribution cannot form an exhaustive review of activities in Europe, but will give a brief overview of what is happening at the European level, followed by a somewhat subjective/personal choice of 'snapshots' of activities in various countries, and concluding with plans and dreams for the future of alcohol and pregnancy in Europe.

European Union policy related to alcohol and pregnancy

The European Union (EU) currently includes 27 countries cooperating in various economic and political activities. The decision-making bodies which are most relevant to alcohol and pregnancy are the European Commission, the Council of the European Union and the European Parliament. The European Commission proposes legislation, which may then be adopted by the Council and the Parliament. The Member States are then responsible for application of legislation into national legislation. The work of the European Commission is prepared by the various departments, the Directorates-General. The department concerned with issues of alcohol and pregnancy is the Health and Consumers Directorate-General, often referred to by its French abbreviation, DG SANCO.

The mandate of the EU in the fields of public health and consumer protection is defined in Articles 168 and 169 of the Treaty on the Functioning of the European Union. Public health is a shared competency of the EU legislature and Member States, so the EU aims to 'complement national policies'. Cooperation among Member States is encouraged. Furthermore, Article 168 specifically states that the EU may adopt 'measures which have as their direct objective the protection of public health regarding tobacco and the abuse of alcohol'. With respect to consumer protection, again the Member States have the main responsibility, but 'the Union shall contribute to protecting the health, safety and economic interests of consumers, as well as to promoting their right to information, education and to organise themselves in order to safeguard their interests'.[1]

Although normally national authorities must take the lead, in some cases, in order to promote coordination among the Member States, the EU can pass binding legislation in order to promote coordination among the Member States.

Let us take tobacco as an example of what the European Union can do. Various binding directives have been issued; for example, with respect to labels on packages. Warning labels are obligatory, and to be rotated. Some of the options are 'Smoking when pregnant harms your baby' and 'Smoking can damage the sperm and reduces fertility'. Tobacco advertising is severely limited, high excise taxes are obligatory and agricultural subsidies for tobacco have been phased out. The Commission monitors national compliance, funds regional projects to reduce smoking, and launched a Europe-wide campaign, 'Ex-smokers are unstoppable'.[2]

In comparison, action on alcohol use has been slower in the EU. Some binding legislation exists – for example, minimum excise duties and certain limitations on television advertising – but regulation has not been as strict as for tobacco.[3] In order to gain an overview of the health problems resulting from alcohol, the Commission produced a report, *Alcohol in Europe*, which was published in 2006 (Anderson and Baumberg 2006), and provided a valuable overview of alcohol-related harm in the EU. Based on this report and the request from Member States (especially Sweden), the Commission prepared *An EU Strategy to Support Member States in Reducing Alcohol Related Harm* (Commission of the European Communities

2006), which was adopted in October 2006. The term alcohol-related harm, of course, covers a broad range of health effects. But most importantly, Section 5.1 made it a priority to 'protect young people, children and the unborn child'. In accordance with treaty Article 168 on Public Health, as mentioned above, the Strategy clearly states that 'there is no intention to substitute Community action to national policies' and 'the Commission does not intend as a consequence of this Communication to propose the development of harmonised legislation in the field of the prevention of alcohol-related harm'. Three levels of action were proposed: the national level, coordination among Member States and actions by the European Commission itself.

The first progress report on the Strategy was published in 2009. The authors found that 'there has been considerable activity on the part of the Commission, the Member States and the wider stakeholders to set up the infrastructure for implementation' and that 'there has been a steady convergence of actions towards those identified as good practice.' Specifically with respect to alcohol and pregnancy, the report notes that almost half of Member States have some kind of campaign to give information on alcohol and pregnancy, whether by the public health services or non-governmental organizations (NGOs). The report also noted the implementation of labelling in France, which took effect in 2007.[4]

The second and final progress report will appear in 2012, at which time the current Strategy expires. Based on the final progress report, the Commission will decide how to proceed. Many stakeholders are now pushing for more definitive action from the EU; for example, with respect to labelling. Indeed, in 2010, a survey of European citizens showed that 79 per cent support labelling to warn pregnant women not to drink.[5]

The World Health Organization and European NGOs

The World Health Organization (WHO) notes that Europe is the heaviest drinking region in the world, and bears the largest burden of alcohol-related harm in the world. Only since May 2010, however, has prenatal exposure become a priority for the WHO, through the adoption of a 'Global strategy to reduce the harmful use of alcohol'. A new action plan has been developed by the European section for 2012 to 2020; this strategy builds upon and strengthens the global strategy. As a result of the global strategy, the WHO, in collaboration with FASD experts, has developed standardized protocols for screening for FASDs and prenatal exposure. In collaboration with international research groups and local health authorities, screening will be carried out in several countries, with the participation of the following European countries currently confirmed: Ukraine, Moldova and Belarus.[6]

Among NGOs concerned with alcohol-related harm in Europe, Eurocare stands out.[7] Eurocare, the European Alcohol Policy Alliance, fosters cooperation among member organizations, engages in dialogue with European policymakers and carries out advocacy campaigns. Since 2006, Eurocare has organized regular events at the Europarliament around international FAS day on 9 September, with the goal of informing policymakers about the dangers of alcohol during pregnancy. The actions seem to be paying off: in 2011, the conference on 'Protecting the unborn baby from alcohol' drew high-level participation, including a speech by the Commissioner for Health and Consumer Affairs, Mr John Dalli. The Commissioner clearly recognized in this speech that there is no safe level for alcohol consumption during pregnancy, and gave his support for warning labels on containers of alcoholic drinks (Dalli 2011).

Finally, the First European Conference on FASDs was held in Kerkrade, the Netherlands, in November 2010. This conference drew 160 attendees from 23 countries within and outside Europe. As a result of the enthusiasm for closer cooperation shown at this conference, the European FASD Alliance was founded in February 2011.[8] The principal goals of this organization are to promote communication and sharing of ideas, via the website as well as the organization of a European conference every two years. The Second European Conference on FASDs was held in Barcelona, in October of 2012, drawing 200 attendees from 24 countries. The next such conference is planned for Rome in October of 2014.

In the next sections of this chapter, I present a brief overview of activities related to FASDs in several countries. This is a personal choice, as it is impossible to treat every country in depth. I attempt, however, to demonstrate the wide range of action in Europe.

France

Since the early publication by Lemoine mentioned above, research on effects of alcohol during pregnancy has been very active in France, though the French language publications remain under-recognized in the anglophone world. Topics of research range from the effects on the digestive tract, reducing the ability to digest protein (Raul *et al.* 1987), and the increased risk of certain childhood cancers (Latino-Martel *et al.* 2010), to studies on psychomotor development (Larroque *et al.* 2000). The first follow-up to adulthood reported the typical facial features and continuing behavioural issues (Lemoine and Lemoine 1992). Regarding drinking during pregnancy, studies in various regions have reported widely divergent figures: in Auvergne, 47 per cent of pregnant women (Malet *et al.* 2006); Paris, 25.3 per cent (Dumas *et al.* 2008); Clermont-Ferrand, 52.2 per cent (de Chazeron *et al.* 2008); Nantes, 63 per cent (Chassevent-Pajot *et al.* 2011). A recent study in the Paris region found that, of mothers who continued drinking during pregnancy, 30 per cent of the births were premature, and about 60 per cent of the babies had to receive special neonatal care (Toutain *et al.* 2010). As for prevalence of FASDs, Dr Philippe Dehaene carried out a first prevalence study in Roubaix, finding 4.8 children per thousand expressing degrees of FAS (Sampson *et al.* 1997). A study in Reunion Island, found a similar rate of 4.3 cases of FAS per thousand (Maillard *et al.* 1999).

France is the only country in Europe to mandate that alcoholic beverages carry labels warning pregnant women not to drink. The story began in 2002, when three women who had given birth to children with FAS approached Benoît Titran, an attorney, about charging manufacturers with failure to warn them of the dangers of their product. Publicity about this case led to the involvement of more players. In March 2004, the National Academy of Medicine made recommendations including labelling on containers of alcoholic drinks. Later that year, the public prosecutor opened an investigation into possible endangerment of the lives of others, deceit in goods and involuntary harm to others. Senator Anne-Marie Payet introduced an amendment which would mandate information for school children, education for health professionals, regular media campaigns and labelling on containers of alcoholic drinks. All the measures became law in 2005 except that on labelling. However, when the Minister of Health put his support behind labelling, that measure was finally enacted into law in 2006.[9]

At the national level, the organization SAF France[10] (founded 2008) has goals to share information and promote research, training, prevention and care of people with FASDs in

France. In various regions there are centres for research, diagnosis and support of people with FASDs. More information on the regional centres is available on the SAF France website.

Sweden

Recognition of the dangers of alcohol and pregnancy began in the 1970s when a paediatrician, Dr Ragnar Olegård, who had read the seminal publication by Lemoine, recognized the problems in a child of an alcoholic mother. In one of his first publications, Dr Olegård named prenatal exposure to alcohol as the 'largest known health hazard by a noxious agent that is preventable' (Olegård *et al.* 1979: 112). Marita Aronson, a psychologist, worked with Olegård on the evaluation of 24 children, publishing one of the first follow-up studies of children of alcoholic mothers. At the ages of 12 to 14 years, there was a high rate of neuropsychological problems, and notably 16 of the 24 were in foster care (Aronson and Hagberg 1998). Ophthalmologist Kerstin Strömland was the first to report ocular damage in FAS (Strömland 1990).

The Swedish National Board of Health and Welfare recommends avoidance of alcohol during pregnancy.[11] Midwives, who see almost all pregnant women in Sweden, are well-informed of the dangers of drinking during pregnancy, but feel less confident about their ability to detect and address harmful drinking (Holmqvist and Nilsen 2010). One study based on the use of standardized interviews found that 15 per cent of pregnant urban women drank to risky levels (Magnusson *et al.* 2005). In Sweden, print advertisements for alcoholic beverages are required to include one of a series of 11 rotating notices about various types of alcohol-related harm, covering at least 20 per cent of the surface of the advertisement.[12]

A fascinating insight into the effects of alcohol use during pregnancy comes from an economic analysis related to a social experiment conducted in 1967 to 1968, when grocery stores in two regions of Sweden were allowed to sell strong beer, the sale of which was normally confined to state-run alcohol monopolies. During the first months of 1968, alcohol consumption in these areas increased ten-fold – such an alarming increase that the experiment was prematurely stopped. Thirty years later, an economic analysis showed that babies *in utero* during the social experiment had become adults with lower educational achievements, lower earnings and a higher rate of welfare dependency than adults of the same age in surrounding regions (Nilsson 2008).

The prevalence of FASDs in Sweden has not been studied. There are no specialist diagnostic clinics. One early study on the causes of mild mental retardation among Swedish school children concluded that 8 per cent of cases were related to prenatal alcohol exposure (Hagberg *et al.* 1981). Due to the fact that many children adopted in Sweden come from Eastern Europe, a recent study examined the incidence of FASDs in these children, finding that 52 per cent (n = 71) had an FASD (Landgren *et al.* 2010).

The FAS Förening (FAS Foundation of Sweden), founded in the year 2000, is the major organization providing information and support on FASDs. One initiative of the FAS Förening, apparently unique in Europe, is a combination of family camps and special week-long camps for teens with FASDs, providing activities and counselling for young people with FASDs from all over Sweden. In 2011, for example, 16 teens attended this camp. The FAS Förening provides books, flyers and a website in Swedish.[13]

Germany

Research on FAS in Germany began early with a series of case studies in both English and German by paediatrician Frank Majewski (Majewski 1978). Paediatricians Spohr and Steinhausen published their first observations in the early 1980s (Nestler *et al.* 1981), with a follow-up 20 years later (Spohr *et al.* 2007). There have been no studies on prevalence of FASDs in the general population in Germany, but several studies suggest that drinking during pregnancy is widespread. One multicentre study of women treated at infertility clinics revealed that only 0.6 per cent of treated women consumed alcohol during pregnancy, but that 23.5 per cent of control women did so (Ludwig *et al.* 2006). A study involving a database of over 170,000 singleton births found that 8.6 per cent of women used alcohol during pregnancy, and that this was a significant factor in physical abnormalities (Baumann *et al.* 2006). A national survey reported that 14 per cent of women drank during pregnancy, with upper socioeconomic group women more likely to report drinking (Bergmann *et al.* 2007). Finally, a shockingly clear demonstration of the effect of alcohol on the developing brain appeared in the journal, *Science*, showing that even transient single exposure triggers apoptosis of thousands of nerve cells in the developing brain (Ikonomidou *et al.* 2000).

The German Drug Commissioner warns that even small amounts of alcohol can be harmful, and that alcohol should be completely avoided during pregnancy. Furthermore she estimates that there are 10,000 births per year of alcohol-damaged children, with 4,000 having full FAS.[14] No warning labels are required by law, though Pernod-Ricard voluntarily puts a warning to pregnant women on their labels.[15]

Germany is unique in having specialized residential and assisted living for adults with FASDs. For adults who need more help with organizing their time and with social skills, there is a home in the Spandau area of Berlin with individual rooms for four adults, who share common areas. Professional supervision is present during most daytime hours. For adults ready to make the step to greater independence, there are several homes and apartments in the area, where regular support can be offered.[16]

FASworld Deutschland, perhaps the oldest of the European FAS support organizations, provides an online support group and 17 regional support groups for parents, as well as raising awareness via publications and a yearly conference. There are two specialist clinics for FASD diagnosis and support, in Münster and Berlin.[17]

Italy

As in many other countries, the first Italian publications on FAS were case reports (De Nigris *et al.* 1981; Scianaro *et al.* 1978). In 1990, Gabrielli and colleagues published what was apparently the first MRI study of a child with FAS. Throughout the 1990s and into the first years of this century, the bulk of reported research involved rat studies on brain development. Beginning in 2003, however, in collaboration with an American group, there began the first active case ascertainment study of FASDs in Europe, in the Lazio region around Rome. In this study, six-year-olds in the local schools were screened for FASDs, resulting in an estimated prevalence of between 2 and 4 per cent FASDs (May *et al.* 2006). In a second wave study in the same geographical region, using slightly refined diagnostic criteria, a prevalence of 2 to 6 per cent was found (May *et al.* 2011). Another active field of study in collaboration with a group in Barcelona, Spain, has been investigation and validation of biomarkers of alcohol consumption in the meconium as a measure of prenatal exposure (Morini *et al.* 2010).

There are no official guidelines on drinking during pregnancy, and few statistics are available as a measure of the problem. There are no representative national studies showing prevalence of FASDs, but a new study analysing meconium samples from seven sites in Italy showed a dramatic regional variation, with exposure ranging from 0 per cent in Verona to 29 per cent in Rome (Pichini *et al.* 2012). A survey of women who telephoned the Teratology Information Services in Rome revealed that about 18 per cent used alcohol during pregnancy (De Santis *et al.* 2011), and alcohol consumption has been identified as a risk factor in spina bifida (De Marco *et al.* 2011). Regarding professionals, a survey among Italian doctors revealed that about 50 per cent advise their pregnant patients that they can drink occasionally, and that neonatologists and paediatricians have low confidence in their ability to diagnose FAS (Vagnarelli *et al.* 2011). Several recent events should help to improve the awareness among professionals, including the recent foundation of the Società Italian sulla Sindrome Feto-Alcolica[18] by Dr Mauro Ceccanti and colleagues to share information among professionals and the release of Italian-language diagnostic guidelines.[19]

A project on alcohol and pregnancy, begun in 2008 and still ongoing, has been carried out in the Treviso area, as a collaboration between researchers and the local public health authorities. First, surveys on attitudes to drinking during pregnancy were carried out in various professional and population groups. Next a social marketing campaign, 'Mamma beve, bimbo beve' (Mamma drinks, baby drinks) was designed in collaboration with Fabrica, the communication agency of Benetton. During the campaign, the controversial posters of a fetus at the bottom of a cocktail glass made world news.[20]

As with other Mediterranean countries, there is no parent group involved in prevention, and no support groups for families or people with FAS.

Netherlands

Until about ten years ago, mention of the issue of alcohol and pregnancy was sporadic in the Netherlands, and prenatal exposure to alcohol was under-recognized as a cause of disability (van Balkom *et al.* 1996). Various professional groups gave different guidelines on drinking during pregnancy, and physicians regularly told pregnant women that 'one glass can't hurt'. The situation began to change with the creation of the Fetal Alcohol Syndrome Foundation of the Netherlands[21] in 2002 and a collaborative public education project with the Dutch Institute for Alcohol Policy[22] (STAP). In 2005 the Health Council of the Netherlands gave clear official advice that neither men nor women should drink during the conception period, and that women should not drink during pregnancy (Health Council of the Netherlands 2005). Preconception counselling now includes advice about alcohol use during pregnancy, and has been shown to be effective in helping women reduce alcohol use during the first trimester of pregnancy (Elsinga *et al.* 2008).

There are no reliable statistics on prevalence of FASDs. There are two dedicated FAS clinics, at the Gelre Hospital, Zutphen,[23] and at the Lentis/Jonx Youth Psychiatric Mental Health Services, Winschoten.[24] Both these clinics see adults as well as children. Many children are adopted from Poland by Dutch families; evidence suggests that many of these children are affected by FASDs (Knuiman *et al.* 2010).

Regarding drinking during pregnancy, the Health Council estimated in 2005 that 35 to 50 per cent of pregnant women continue using alcohol during pregnancy. The Amsterdam Born Children and their Development study found that about 30 per cent of ethnic Dutch women reported alcohol use around the thirteenth week of pregnancy (Goedhart *et al.* 2008), and a recent study in Rotterdam among 7,333 subjects showed that 37 per cent of pregnant women continued to use alcohol throughout pregnancy; these women were primarily highly educated ethnic Dutch and other Europeans (Bakker *et al.* 2010).

Parents raising children with FASDs can get professional advice from the FAS policlinics. Furthermore, the FAS Foundation provides books and other literature in Dutch, a website, newsletter and an email support group for parents. Both the FAS Foundation and STAP provide information and flyers to midwives for use in counselling pregnant women.

Conclusion

This chapter has given only a brief overview of some of the action surrounding the issues of alcohol and pregnancy in Europe, primarily focusing on the European Union. It is impossible to close this chapter without at least a brief mention of the public education campaigns held by the Polish State Agency for Prevention of Alcohol Related Problems,[25] by the Estonian Temperance Union,[26] the long-standing research in Finland (Fang *et al.* 2008), and so much activity now in European countries outside the EU, including the Ukraine and Russia. With increased awareness of the dangers of alcohol during pregnancy both at the national and European levels, we hope to both reduce prenatal exposure to alcohol and improve quality of life of children and adults affected by FASDs and their families.

Notes

1 Treaty on the Functioning of the European Union, available at: http://eur-lex.europa.eu/LexUriServ/LexUriServ.do?uri=OJ:C:2010:083:0047:0200:EN:PDF
2 http://ec.europa.eu/health/tobacco/policy/index_en.htm
3 http://ec.europa.eu/health/alcohol/policy/index_en.htm
4 http://ec.europa.eu/health/archive/ph_determinants/life_style/alcohol/documents/alcohol_progress.pdf
5 http://ec.europa.eu/health/alcohol/docs/ebs_331_en.pdf
6 www.who.int/topics/alcohol_drinking/en/
7 www.eurocare.org
8 www.eufasd.org
9 The full story can be read in English at: www.eurocare.org/library/resources/special_topics/alcohol_and_pregnancy/labeling_and_fasd_prevention_in_france_anpaa
10 Syndrome d'Alcoolisation Foetale France: www.saffrance.fr
11 www.socialstyrelsen.se/missbrukochberoende/missbrukundergraviditeten, consulted 27 July 2011
12 www.notisum.se/rnp/sls/sfs/20101636.pdf, para. 14, consulted 27 July 2011.
13 www.fasforeningen.nu
14 http://drogenbeauftragte.de/drogen-und-sucht/alkohol/alkohol-und-schwangerschaft.html
15 http://pernod-ricard.com/724/csr/responsible-drinking/pregnant-women
16 www.ev-sonnenhof.de/wg-bew-fasd.html
17 Münster: www.fetales-alkoholsyndrom.de/index.html; Berlin: www.fasd-zentrum.blogspot.com/
18 www.sifasd.it
19 www.sifasd.it/media/fa_linee_guida.pdf
20 www.fabrica.it/news/2010?page=6; and www.kambiomarcia.it/home1/mamma/index.php
21 www.fasstichting.nl
22 www.stap.nl

23 www.gelreziekenhuizen.nl/Gelreziekenhuizen/Zutphen-Specialismen-Afdelingen-Zutphen-Specialismen-Afdelingen-Polikliniek-Kindergeneeskunde/FAS-polikliniek.html
24 www.jonx.nl/Locaties/Locatieitem/tabid/741/articleType/ArticleView/articleId/1383/Jonx%20-%20FASD%20Polikliniek%20Winschoten.aspx 25   http://fas.nazwa.pl/parpa_en/
26 www.ave.ee/fas/

References

Anderson, P. and Baumberg, B. (2006) *Alcohol in Europe: a public health perspective*, a report for the European Commission, London: Institute of Alcohol Studies [online at: http://ec.europa.eu/health/archive/ph_determinants/life_style/alcohol/documents/alcohol_europe_en.pdf; accessed: 29 November 2012].

Aronson, M. and Hagberg, B. (1998) 'Neuropsychological disorders in children exposed to alcohol during pregnancy: a follow-up study of 24 children to alcoholic mothers in Goteborg, Sweden', *Alcoholism: Clinical and Experimental Research*, 22(2): 321–4.

Bacon, F. (1627) *Sylva Sylvarum: or a naturall historie in ten centuries*, London: William Lee.

Bakker, R., Pluimgraaff, L.E., Steegers, E.A., Raat, H., Tiemeier, H., Hofman, A. and Jaddoe, V.W. (2010) 'Associations of light and moderate maternal alcohol consumption with fetal growth characteristics in different periods of pregnancy: the Generation R Study', *International Journal of Epidemiology*, 39(3): 777–89.

Baumann, P., Schild, C., Hume, R.F. and Sokol, R.J. (2006) 'Alcohol abuse – a persistent preventable risk for congenital anomalies', *International Journal of Gynaecology and Obstetrics*, 95(1): 66–72.

Bergmann, K.E., Bergmann, R.L., Ellert, U. and Dudenhausen, J.W. (2007) '[Perinatal risk factors for long-term health. Results of the German Health Interview and Examination Survey for Children and Adolescents (KiGGS)]', *Bundesgesundheitsblatt Gesundheitsforschung Gesundheitsschutz*, 50(5/6): 670–6.

Chassevent-Pajot, A., Guillou-Landréat, M., Grall-Bronnec, M., Wainstein, L., Philippe, H.J., Lombrail, P. and Venisse, J.L. (2011) '[Epidemiological study on addictive behaviours during pregnancy in a university department]', *Journal de gynécologie, obstétrique et biologie de la reproduction*, 40(3): 237–45.

Commission of the European Communities (2006) *An EU Strategy to Support Member States in Reducing Alcohol Related Harm: Communication from the Commission to the Council, the European Parliament, the European Economic and Social Committee and the Committee of the Regions*, Luxembourg: Office for Official Publications of the European Communities.

Dalli, J. (2011) 'Way forward at the EU level', keynote address to the conference, 'Protecting the unborn baby from alcohol', European Parliament, Brussels, 7 September [online at: www.eurocare.org/media_centre/previous_eurocare_events/protecting_the_unborn_baby_from_alcohol_7_september_2011_european_parliament_brussels; accessed: 9 June 2013].

de Chazeron, I., Llorca, P.M., Ughetto, S., Vendittelli, F., Boussiron, D., Sapin, V., Coudore, F. and Lemery, D. (2008) 'Is pregnancy the time to change alcohol consumption habits in France?', *Alcoholism: Clinical and Experimental Research*, 32(5): 868–73.

De Marco, P., Merello, E., Calevo, M.G., Mascelli, S., Pastorino, D., Crocetti, L., De Biasio P., Piatelli, G., Cama, A. and Capra, V. (2011) 'Maternal periconceptional factors affect the risk of spina bifida-affected pregnancies: an Italian case-control study', *Child's Nervous System*, 27(7): 1073–81.

De Nigris, C., Awabdeh, F., Tomassini, A. and Remotti, G. (1981) '[Alcohol and pregnancy: incidence of the phenomenon and effects on the newborn infant in the population of a Varese hospital]', *Annali di ostetricia, ginecologia, medicina perinatale*, 102: 419–30.

De Santis, M., De Luca, C., Mappa, I., Quattrocchi, T., Angelo, L. and Cesari, E. (2011) 'Smoke, alcohol consumption and illicit drug use in an Italian population of pregnant women', *European Journal of Obstetrics, Gynecology and Reproductive Biology*, 159(1): 106–110.

Dumas, A., Lejeune, C., Simmat-Durand, L., Crenn-Hebert, C. and Mandelbrot, L. (2008) '[Pregnancy and psychoactive substances: prevalence study based on the declared consumption]', *Journal de Gynécologie Obstétrique et Biologie de la Reproduction*, 37(8): 770–8.

Elsinga, J., de Jong-Potjer, L.C., van der Pal-de Bruin K.M., le Cessie S., Assendelft, W.J. and Buitendijk, S.E. (2008) 'The effect of preconception counselling on lifestyle and other behaviour before and during pregnancy', *Women's Health Issues*, 18(6Suppl): S117–25.

Fang, S., McLaughlin, J., Fang, J., Huang, J., Autti-Rämö, I., Fagerlund, A., Jacobson, S.W., Robinson, L.K., Hoyme, H.E., Mattson, S.N., Riley, E., Zhou, F., Ward, R., Moore, E.S. and Foroud, T. (2008) 'Automated diagnosis of fetal alcohol syndrome using 3D facial image analysis', *Orthodontics and Craniofacial Research*, 11(3): 162–71.

Gabrielli, O., Salvolini, U., Coppa, G.V., Catassi, C., Rossi, R., Manca, A., Lanza, R. and Giorgi, P.L. (1990) 'Magnetic resonance imaging in the malformative syndromes with mental retardation', *Pediatric Radiology*, 21(1): 16–19.

Goedhart, G., van Eijsden, M., van der Wal, M.F. and Bonsel, G.J. (2008) 'Ethnic differences in term birthweight: the role of constitutional and environmental factors', *Paediatric and Perinatal Epidemiology*, 22(4): 360–8.

Haddon, J. (1876) 'On intemperance in women, with special reference to its effects on the reproductive system', *British Medical Journal*, 1(807): 748–50.

Hagberg, B., Hagberg, G., Lewerth, A. and Lindberg, U. (1981) 'Mild mental retardation in Swedish school children. II. etiologic and pathogenetic aspects', *Acta paediatrica Scandinavica*, 70(4): 445–52.

Health Council of the Netherlands (2005) *Risks of Alcohol Consumption Related to Conception, Pregnancy and Breastfeeding*, publication no. 2004/22, The Hague: Health Council of the Netherlands.

Holmqvist, M. and Nilsen, P. (2010) 'Approaches to assessment of alcohol intake during pregnancy in Swedish maternity care – a national-based investigation into midwives' alcohol-related education, knowledge and practice', *Midwifery*, 26(4): 430–4.

Ikonomidou, C., Bittigau, P., Ishimaru, M.J., Wozniak, D.F., Koch, C., Genz, K., Price, M.T., Stefovska, V., Hörster, F., Tenkova, T., Dikranian, K. and Olney, J.W. (2000) 'Ethanol-induced apoptotic neurodegeneration and fetal alcohol syndrome', *Science*, 287(5455): 1056–60.

Jones, K.L. and Smith, D.W. (1973) 'Recognition of the fetal alcohol syndrome in early infancy', *Lancet*, 302(7836): 999–1001.

Knuiman, S., Rijk, C.H.A.M., Hoksbergen, R. and van Baar, A.L. (2010) 'FASD in children adopted from Poland', poster presented at the First European Conference on FASD, Kerkrade, Netherlands, 3–5 November.

Landgren, M., Svensson, L., Strömland, K. and Andersson Grönlund, M. (2010) 'Prenatal alcohol exposure and neurodevelopmental disorders in children adopted from Eastern Europe', *Pediatrics*, 125(5): e1178–85.

Larroque, B., Kaminski, M., Dehaene, P., Subtil, D. and Querleu, D. (2000) 'Prenatal alcohol exposure and signs of minor neurological dysfunction at preschool age', *Developmental Medicine and Child Neurology*, 42(8): 508–14.

Latino-Martel, P., Chan, D.S., Druesne-Pecollo, N., Barrandon, E., Hercberg, S. and Norat, T. (2010) 'Maternal alcohol consumption during pregnancy and risk of childhood leukemia: systematic review and meta-analysis', *Cancer Epidemiology, Biomarkers and Prevention*, 19(5): 1238–60.

Lemoine, P. and Lemoine, P. (1992) '[Outcome of children of alcoholic mothers (study of 105 cases followed to adult age) and various prophylactic findings]', *Annales de pédiatrie*, 39(4): 226–35.

Lemoine, P., Harousseau, H., Borteyru, J.-P. and Menuet, J.-C. (1968) 'Les enfants de parents alcooliques: anomalies observées', *Ouest-Médical*, 21: 476–482.

Ludwig, A.K., Katalinic, A., Steinbicker, V., Diedrich, K. and Ludwig, M. (2006) 'Antenatal care in singleton pregnancies after ICSI as compared to spontaneous conception: data from a prospective controlled cohort study in Germany', *Human Reproduction*, 21(3): 713–20.

Magnusson, A., Göransson, M. and Heilig, M. (2005) 'Unexpectedly high prevalence of alcohol use among pregnant Swedish women: failed detection by antenatal care and simple tools that improve detection', *Journal of Studies on Alcohol*, 66(2): 157–64.

Maillard, T., Lamblin, D., Lesure, J.F. and Fourmaintraux, A. (1999) 'Incidence of fetal alcohol syndrome on the southern part of Reunion Island (France)', *Teratology*, 60(2): 51–2.

Majewski, F. (1978) '[Alcoholic embryopathy]', *Fortschritte der Medizin*, 96(43): 2207–13.

Malet, L., de Chazeron, I., Llorca, P.M. and Lemery, D. (2006) 'Alcohol consumption during pregnancy: a urge to increase prevention and screening', *European Journal of Epidemiology*, 21(10): 787–8.

May, P.A., Fiorentino, D., Gossage, J.P., Kalberg, W.O., Hoyme, E.H., Robinson, L.K., Coriale, G., Jones, K.L., del Campo, M., Tarani, L., Romeo, M., Kodituwakku, P.W., Deiana, L., Buckley,

D. and Ceccanti, M. (2006) 'Epidemiology of FASD in a province in Italy: Prevalence and characteristics of children in a random sample of schools', *Alcoholism: Clinical and Experimental Research*, 30(9): 1562–75.

May, P.A., Fiorentino, D., Coriale, G., Kalberg, W.O., Hoyme, H.E., Aragon, A.S., Buckley, D., Stellavato, C., Gossage, J.P., Robinson, L.K., Jones, K.L., Manning, M. and Ceccanti, M. (2011) 'Prevalence of children with severe fetal alcohol spectrum disorders in communities near Rome, Italy: new estimated rates are higher than previous estimates', *International Journal of Environmental Research and Public Health*, 8(6): 2331–51.

Morini, L., Marchei, E., Vagnarelli, F., Garcia Algar, O., Groppi, A., Mastrobattista, L. and Pichini, S. (2010) 'Ethyl glucuronide and ethyl sulfate in meconium and hair-potential biomarkers of intrauterine exposure to ethanol', *Forensic Science International*, 196(1/3): 74–7.

Nestler, V., Spohr, H.L. and Steinhausen, H.C. (1981) '[Studies on alcohol embryopathy (author's transl.)]', *Monatsschrift fur Kinderheilkunde*, 129(7): 404–9.

Nilsson, J.P. (2008) *Does a Pint a Day Affect Your Child's Pay? The effect of prenatal alcohol exposure on adult outcomes*, Uppsala: Institute for Labor Market Policy Evaluation.

Olegård, R., Sabel, K.G., Aronsson, M., Sandin, B., Johansson, P.R., Carlsson, C., Kyllerman, M., Iversen, K. and Hrbek, A. (1979) 'Effects on the child of alcohol abuse during pregnancy: retrospective and prospective studies', *Acta pædiatrica Scandinavica*, 275(Supplement): 112–21.

Pichini, S., Marchei, E., Vagnarelli, F., Tarani, L., Raimundi, F., Maffucci, R., Sacher, B., Bisceglia, M., Rapisardi, G., Elicio, M., Biban, P., Zuccaro, P., Pacifici, R., Pierantozzi, A. and Morini, L. (2012) 'Assessment of prenatal exposure to ethanol by meconium analysis: results of an Italian multicenter study', *Alcoholism: Clinical and Experimental Research*, 36(3): 417–24.

Raul, F., Ledig, M., Gosse, F., Galluser, M. and Doffoel, M. (1987) 'Prenatal exposure to alcohol in rats: effect on intestinal enzymes in offspring', *Alcohol*, 4(5): 405–8.

Sampson, P.D., Streissguth, A.P., Bookstein, F.L., Little, R.E., Clarren, S.K., Dehaene, P., Hanson, J.W. and Graham, J.M., Jr. (1997) 'Incidence of fetal alcohol syndrome and prevalence of alcohol-related neurodevelopmental disorder', *Teratology*, 56(5): 317–26.

Scianaro, L., Prusek, W. and Loiodice, G. (1978) '[The fetal alcohol syndrome: clinical observations]', *Minerva Pediatrica*, 30(20): 1585–8.

Spohr, H.L., Willms, J. and Steinhausen, H.C. (2007) 'Fetal alcohol spectrum disorders in young adulthood', *The Journal of Pediatrics*, 150(2): 175–9.

Strömland, K. (1990) 'Contribution of ocular examination to the diagnosis of foetal alcohol syndrome in mentally retarded children', *Journal of Mental Deficiency Research)^$*, 34(5): 429–35.

Toutain, S., Simmat-Durand, L., Crenn-Hébert, C., Simonpoli, A.M., Vellut, N., Genest, L., Miossec, E. and Lejeune, C. (2010) '[Consequences for the newborn of alcohol consumption during pregnancy]', *Archives de pédiatrie*, 17(9): 1273–80.

Vagnarelli, F., Palmi, I., Garcia-Algar, O., Falcon, M., Memo, L., Tarani, L., Spoletini, R., Pacifici, R., Mortali, C., Pierantozzi, A. and Pichini, S. (2011) 'A survey of Italian and Spanish neonatologists and paediatricians regarding awareness of the diagnosis of FAS and FASD and maternal ethanol use during pregnancy', *BMC Pediatrics*, 11: 1–5.

van Balkom, I.D., Gunning, W.B. and Hennekam, R.C. (1996) '[Fetal alcohol syndrome: an unrecognized cause of intellectual handicap and problem behavior in The Netherlands]', *Nederlands Tijdschrift voor Geneeskunde*, 140(11): 592–5.

22

FETAL ALCOHOL SPECTRUM DISORDERS

The current situation in South Africa

Denis Viljoen

Brief historical perspective

South Africa has endured a convoluted and unfortunate political history since the coastal exploration in the fifteenth and sixteenth centuries by mainly Portuguese mariners such as Vasco da Gama and Bartholomew Diaz. Prior to the construction of the Suez Canal, the Cape sea route was the most accessible commercial means for trade between European nations and the Spice Islands of the East Indies. Cape Town then became a refurbishing station for this trade, and the facility was initially established by the Dutch East India Company. The French Huguenots settled in the Cape in the mid- to late seventeenth century after fleeing religious persecution in France and brought viticulture into the nearby hinterland to resupply ships travelling to and from the seafaring nations in Europe.

As outlined by Ron Gray (Chapter 3, this publication), the saga of wine production with all its social implications, the slave importation, *dop* or 'tot' system and legacy thereof (discussed below) and currently, the societal impacts of generalized alcohol abuse, has evolved over a period of 300 years since the first colonial settlements. One of the most damaging outcomes is the 'epidemic' of fetal alcohol spectrum disorders (FASDs) in South Africa.

Background

The Foundation for Alcohol Related Research (FARR) is a non-governmental organization (NGO) constituted in 1997 and registered specifically to address the challenges relating to substance abuse, especially that of alcohol, in South Africa. A site visit comprising several experts from the National Institutes for Alcoholism and Alcohol Abuse (NIAAA), Bethesda, Washington was arranged in 1997 to assess the situation in the Western Cape relating to fetal alcohol syndrome (FAS). Multiple collaborative studies between FARR and academic institutions in the United States were set up and funded by the NIAAA:

- an epidemiological study in collaboration with the Center on Alcholism, Substance Abuse, and Addictions (CASAA), University of New Mexico (May *et al.* 2000);

- studies of genetic polymorphisms of alcohol-related metabolic enzymes, a prenatal ultrasound study with Indiana State University (Viljoen *et al.* 2001);
- an investigation into neuro-developmental aspects of FAS-affected children (Adnams *et al.* 2001; Croxford *et al.* 2002; Jacobson *et al.* 2002; Kodituwakku *et al.* 2001);
- studies determining epidemiological and prevalence rates of FAS in four communities in Johannesburg, Gauteng Province (Viljoen *et al.* 2003) and two centres in the Northern Cape Province (Urban *et al.* 2008) with the Centers for Disease Control and Prevention (CDC) also becoming a collaborating agency with FARR;
- a prevention study in Upington and De Aar, Northern Cape (Chersich *et al.* 2012), also with CDC, was the first to demonstrate a major reduction in the prevalence of FASDs in any population worldwide.

Subsequently, other investigations of populations in the Witzenberg region, Aurora and Karatara in the Western Cape Province have revealed many maternal risk factors for FASDs. In the Northern Cape Province several innovative prevention models have been a consequence of these findings, and more recently these have been refined in projects in the Western Cape Province. These are described in greater detail below.

The activities of FARR have resulted in more than 50 reports and abstracts in peer-reviewed journals, as well as informing the South African public health, social development, educational and agricultural leadership of the massive implications of FASDs for all communities. The South African Minister of Health has since moved to include FAS as one of the four major birth defects in South Africa. Two Substance Abuse Congresses have been promoted by the South African Department of Social Development and all nine provincial and national departments intersecting with the challenges of substance abuse have been encouraged to devote resources to alleviating these problems. In addition, at least ten other NGOs have emerged to assist in tackling these challenges. FARR has led the research, awareness-raising, education and prevention of FASDs. Brief summaries of the current status of these activities follow below.

The dop system

In order to understand some of the social issues involved with heavy alcohol consumption in South Africa communities, it is necessary to discuss the so-called *dop* system. The *dop* or 'tot' system comprises part-payment of farm workers' wages through the dispensing of various amounts of alcohol either daily or at weekends in lieu of payment. The origins of *dop* arose from early viticultural activities in the late sixteenth century by farmers, many of Huguenot origins. The use of *dop* followed practices of part-payment of wages in goods which were common in Europe at that time and are still practised in a minority of European settings. *Dop* is outlawed in South Africa, although it is still claimed to be used on a small minority of wine farms. In epidemiological studies undertaken by FARR and involving several thousand mothers working in the agricultural sector, less than 3 per cent have ever been exposed to *dop*. That *dop* remains a major driver of alcohol abuse on farms and in other disadvantaged groups of workers is thus very unlikely, although the legacy of binge drinking in many underprivileged, uneducated, pregnant mothers, particularly at weekends, probably has its origins in this practice.

Prevalence studies of FASDs

Prevalence studies for FASDs in whole populations are problematic and expensive. In order to arrive at meaningful results which can then be extrapolated into populations at large, the capture of children in such communities must be complete, and the subjects have to undergo detailed evaluations. Prevalence studies in South Africa have focused on school-entry children to maximize complete 'capture' of that age group and to ensure that the biological features of FASDs are most easily recognizable. Care is taken to inform leaders, church groups, politicians and teachers within the community and to obtain informed consent from parents or guardians. The latter is most important so that ethical guidelines from funding groups and research organizations are fulfilled.

A prevalence study involves three major elements:

- a detailed physical examination by a dysmorphologist skilled in the diagnosis of FASDs;
- a neuro-developmental profile;
- a detailed maternal history particularly relating to substance abuse.

As alluded to previously, prevalence studies have been undertaken in various communities within three provinces of South Africa, namely the Western and Northern Cape Provinces and Gauteng. The initial study done in 1996–1997 in the town of Wellington, Western Cape Province, consisted of a two-stage process involving children from 13 primary schools:

- An anthropometric and physical evaluation of 400 randomly selected children was followed by a maternal history of alcohol ingestion during pregnancy. Cut off parameters from these assessments were then calculated.
- Children with the pathognomonic features of FASDs were then identified. In those with confirmed FASDs, all had measurements on or below the tenth percentiles for mass, height and head circumference.
- The remaining children from 13 primary schools were then initially screened for these growth parameters and all on or below the tenth percentile were deemed 'screen-positive' and were fully evaluated physically and neurologically for signs of FASDs. A maternal history was also derived for all screen-positive children.

In subsequent prevalence studies of school-entry children in other provinces, the same screening procedure was also employed. Table 22.1 summarizes the results of these studies, the years of evaluation and their location. At-risk populations were determined as occurring in both the Northern and Western Cape Provinces, whereas four communities in Gauteng had, by comparison, much lower prevalence figures.

Other studies undertaken in Karatara and Aurora, Western Cape Province, are currently being analysed.

Following the aforementioned population evaluations, it became imperative, for moral and ethical reasons, to study younger populations of children and to commence urgent prevention/intervention activities in these at-risk communities. Further analysis of the data had shown that heavy-drinking women in the childbearing age group may sometimes have conceived two to three additional pregnancies if the age group of study subjects remained at school-entry age or, in the South African context, seven years of age, and many of these

TABLE 22.1 FASDs in school-entry children

Province	Location	Date	Prevalence rate per 1,000
Western Cape Province	Wellington I	1997	45
	Wellington II	1999	65
	Wellington III	2001	85
Northern Cape Province	Upington	2001	76
	De Aar	2002	119
Gauteng Province	Soweto	2006	19
	Lenasia South	2006	11
	Diepsloot	2006	0
	Westburg	2006	40
Western Cape	Witzenberg	2010	75

later siblings would also have FASDs. Thus, evaluation of nine-month-old subjects was undertaken before and after prevention activities.

In De Aar, where prevalence data were the highest ever previously reported in any population worldwide (119 per 1,000), the study of nine-month-old babies gave very similar results (112 per 1,000) (Viljoen *et al.* 2007). However, a prevention programme incorporating mainly universal methodologies and using brief educational or motivational interventions succeeded in reducing FASD rates by 30 per cent (Chersich *et al.* 2012). Such activities have been broadened in these Northern Cape regions and preliminary data (currently unpublished) indicate a further reduction in FASD rates in these communities.

Epidemiological studies

In socio-economically impoverished communities in the Northern and Western Cape Provinces of South Africa, 'risk' or 'associated' factors have been determined to assist in prevention activities. A host of associations have been described differentiating those women most likely to produce more children with FASDs from the general population, namely:

- *Having a previous child with an FASD.* This was the most important marker of risk discovered from South African studies. In communities in which successive and longitudinal evaluations of at-risk women were undertaken (e.g. Wellington, Western Cape, and De Aar, Northern Cape), women who had previously had a child with an FASD were three to five times more likely to have another affected child than age-related mothers from the same ethnic and socio-economic background. Interventions for such individuals are thus urgent and imperative.
- *Poor education.* Women with an FASD-affected child on average had five years of schooling compared to those with unaffected children who had received an average of eight years of schooling.
- *Religiosity.* Women who undertook spiritual activities, regardless of faith or denomination, were at less risk of producing a child with FASDs than abstainers from religious participation or practices.

- *Family income.* Earnings of US$100 or less per month per family member were associated with increased risk of FASDs.
- *Heavy, binge-pattern alcohol consumption.* The normal drinking pattern of women in poor socio-economic circumstances in South Africa comprised, almost entirely, a binge pattern of weekend consumption. Drinking to a high level of intoxication (a blood alcohol content equal to or greater than 100 mg alcohol per 100 ml blood) is the norm among these persons in at-risk communities (Khaole et al. 2004) with more than five drinks (more than 60 mg of alcohol) per occasion being usual. Such activities coupled with body masses of 40–50 kg and poor diets probably accounts for the poor fetal and infantile outcomes in these instances.
- Other risk factors which were determined were maternal depression, high rates of tuberculosis and HIV/AIDS infection, poor work opportunities and advancing maternal age and having previously borne children (Viljoen et al. 2007).

Genetic and biomarkers of fetal exposure to alcohol

FARR was the first to ascribe susceptibility to FASDs due to inheritance of various polymorphisms of maternal alcohol dehydrogenase (ADH) (Khaole et al. 2004). This was later confirmed by other investigators.

The higher kinetic activity of the maternal ADH 2★2 allele appeared to confer protection on fetuses for the adverse effects of heavy maternal alcohol consumption.

Similarly, the validation of a new biomarker for fetal exposure was determined through the study of ethyl oleate concentration in fetal meconium samples in alcohol-exposed newborns (Bearer et al. 2003). This ground-breaking research enables at-risk infants to be identified early in life thereby allowing prevention activities to be set in place to avoid secondary disabilities. Also, professional support of the mother can be planned so that future pregnancies may not be similarly affected.

Summary

The identification of extreme frequencies of FASDs in South African populations has allowed health and social services providers to address the challenges of health education, the need for surveillance of at-risk populations, the introduction of substance abuse management facilities, fiscal and legal considerations, and many other ramifications. It has also introduced the study of FASDs as frequent birth defects in many countries in which, hitherto, the disorder had been previously unrecognized.

References

Adnams, C.M., Kodituwakku, P.W., Hay, A., Molteno, C.D., Viljoen, D. and May, P.A. (2001) 'Patterns of cognitive-motor development in children with fetal alcohol syndrome from a community in South Africa', *Alcoholism: Clinical and Experimental Research*, 25(4): 557–62.

Bearer, C.F., Jacobson, J.L., Jacobson, S.W., Barr, D., Croxford, J., Molteno, C.D., Viljoen, D.L., Marais, A.S., Chiodo, L.M. and Cwik, A.S. (2003) 'Validation of a new biomarker of fetal exposure to alcohol', *Journal of Pediatrics*, 143(4): 463–9.

Chersich, M.F., Urban, M., Olivier, L., Davies, L.-A., Chetty, C. and Viljoen, D. (2012) 'Universal prevention is associated with lower prevalence of fetal alcohol spectrum disorders in Northern Cape, South Africa: a multicentre before-after study', *Alcohol and Alcoholism*, 47(1), 67–74.

Croxford, J.A., Jacobson, S.W., Viljoen, D.L., Chiodo, L.M., Marais, A.S., Corobama, R. and Jacobson, J.L. (2002) 'Impact of years of maternal alcohol use on infants born heavy drinking South African mothers', *Alcoholism: Clinical and Experimental Research*, 26(5): 1045A.

Jacobson, S.W., Hay, A., Molteno, C., Marais, A.S., Carter, R.C., September, M., Chiodo, L.M., Wynn, K., Jones, K.L., Khaole, N., Viljoen, D. and Jacobson, J.L. (2002) 'FAS and neurobehavioral deficits in alcohol-exposed South African infants', *Alcoholism: Clinical and Experimental Research*, 26(5): 175A.

Khaole, N.C.O., Ramchandani, V.A., Viljoen, D.L. and Li, T.-K. (2004) 'A pilot study of alcohol exposure and pharmakinetics in women with or without children with fetal alcohol syndrome', *Alcohol and Alcoholism*, 39(6): 503–8

Kodituwakku, P.W., Adnams, C.M., Hay, A., Kitching, A., Adams, R., Viljoen, D. and May, P.A. (2001) 'Handedness in children with fetal alcohol syndrome', *Alcoholism: Clinical and Experimental Research*, 25(5): 75A.

May, P.A., Brooke, L., Gossage, J.P., Croxford, J., Adnams, C., Jones, K.L., Robinson, L. and Viljoen, D. (2000) 'The epidemiology of fetal alcohol syndrome in a South African community in the Western Cape Province', *American Journal of Public Health*, 90(12): 1905–12.

Urban, M., Chevsich, M.F., Fourie, L-A., Chetty, C., Olivier, L. and Viljoen, D. (2008) 'Fetal alcohol syndrome among Grade 1 school children in the Northern Cape Province: prevalence and risk factors', *South African Medical Journal*, 98: 877–82.

Viljoen, D., Craig, P., Hymbaugh, K. and Boyle, C./Centers for Disease Control and Prevention (2003) 'Fetal alcohol syndrome – South Africa, 2001', *Morbidity and Mortality Weekly*, 52(28): 660–2.

Viljoen, D., Fourie, L., Chetty, C.M., Urban, M., Nero, M., Josephs, J. and Rosenthal, J. (2007) 'The epidemiology of fetal alcohol spectrum disorders in the Northern Cape Province of South Africa', *Alcoholism: Clinical and Experimental Research*, 31(6): 188A.

Viljoen, D.L., Carr, L.G., Foroud, T.M., Brooke, L., Ramsay, M. and Li, T-K. (2001) 'Alcohol dehydrogenase 2*2 allele is associated with decreased prevalence of fetal alcohol syndrome in the mixed-ancestry population of the Western Cape Province, South Africa', *Alcoholism: Clinical and Experimental Research*, 25(12): 1719–22.

23
FETAL ALCOHOL SPECTRUM DISORDERS
Australian perspectives

Elizabeth J. Elliott

Introduction

Despite Australia's slow entrée into the world of fetal alcohol spectrum disorders (FASDs), interest in the subject has increased dramatically over the last ten years. The need for research, advocacy and clinical services has been enthusiastically embraced by medical and allied health clinicians, researchers, Indigenous communities, parents and caregivers, lawyers and teachers, philanthropists, non-government organizations and, importantly, governments. Interest in FASDs, initially led by researchers, was propelled by the establishment, in 2006, of an Intergovernmental Committee on Drugs Working Party into FASDs. The working party, an initiative of the Ministerial Council on Drugs Strategy, convened the first national conference on FASDs in Australia in 2008 and conducted several significant research projects addressing services and treatments for FASDs. In 2009 the Working Group wrote a Monograph, *FASD in Australia: An update*. Recent provision of government funding for: an FASDs prevalence study in remote WA; development of a screening and diagnostic tool for FASDs; activities of the National Organization for FAS and related disorders (NOFASARD); and an audit of existing databases and educational materials has been most welcome. Escalating activity over the last decade culminated in the recognition of the importance of FASDs by the federal government, as demonstrated by the House of Representatives initiating an Inquiry into the prevention and management of FASDs in November 2011 which was reported to the Federal Parliament in late 2012 and is currently under consideration (Parliament of Australia *et al.* 2012). In September 2012, a draft national plan of action for FASDs was launched in Parliament House and submitted to the Inquiry. This chapter outlines the use of alcohol in Australian women and in pregnancy and showcases current Australian research that has contributed to our understanding of the epidemiology, diagnosis, management and prevention of FASDs in Australia.

Alcohol use in Australia

According to the World Health Organization, Australia has one of the highest rates of alcohol consumption worldwide, at about ten litres of pure ethyl alcohol per head per year for every person aged 15 years or more (WHO 2011). Recent media attention about the harms of alcohol and its negative impacts on social cohesion, health, education, acute injury and later risks of chronic liver disease and malignancy, have had little impact on drinking behaviour. *Australian Guidelines to Reduce Health Risks from Drinking Alcohol* suggest that risks associated with alcohol can be minimized if both men and women limit their intake to two standard drinks (SD) per day, or to four SD in a single drinking session (NHMRC 2009). Yet, a recent survey by the Foundation for Alcohol Research and Education, involving young people aged 14–25 years, indicates that this public health message has been poorly disseminated (FARE 2012a). When asked what they considered to be a safe intake for a single drinking session, young men aged 14–19 years said 8.8 drinks and women aged 14–17 years said 6.5 drinks (FARE 2012a).

The steady increase in rates of alcohol use in women is of particular concern: between 1995 and 2006 the rate of risky and high risk drinking in women more than doubled to 12 per cent (Australian Bureau of Statistics 2006). In 2011, 78 per cent of women reported drinking alcohol in the previous year, over 30 per cent reported drinking each week and 5 per cent reported daily use of alcohol (Australian Institute of Health and Welfare 2011). The changing pattern of alcohol consumption in Australian society reflects the changing role of women and the ready access to alcohol, including to pre-mixed, spirit-based drinks that are marketed to young women. Traditionally, alcohol was the preserve of men; however, drinking in women, including to the point of intoxication, is increasingly tolerated (Roche 2009). To prevent FASDs, these entrenched societal attitudes and patterns of drinking must be addressed.

Alcohol and pregnancy

Considering the high rates of alcohol use in women, and that about half of all pregnancies in Australia are unplanned (Naimi *et al*. 2003), there is a risk of women inadvertently damaging their unborn children before realizing they are pregnant. Although drinking rates are similar in Indigenous and non-Indigenous Australian women, the pattern of drinking differs: 67 per cent of Indigenous women compared to 11 per cent of non-Indigenous women who drink do so at levels considered to pose a risk of acute and chronic harm or alcohol dependence (Commonwealth Department of Human Services and Health 1996). Despite current public health recommendations that 'for women who are pregnant or planning a pregnancy, not drinking is the safest option' (NHMRC 2009) alcohol consumption during pregnancy is common in Australia, ranging from 34 per cent to 59 per cent (Colvin *et al*. 2007; Peadon *et al*. 2010; O'Callaghan *et al*. 2007). Although many women decrease their alcohol consumption during pregnancy, 20 per cent of women in one study reported 'binge' drinking on at least one occasion in early pregnancy (O'Callaghan *et al*. 2007) and in another study 2 per cent reported a 'binge' in the second and third trimesters (Colvin *et al*. 2007).

Survey results suggesting that Indigenous (Australian and Torres Strait Islander) women have a different pattern of drinking and are more likely to drink at risky levels are supported by data from Western Australia. Eades reported that 44 per cent of Aboriginal women studied in Perth had consumed alcohol during pregnancy and that 23 per cent of them had become intoxicated (Eades *et al*. 2008). Elliott *et al*. reported that 50 per cent women from the remote Fitzroy Valley drank alcohol during pregnancy and that 93 per cent of these women drank at risky levels according to AUDIT-C (Elliott *et al*. 2012; Fitzpatrick *et al*. 2012).

Burns *et al.* (2011) identified all (417,464) live births in New South Wales in 2000 to 2006 and linked these to records of alcohol-related admissions for mothers using ICD-10-AM codes. Cases (488 women who had at least one alcohol-related hospital admission during pregnancy or at birth) were compared with controls. Cases were more likely to live in a remote/very remote area, have smoked during pregnancy, have received limited antenatal care and were less likely to have attended a specialist obstetric hospital. Their pregnancies were associated with poorer obstetric and neonatal outcomes. This study highlights the need for systematic screening to identify mothers and pregnancies at risk – as early as possible during pregnancy – and for clear guidelines for management and referral. Regrettably, few services or evidence-based therapies are available for pregnant women who drink (Burns and Woods 2009). Existing services often include women who use illicit drugs, and are unpopular with women who do not use drugs. Muggli *et al.* have reviewed and trialled methods to ask about alcohol use in pregnancy (Muggli *et al.* 2010) and are using the tools developed in a birth cohort study (Halliday *et al.* 2011–2015). Birth offers another opportunity to recognize and assist woman who have been drinking during pregnancy and to examine and follow-up their children. Reluctance of health professionals to ask about alcohol use (Elliott *et al.* 2006; Payne *et al.* 2005) and lack of questions about alcohol use in pregnancy in the *National Perinatal Data Collection* (alcohol is recorded in only three of eight Australian states and territories) limits this opportunity (Burns *et al.* 2009b).

Why women drink

Several studies give an insight into why Australian women drink during pregnancy. Women with a high family income are more likely to use alcohol before and during pregnancy (Zammit *et al.* 2008) and women in their first pregnancy are more likely to drink (Hotham *et al.* 2008). In a cross-sectional, nationally representative survey of predominantly non-Indigenous women of child-bearing age, Peadon and colleagues (2011) found that current risky drinking behaviour, use of alcohol in a previous pregnancy, and a tolerant or neutral attitude to alcohol use in pregnancy (indicated by 20 per cent of women surveyed) were associated with alcohol use in a previous pregnancy and predicted intention to drink during a future pregnancy. Intention to drink was not related to knowledge about the potential harms to the fetus from alcohol. Drinking in pregnancy was also associated with smoking and having a partner who drinks (Peadon *et al.* 2010; Peadon *et al.* 2011). D'Antoine and colleagues (2008) reported that many Australian Aboriginal women continue their pre-pregnancy drinking behaviour during pregnancy because they are unaware of the potential harms to the fetus. Women also cited several social factors that underpin their alcohol use, including being subject to domestic violence, victims of the stolen generation, dispossessed of traditional land, and having lost language and culture. Women from remote settings also cited the lack of drug and alcohol services and the need to travel up to 500 km to spend the final stages of pregnancy and delivery away from their family and community as stressors that might result in alcohol consumption (D'Antoine *et al.* 2008).

These studies identify women at risk of drinking during pregnancy and thus are informative for clinicians and those developing public health policies (Elliott and Bower 2008). They suggest that education alone will not change drinking behaviour and that both community attitudes to alcohol use and socio-economic determinants on the FASDs causal pathway must be addressed – a difficult challenge (Elliott and Bower 2004). Analogous to the successful campaign to decrease smoking in Australia, evidence-based strategies must be introduced to decrease alcohol consumption across society, including legislation to limit advertising and to restrict access to alcohol through taxation, minimum pricing, restrictions on the number and opening hours of alcohol outlets, and support of Indigenous-led alcohol restrictions.

FASDs in Australia: an historical perspective

In 1980 the first Australian publication relating to fetal alcohol syndrome (FAS) (Collins and Turner 1978) appeared in the *Medical Journal of Australia*, five years after the landmark 1973 *Lancet* publications by Jones et al. describing 'the recognizable pattern of malformations in the offspring of chronic alcoholic mothers' (Jones et al. 1973) and 'the Fetal Alcohol Syndrome' (Jones and Smith 1973). In their publication, Collins and Turner (1978) described six children born to alcoholic mothers, in order 'to increase awareness of the FAS in Australia, whose population has a high and changing pattern of alcohol consumption.' In 1980, Walpole and Hockey described the implications of FAS for Australian society (Walpole and Hockey 1980) and in 1994 Lipson (1994) published a case series. Walpole's later studies failed to show any significant relationship between low to moderate pre-pregnancy maternal alcohol intake and either newborn clinical or neurological status (Walpole et al. 1990, 1991). This led to the conclusion that it is inaccurate to advise pregnant women that any alcohol in pregnancy is potentially harmful to the fetus and may be counterproductive (Walpole et al. 1990) and may have reassured clinicians that advising abstinence during pregnancy was unnecessary.

Prevalence of FASDs

Interest in FASDs was renewed in 2000, when Bower attempted to determine FAS prevalence (Bower et al. 2000) using two data sources from Western Australia to maximize case ascertainment, a State-wide birth defects register and the Rural Paediatric Service database. She concluded that FAS prevalence (0.18 per 1,000 live births) was an underestimate, due to both under-recognition and under-reporting. A striking result was the 100-fold increase in the rate of FAS in Indigenous versus non-Indigenous children (2.76 versus 0.02 per 1,000 respectively). In the same year Elliott and Bower initiated an active, national surveillance study using the Australian Paediatric Surveillance Unit, with monthly reporting of incident (newly diagnosed) cases of FAS by paediatricians (Elliott et al. 2008). The overall birth prevalence (based on 92 cases reported between 2001 and 2004 inclusive) was 0.06/1,000 live births. The incidence in children under five years was 0.58 per 10^5 children per annum (0.18 per 10^5 in non-Indigenous and 14.6 per 10^5 in Indigenous children) (ibid.).

A ten-year, retrospective case note review of all admissions to Darwin hospital in the Northern Territory (Harris and Bucens 2003), included children with clinical features consistent with FAS and their siblings. All children identified were Indigenous and the birth prevalence was estimated at 1.7 per 1,000 live births overall and 4.7 per 1,000 Indigenous births. In a Victorian study, birth prevalence was estimated from perinatal and birth defects databases at 0.01–0.03 per 1,000 live births but no Indigenous children were identified (Allen et al. 2007). All Australian estimates are significantly lower than those recorded overseas, which may reflect study design, use of different diagnostic criteria or under-recognition and under-reporting of FAS. No population-based data are available for any of the FASDs and no prevalence data are available for the full spectrum of neurodevelopmental disorders.

In 2009 the Aboriginal communities of Fitzroy Crossing in remote north-western Australia initiated Australia's first population-based study of FASDs prevalence, in primary school-aged children, using active case ascertainment and an interdisciplinary diagnostic approach (Elliott *et al.* 2012; Fitzpatrick *et al.* 2012; Latimer *et al.* 2010). Data from this study, in which over 50 per cent children were exposed to high levels of alcohol *in utero* are currently being analysed. Two birth cohort studies are currently underway in Australia: one in Victoria examining the effects of low to moderate alcohol use in pregnancy on infant outcomes (Halliday *et al.* 2011–2015) and the other in New South Wales and Western Australia examining the effects of parental substance use on maternal, infant and child outcomes (Hutchinson *et al.* 2010–2014).

Characteristics of children with FAS

The Australian Paediatric Surveillance Unit study provides the only detailed clinical description of FAS in Australia (Elliott *et al.* 2008). Among the 92 cases identified 53 per cent were male, 35 per cent were preterm and 65 per cent low birth weight. The median age at diagnosis was 3.3 years (range birth to 11.9 years) and only 7 per cent were diagnosed at birth. Half (53 per cent) the children had microcephaly, a quarter (24 per cent) had significant birth defects in addition to facial dysmorphology, 5 per cent had sensorineural hearing loss and 5 per cent had visual impairment. Behavioural problems were reported in the majority (85 per cent). Only 40 per cent of children lived with a biological parent, 60 per cent were in foster care and 51 per cent had an affected sibling, indicating missed opportunities for prevention. Consistent with the literature, these data highlight the complex needs of children with FAS and the need for prevention strategies. O'Leary *et al.* (2010) proposed a new method of classification for prenatal alcohol exposure that accounts for dose, pattern and timing of exposure. They then investigated a large population-based cohort from Western Australia, linking data from multiple sources (medical, education, justice), to examine child outcomes. In this cohort high-level maternal alcohol intake during pregnancy resulted in increased rates of stillbirth (O'Leary *et al.* 2012a), fetal growth impairment and prematurity (O'Leary *et al.* 2009b), birth defects (O'Leary *et al.* 2011), cerebral palsy (O'Leary *et al.* 2012b) and language delay (O'Leary *et al.* 2009a).

Diagnostic tools for FASDs

In order to improve identification of FASDs and standardize the approach to diagnosis, the Commonwealth Department of Health and Ageing provided funding for development of a diagnostic instrument for Australia. Health professionals' perceptions were sought regarding existing diagnostic guidelines (Watkins *et al.* 2012a) as was consensus on the components most suitable for Australia (Watkins *et al.* 2012b).

Services for the diagnosis and management of FASDs

Early diagnosis and appropriate health and educational interventions will maximize a child's chances of reaching their full potential. Peadon *et al.* identified the urgent need for health professional (HP) training and dedicated services to facilitate the diagnosis and care of children with FASDs in Australia (Peadon et al. 2008). An international audit involving 34 FASDs clinics in North and South America, Africa and Europe, confirmed the preference for multidisciplinary services, highly skilled practitioners, standardized diagnostic criteria, and a screening and referral strategy that is appropriate to the local setting and sustainable. In the clinic audit, five different sets of diagnostic criteria (alone or in combination) were used; most took referrals from multiple sources including parents; the majority of children assessed lived in out-of-home care; the average consultation time was 3.25 hours; few offered long-term management; and funding was rarely sustainable and often dependent on research grants (ibid.).

For Australia, the optimal service model might include specialized clinics, teams of trained professionals providing outreach services, up-skilling of professionals working within existing services e.g. child development clinics or pediatric facilities, or a combination of these options. A pilot clinic in Sydney has recently been funded by FARE. An interdisciplinary team was trained to work on the Lililwan (FASDs prevalence) Project in the remote Fitzroy Valley (Fitzpatrick et al. 2012). In this project the multidisciplinary team, blinded to alcohol exposure, held a 'case conference' to review all assessments, to jointly allocate a diagnosis, and to develop a management plan for immediate feedback to parents, teachers and local HPs.

Interventions for FASDs

A systematic review of the literature exposed the lack of high-quality evidence for interventions for management of FASDs (Peadon et al. 2009). From nearly 6,000 studies identified, only 11, seven of which were randomized controlled trials (RCTs), met inclusion criteria. Most of these suffered methodological problems, particularly small sample size. For children with ADHD, there is limited evidence of benefit from stimulant medication for hyperactivity and impulsivity but not attention, but a risk of adverse effects including decreased appetite, headache and insomnia. Use of a virtual reality computer game but not modelling of a task enabled children with FASDs to learn new skills. Classroom interventions may improve mathematical and language skills, adaptive behaviour and classroom behaviour. Social communication interventions improve social skills, and attention process training significantly improves attention. We eagerly await results of a number of large RCTs funded by the Centers for Disease Control in Atlanta and evaluating a range of interventions for FASDs. A protocol for a systematic review of pharmacological interventions for ADHD in FASDs has been published in the Cochrane Library (Peadon et al. 2012) and a protocol for non-pharmacological interventions for FASDs drafted. In the absence of good evidence for effective therapies, children with FASDs are best managed by a developmental or general pediatrician or within a child development service. Age-appropriate physical and neurodevelopmental assessment is recommended to identify dysmorphic features and domains of central nervous system dysfunction, to inform the exclusion or diagnosis of one of the FASDs, to identify strengths and to guide appropriate medical, allied health, educational and community support.

Health professionals and FASDs

Barriers to the diagnosis of FASDs include scepticism among HP, as highlighted in a 2004 editorial asking whether FAS in Australia was 'fact or fiction' (Elliott and Bower 2004). The likelihood of under-recognition of FAS was explored in surveys of 1,143 general practitioners, obstetricians, allied HPs, Aboriginal health workers and community nurses in Western Australia conducted in 2002 (Payne et al. 2005). Of those who cared for pregnant women, only 45 per cent routinely asked about alcohol use during pregnancy and 12 per cent never asked. This is contrary to the view of over 95 per cent of women who believe that doctors should ask about alcohol use during pregnancy (Peadon et al. 2011). Most HP were unaware of the then current (2002) NHMRC Australia Alcohol guidelines regarding alcohol use in pregnancy, few knew what to advise women, and only 25 per cent provided advice (Payne et al. 2005). There was also lack of knowledge about how to make the diagnosis of FAS. Over 30 per cent of HP admitted they'd failed to record a suspected FAS diagnosis for fear of upsetting women or stigmatizing children and families. Results were similar in a 2004 survey of pediatricians (Elliott et al. 2006) and these data provide a possible explanation for the low rates of FAS recorded in Australia. Most HP surveyed indicated their need for educational materials, which were developed in 2006, informed by focus groups involving HP that explored barriers to talking about alcohol use with pregnant women (France et al. 2010). The resources, distributed in 2006, are available online.[1]

In a repeat survey in 2007 (Payne et al. 2011a) about 70 per cent of HP said they had seen the educational resources. Of these, 77 per cent had used the resources and 49 per cent indicated they had changed their practice as a result. More HP than previously knew the diagnostic features of FAS, had diagnosed FAS, and felt adequately informed and confident in dealing with FAS. However, a larger proportion failed to record the diagnosis in a suspected case. Although the proportion overall who routinely asked about alcohol use in pregnancy did not increase, an increase was reported by obstetricians. In the 2007 pediatrician survey (Payne et al. 2011a) there was no change in the proportion that knew the diagnostic features or had suspected or diagnosed FAS. However, pediatricians did indicate they felt more prepared to deal with FAS and to refer children for confirmation of the diagnosis. In 2007 the proportion of pediatricians asking about alcohol use in pregnancy did not increase, although there was an increase in the number who provided women with advice about potential harms of alcohol. As in 2004, nearly 70 per cent of both HP groups in 2007 believed that an FAS diagnosis might stigmatize a child and family (Payne et al. 2011a, 2011b). However, an increased proportion of HP (98 per cent) and pediatricians (82 per cent) now gave the advice that 'no alcohol in pregnancy is the safest choice' (Payne et al. 2011a, 2011b). There remain barriers to the diagnosis of FASDs, including lack of HP knowledge and confidence in making the diagnosis and managing the child. There is persistent reluctance by HP to ask about alcohol use in pregnancy and to provide advice to women about potential harms from alcohol. A majority view the diagnosis as stigmatizing. In order to change HP behaviour, research is needed to understand the factors underpinning current attitudes and practice.

Other professionals

There is an urgent need for educational opportunities for teachers, lawyers, correction services and other professionals to increase understanding of FASDs and the needs of affected individuals. In August 2012 the Department of Education and Child Development in South Australia held a conference attended by several hundred teachers and has since developed a fact sheet, *Facilities for Children and Young People with FASD*.[2] Australian researchers are exploring the attitudes and knowledge of the legal profession about FASDs.

Support for families

The National Organization for Fetal Alcohol Syndrome and Related Disorders (NOFASARD), under the leadership of Ms Sue Miers AM, has provided information and support to parents and caregivers, professionals and communities since it was established in 1998 with the objectives to: promote and resource good practice in the management of FAS and related disorders; provide information, advocacy, education and support that will assist carers and those working with and affected by FAS and related disorders; and work towards prevention of FAS and related disorders.[3] NOFASARD has recently received Federal Health Funding to support its activities. The National Indigenous Australian Fetal Alcohol Syndrome Education Network (NIAFASEN)[4] led by Ms Lorian Hayes and the Russell Family Fetal Alcohol Disorders Foundation[5] led by Ms Anne Russell also provide education and caregiver support (Russell 2005).

Policy

A 2007 review of policy published by state and federal health departments and professional organizations in Australia revealed a lack of evidence-based policy and lack of consistency, which could result in a mixed message (O'Leary *et al.* 2006). The current *Australian Guidelines to Reduce Health Risks from Drinking Alcohol* (NHMRC 2009: 1) recommend that 'for women who are pregnant or planning a pregnancy, not drinking is the safest option.' This recommendation represents a significant change from the previous guidelines which provided a mixed message to women, were poorly disseminated and were not known to HP (Elliott *et al.* 2006; Payne *et al.* 2005). The current (2009) Australian guideline is based on the precautionary principle, and provides a clear message (NHMRC 2009).

The need for research into FASDs in Australia has been recognized by medical and allied health clinicians, the federal government, and the NHMRC. Interest was propelled by the establishment, in 2006, of an Intergovernmental Committee on Drugs Working Party into FASDs, comprising clinicians, jurisdictional representatives and public health experts. This working party initiated several significant research projects (Peadon *et al.* 2008, 2009) convened the first national conference on FASDs (2008), and wrote a Monograph on FASDs in Australia (2009) (Burns *et al.* 2009a) which included priorities for action on FASDs. Several of these have been taken up by government including support for: an FASDs prevalence study in remote WA; development of a diagnostic tool for FASDs; an audit of existing FASDs databases, educational materials and midwife data collections. Escalating activity over the last decade culminated in recognition of the importance of FASDs by the federal government, as demonstrated by the House of Representatives initiating an Inquiry into the prevention and management of FASDs in November 2011. In September 2012, a draft national plan of action for FASDs was launched in the Federal Parliament (FARE 2012b). The Federal Inquiry report was presented to the Federal Parliament in late 2012 and hopefully will be followed by funding for research and for programs to prevent and services to diagnose and manage FASDs (Parliament of Australia *et al.* 2012).

Notes

1 http://alcoholpregnancy.childhealthresearch.org.au/alcohol-pregnancy-resources.aspx
2 Fact Sheet SU001 from: www.decd.sa.gov.au/assetservices/pages/topiclisting/44801/
3 www.nofasard.org
4 www.nicfasen.org.au/
5 www.rffada.org

References

Allen, K., Riley, M., Goldfeld, S. and Halliday, J. (2007) 'Estimating the prevalence of fetal alcohol syndrome in Victoria using routinely collected administrative data', *Australian and New Zealand Journal of Public Health*, 31(1): 62–6.

Australian Bureau of Statistics (2006) *Alcohol Consumption in Australia: A snapshot, 2004–05. Report No. 4832.0.55.001*, Canberra, ACT: Australian Bureau of Statistics [online at: www.abs.gov.au/ausstats/abs@.nsf/Previousproducts/4832.0.55.001Main%20Features99992004-05?opendocument&tabname=Summary&prodno=4832.0.55.001&issue=2004-05&num=&view=; accessed: 14 January 2013].

Australian Institute of Health and Welfare (2011) *Alcohol and Other Drug Treatment Services in Australia 2009–2010: Report on the National Minimum Data Set. Drug treatment series No.14. Cat. No. HSE 114*. Canberra, ACT: AIHW.

Bower, C., Silva, D., Henderson, T.R., Ryan, A. and Rudy, E. (2000) 'Ascertainment of birth defects: the effect on completeness of adding a new source of data', *Journal of Pediatrics and Child Health*, 36(6): 574–6.

Burns, L. and Woods, A. (2009) 'Services for pregnant women', Chapter 4 in L. Burns, E. Black and E. Elliott (eds) *Monograph of the Intergovernmental Committee on Drugs Working Party on Fetal Alcohol Spectrum Disorders. Fetal Alcohol Spectrum Disorders in Australia: An Update*, Canberra, ACT: Commonwealth Department of Health and Ageing.

Burns, L., Black, E. and Elliott, E. (eds) (2009a) *Monograph of the Intergovernmental Committee on Drugs Working Party on Fetal Alcohol Spectrum Disorders. Fetal Alcohol Spectrum Disorders in Australia: An Update*, Canberra, ACT: Commonwealth Department of Health and Ageing [online at: www.nationaldrugstrategy.gov.au/internet/drugstrategy/publishing.nsf/Content/30712AE1430616C6CA257A2A000B7D8A/$File/FASDMonogrph2009.pdf; accessed: 14 January 2013].

Burns, L., Black, E., Powers, J., Loxton, D., Elliott, E., Shakeshaft, A. and Dunlop, A. (2011) 'Geographic and maternal characteristics associated with alcohol use in pregnancy', *Alcoholism: Clinical and Experimental Research*, 35(7): 1230–7.

Burns, L., O'Leary, C., Peadon, E., Black, E. and D'Antoine, H. (2009b) 'Prevalence and correlates of alcohol use in pregnancy', Chapter 2 in L. Burns, E. Black and E. Elliott (eds) *Monograph of the Intergovernmental Committee on Drugs Working Party on Fetal Alcohol Spectrum Disorders. Fetal Alcohol Spectrum Disorders in Australia: An Update*, Canberra, ACT: Commonwealth Department of Health and Ageing.

Collins, E. and Turner, G. (1978) 'Six children affected by maternal alcoholism', *Medical Journal of Australia*, 2(14): 606–8.

Colvin, L., Payne, J., Parsons, D., Kurinczuk, J. and Bower, C. (2007) 'Alcohol consumption during pregnancy in non-Indigenous West Australian women', *Alcoholism: Clinical and Experimental Research*, 32(2): 276–84.

Commonwealth Department of Human Services and Health (1996) *National Drug Strategy Household Survey: Urban Aboriginal and Torres Strait Islander Peoples Supplement 1994*, Canberra, ACT: Australian Government Publishing Service.

D'Antoine, H., Henley, N., Payne, J., Elliott, E., Bower, C. and Bartu, A. (2008) 'Alcohol and pregnancy: Aboriginal women's knowledge, attitudes and practice' (unpublished).

Eades, S., Read, A.W., Stanley, F.J., Eades, F.N., McCaullay, D. and Williamson, A. (2008) 'Bibbulung Gnarneep (solid kid): Causal pathways to poor birth outcomes in an urban Aboriginal birth cohort', *Journal of Pediatrics and Child Health*, 44(6): 342–6.

Elliott, E., Latimer, J., Fitzpatrick, J., Oscar, J. and Carter, M. (2012) 'There's hope in the valley', *Journal of Paediatrics and Child Health*, 48(3): 190–2.

Elliott, E.J and, Bower, C. (2004) 'FAS in Australia: fact or fiction?', *Journal of Pediatrics and Child Health*, 40(1/2): 8–10.

Elliott, E.J. and Bower, C. (2008) 'Alcohol and pregnancy: the pivotal role of the obstetrician', *Australian and New Zealand Journal of Obstetrics and Gynaecology*, 48(3): 236–9.

Elliott, E.J., Payne, J., Haan, E. and Bower, C. (2006) 'Diagnosis of fetal alcohol syndrome and alcohol use in pregnancy: a survey of paediatricians' knowledge, attitudes and practice', *Journal of Pediatrics and Child Health*, 42(11): 698–703.

Elliott, E.J., Payne, J., Morris, A., Haan, E. and Bower, C. (2008) 'Fetal alcohol syndrome: a prospective national surveillance study', *Archives of Disease in Childhood*, 93(9): 732–7.

FARE (Foundation for Alcohol Research and Education) (2012a) 'Three years on: alcohol guidelines invisible and unknown' (media release) [online at: www.fare.org.au/wp-content/uploads/2011/07/Media-release-060312-Three-years-on-alcohol-guidelines-invisible-and-unknown.pdf; accessed: 14 January 2013].

FARE (Foundation for Alcohol Research and Education) (2012b) 'The Australian Fetal Alcohol Spectrum Disorders Action Plan 2013–2016' [online at: www.fare.org.au/wp-content/uploads/2011/07/FARE-FASD-Plan.pdf; accessed: 13 January 2013].

Fitzpatrick, J., Elliott, E., Latimer, J., Carter, M., Oscar, J., Ferreira, M., Carmichael Olson, H., Lucas, B., Doney, R., Salter, C., Peadon, E., Hawkes, G. and Hand, M. (2012) 'The Lililwan Project: study protocol for a population based, active case ascertainment study of the prevalence of Fetal Alcohol Spectrum Disorders (FASD) in remote Australian Aboriginal communities', *BMJ Open*, 2: 1–12 [online at: http://bmjopen.bmj.com/content/2/3/e000968.full.pdf+html; accessed: 14 January 2013].

France, K., Henley, N., Payne, J., D'Antoine, H., Bartu, A., O'Leary, C., Elliott, E. and Bower, C. (2010) 'Health professionals addressing alcohol use with pregnant women in Western Australia: barriers and strategies for communication', *Substance Use and Misuse*, 45(10): 1474–90.

Halliday, J., O'Leary, C., Forster, D., Carlin, J., Donath, S., Elliott, E., Lewis, S., Nagle, C., Wake, M., Muggli, E. and Cook, B. (2011–2015) 'Asking questions about alcohol' (AQUA): National Health and Medical Research Council (NHMRC) funded project.

Harris, K.R. and Bucens, I.K. (2003) 'Prevalence of fetal alcohol syndrome in the Top End of the Northern Territory', *Journal of Pediatrics and Child Health*, 39(7): 528–33.

Hotham, E., Ali, R., White, J. and Robinson, J. (2008) 'Pregnancy-related changes in tobacco, alcohol and cannabis use reported by antenatal patients at two public hospitals in South Australia', *Australian and New Zealand Journal of Obstetrics and Gynaecology*, 48(3): 248–54.

Hutchinson, D., Mattick, R.P., Allsop, S., Hutchinson, D.M., Burns, L., Ross, J., Jacobs, S. and Elliott, E. (2010–2014) 'Impact of parental substance use on infant development and family functioning': National Health and Medical Research Council (NHMRC) funded project.

Jones, K.L. and Smith, D.W. (1973) 'Recognition of the fetal alcohol syndrome in early infancy', *Lancet*, 302(7836): 999–1001.

Jones, K.L., Smith, D.W., Ulleland, C.N. and Streissguth, P. (1973) 'Pattern of malformation in offspring of chronic alcoholic mothers', *Lancet*, 1(7815): 1267–71.

Latimer, J., Elliott, E., Fitzpatrick, J., Ferreira, M., Carter, M., Oscar, J. and Kefford, M. (2010) *Marulu: The Lililwan Project. Fetal Alcohol Spectrum Disorders (FASD) Prevalence Study in the Fitzroy Valley. A Community Consultation*, Sydney, New South Wales: The George Institute for Global Health.

Lipson, T. (1994) 'The fetal alcohol syndrome in Australia', *Medical Journal of Australia*, 161(8): 461–2.

Muggli, E., Cook, B., O'Leary, C., Forster, D. and Halliday, J. (2010) *Alcohol in Pregnancy: What questions should we be asking? Report to the Commonwealth Department of Health and Ageing*, Parkville, Victoria: Murdoch Children's Research Institute.

Naimi, T., Lipscomb, L., Brewer, R. and Gilbert, B. (2003) 'Binge drinking in the preconception period and the risk of unintended pregnancy: implications for women and their children', *Pediatrics*, 111(5): 1136–41.

NHMRC (National Health and Medical Research Council) (2009) *Australian Guidelines to Reduce Health Risks from Drinking Alcohol*, Canberra, ACT: Commonwealth of Australia.

O'Callaghan, F.V., O'Callaghan, M., Najman, J.M., Williams, G.M. and Bor, W. (2007) 'Prenatal alcohol exposure and attention, learning and intellectual ability at 14 years: a prospective longitudinal study', *Early Human Development* 83(2): 115–23.

O'Leary, C., Jacoby, P., D'Antoine, H., Bartu, A. and Bower, C. (2012a) 'Heavy prenatal alcohol exposure and increased risk of stillbirth', *BJOG: An International Journal of Obstetrics and Gynaecology*, 119(8): 945–52.

O'Leary, C., Zubrick, S., Taylor, C., Dixon, G. and Bower, C. (2009a) 'Prenatal alcohol exposure and language delay in two-year-old children: the importance of dose and timing on risk', *Pediatrics*, 123(2): 547–54.

O'Leary, C.M., Bower, C., Zubrick, S.R., Geelhoed, E., Kurinczuk, J.J. and Nassar, N. (2010) 'A new method of prenatal alcohol classification accounting for dose, pattern and timing of exposure: improving our ability to examine fetal effects from low to moderate alcohol', *Journal of Epidemiology and Community Health*, 64(11): 956–62.

O'Leary, C.M., Heuzenroeder, L., Elliott, E. and Bower, C. (2006) 'A review of policies on alcohol use during pregnancy in Australia and other English-speaking countries', *Medical Journal of Australia*, 186(9): 466–71.

O'Leary, C.M., Nassar, N., Kurinczuk, J.J. and Bower, C. (2009b) 'The effect of maternal alcohol consumption on fetal growth and preterm birth', *British Journal of Obstetrics and Gynaecology*, 116(3): 390–400.

O'Leary, C.M., Nassar, N., Kurinczuk, J.J., de Klerk, N., Geelhoed, E., Elliott, E.J. and Bower, C. (2011) 'Prenatal alcohol exposure and risk of birth defects', *Obstetrical and Gynecological Survey*, 66(2): 88–90.

O'Leary, C.M., Watson, L., D'Antoine, H., Stanley, F. and Bower, C. (2012b) 'Heavy maternal alcohol consumption and cerebral palsy in the offspring', *Developmental Medicine and Child Neurology*, 54(3): 224–30.

Parliament of Australia, House of Representatives Standing Committee on Social Policy and Legal Affairs and Perrett, G. (2012) *FASD: The hidden harm. Inquiry into the prevention, diagnosis and management of fetal alcohol spectrum disorders*, Canberra, ACT: Commonwealth of Australia [Inquiry website: www.aph.gov.au/Parliamentary_Business/Committees/House_of_Representatives_Committees?url=spla/fasd/index.htm; accessed: 14 January 2013].

Payne, J., Elliott, E., D'Antoine, H., O'Leary, C., Mahony, A., Haan, E. and Bower, C. (2005) 'Health professionals' knowledge, practice and opinions about fetal alcohol syndrome and alcohol consumption in pregnancy', *Australian and New Zealand Journal of Public Health*, 29(6): 558–64.

Payne, J., France, K., Henley, N., D'Antoine, H., Bartu, A., O'Leary, C., Elliott, E. and Bower, C. (2011a) 'Changes in health professionals' knowledge, attitudes and practice following provision of educational resources about prevention of prenatal alcohol exposure and fetal alcohol spectrum disorder', *Paediatric and Perinatal Epidemiology*, 25(4): 316–27.

Payne, J.M., France, K.E., Henley, N., D'Antoine, H.A., Bartu, A.E., Mutch, R.C., Elliott, E.J. and Bower, C.(2011b) 'Paediatricians' knowledge, attitudes and practice following provision of educational resources about prevention of prenatal alcohol exposure and fetal alcohol spectrum disorder', *Journal of Paediatrics and Child Health*, 47(10): 704–10.

Peadon, E., Fremantle, E., Bower, C. and Elliott, E.J. (2008) 'International survey of diagnostic services for children with FASD', *BMC Pediatrics*, 8: 12 [online at: http://dx.doi.org/10.1186/1471-2431-8-12; accessed: 13 January 2013].

Peadon, E., Payne, J., Henley, N., D'Antoine, H., Bartu, A., O'Leary, C., Bower, C., Elliott, E. (2010) 'Women's knowledge and attitudes regarding alcohol consumption in pregnancy: a national survey', *BMC Public Health*, 10: 510 [online at: http://dx.doi.org/10.1186/1471-2458-10-510; accessed: 13 January 2013].

Peadon, E., Payne, J., Henley, N., D'Antoine, H., Bartu, A., O'Leary, C., Bower, C., Elliott, E.J. (2011) 'Attitudes and behaviour predict women's intention to drink alcohol during pregnancy: the challenge for health professionals', *BMC Public Health*, 11: 584 [online at: www.biomedcentral.com/1471-2458/11/584/; accessed: 6 June 2013].

Peadon, E., Rhys-Jones, B., Bower, C. and Elliott, E. (2009) 'Systematic review of interventions for children with FASD', *BMC Pediatrics*, 9: 35 [online at: http://dx.doi.org/10.1186/1471-2431-9-35; accessed: 13 January 2013].

Peadon, E., Thomas, D. and Elliott, E. (2012) 'Pharmacological interventions for ADHD symptoms in children with fetal alcohol spectrum disorders (FASD)', *Cochrane Database of Systematic Reviews*, 3 [online at: http://dx.doi.org/10.1002/14651858.CD009724; accessed: 14 January 2013].

Roche, A. (2009) 'Women, workers and systems change: professional education and workforce development in FASD', Chapter 9 in, L. Burns, E. Black and E. Elliott (eds) *Monograph of the Intergovernmental Committee on Drugs Working Party on Fetal Alcohol Spectrum Disorders. Fetal Alcohol Spectrum Disorders in Australia: An Update*, Canberra, ACT: Commonwealth Department of Health and Ageing.

Russell, E. (2005) *Alcohol and Pregnancy: A mother's responsible disturbance*, Mermaid Waters, Queensland: Zeus Publications.

Walpole, I., Zubrick, S. and Pontré, J. (1990) 'Is there a fetal effect with low to moderate alcohol use before or during pregnancy?' *Journal of Epidemiology and Community Health*, 44 (4): 297–301.

Walpole, I., Zubrick, S., Pontré, J. and Lawrence, C. (1991) 'Low to moderate maternal alcohol use before and during pregnancy, and neurobehavioural outcome in the newborn infant', *Developmental Medicine and Child Neurology*, 33(10): 875–83.

Walpole, I.R. and Hockey, A. (1980) 'Fetal alcohol syndrome: implications to family and society in Australia', *Australian Paediatric Journal*, 16(2): 101–5.

Watkins, R.E., Elliott, E.J., Mutch, R.C., Latimer, J. Wilkins, A., Payne, J.M., Jones, H.M., Miers, S., Peadon, E., McKenzie, A., D'Antoine, H.A., Russell, E., Fitzpatrick, J., O'Leary, C.M., Halliday, J., Hayes, L., Burns, L., Carter, M. and Bower, C.(2012a) 'Health professionals' perceptions about the adoption of existing guidelines for the diagnosis of fetal alcohol spectrum disorders in Australia', *BMC Pediatrics*, 12: 69.

Watkins, R.E., Elliott, E.J., Mutch, R.C., Payne, J.M., Jones, H.M., Latimer, J., Russell, E., Fitzpatrick, J.P., Hayes, L., Burns, L., Halliday, J., D'Antoine, H.A., Wilkins, A., Peadon, E., Miers, S., Carter, M., O'Leary, C.M., McKenzie, A. and Bower, C. (2012b) 'Consensus diagnostic criteria for fetal alcohol spectrum disorders in Australia: a modified Delphi study', *BMJ Open*, 2(5): 1–10.

WHO (World Health Organization) (2011) *Alcohol Consumption by Country: Global status report on alcohol and health*, Geneva: World Health Organization.

Zammit, S., Skouteris, H., Werteim, E., Paxton, S. and Milgrom, J. (2008) 'Pregnant women's alcohol consumption: the predictive utility of intention to drink and pre-pregnancy drinking behaviour', *Journal of Women's Health*, 17(9): 1513–22.

24

THE WAY FORWARD FOR FETAL ALCOHOL SPECTRUM DISORDERS

Diverting bleak outcomes

Barry Carpenter, Carolyn Blackburn and Jo Egerton

If we look at the life trajectories of the majority of people with fetal alcohol spectrum disorders (FASDs) then, currently, we see a series of bleak outcomes. There are multiple reports, in this text and elsewhere, of children and young people who, as adults with FASDs, suffer chronic unemployment, persistent offending and tragic homelessness.

Why is this? Why have our health, education, social care and welfare systems so systematically failed this particular group of people with complex needs? We are of the belief that there is a fundamental lack of understanding of FASDs at all levels, and in all facets of our societal systems.

Our schools, in particular, have been bereft of the knowledge about this group of children and young people that would have enabled them to evolve a pedagogy and successfully design a curriculum which was responsive to their needs. The health professions are still divided about fetal alcohol syndrome (FAS)/FASD diagnosis, intervention and support. We hope that the chapters from leading health/medical practitioners in this text will help to convince them that there is a strong, watertight case for coherent and comprehensive service development in relation to those affected by FASDs (see particularly Chapters 2, 3, 13, 19 and 23 by Elliott, Gray, Mukherjee and O'Malley).

No one service can transform the life chances of people with FASDs. An interdisciplinary approach, blending together the rich and varied skills of each discipline in a unified model of service delivery is crucial (see Rogan and Crawford, Chapter 14). That is the thrust and purpose of this text: to bring together representatives of a range of disciplines, for each to articulate their insights, their contributions, their aspirations, and demonstrate how we can evolve a coherent interdisciplinary model of practice that will, for future generations of people affected by FASDs, divert those bleak outcomes, improve their life chances and allow them to experience a quality of life now often enjoyed by other groups with a variety of disabilities.

We are concluding this publication with overviews of each chapter, reprising key messages and aspirations, which we hope will inspire future societal agendas for individuals with FASDs.

Elizabeth J. Elliott articulated the international FASD context. She described the historic professional observations and academic research that documented a growing awareness, across centuries, of the devastating impact of prenatal alcohol exposure on children. Commentators ranged from Aristotle through the conceptualization of 'alcoholic embryopathy' by Frenchman Lemoine (1968) and the diagnostically significant 'fetal alcohol syndrome' by Americans Jones and Smith (1973) to contemporary, multidisciplinary research findings on FASDs in worldwide populations.

Based on troubling FASD statistics, the chapter sets out fundamental challenges towards eradication of FASDs – a 100 per cent preventable disability. Governments must seize the initiative and fund research, share information, drive intervention and ultimately prevent FASDs so no child needlessly experiences the lifelong debilitating consequences of prenatal alcohol exposure.

Ron Gray focused on how alcohol in three populations has given rise to increased risk of FAS, and a cycle of deprivation and disadvantage. He has identified some of the social determinants which give rise to heavy/binge drinking in these communities with high levels of FASDs. The social, political and intergenerational practices and factors heavily influence the behaviour of these populations towards alcohol consumption.

There are major health inequalities which are causing social injustice in these communities, alongside considerable childhood disability, and family fragmentation. Preventative approaches need to appreciate the history and culture of these communities – the social determinants – and use them to contextually educate women about the dangers of drinking during pregnancy.

Moira Plant highlights how the typical UK heavy episodic drinking pattern, popularly known as 'binge drinking', is known to be the most risky for the unborn child. Many women are pregnant for a number of weeks before their pregnancy is confirmed particularly if the pregnancy is unplanned. The UK has one of the highest teenage pregnancy rates in Europe, but many women in their thirties are drinking more now than they did before and more than younger women.

She advocates education for women of all ages about the impact of maternal alcohol consumption on an unborn child, and the risks of heavy episodic drinking for both their own health and that of any resulting unplanned pregnancy. She argues for a priority campaign in line with similar government actions related to pregnancy (e.g. tobacco use).

Peter G. Hepper's research into fetal startle responses has indicated that as little as one glass of wine consumed by a pregnant mother can suppress fetal behaviour and that this can persist even after alcohol has cleared from the mother's bloodstream. Not enough is known about the impact of this suppressed behaviour on the developing limbs, sensory system and brain of the fetus. In addition to crossing the placenta, alcohol may be swallowed along with amniotic fluid by the fetus from 15 weeks gestation leading to a craving for the smell and taste of alcohol later in life.

Women need to be advised that drinking even small amounts of alcohol during pregnancy has the potential to harm their unborn baby and may increase the potential for their child to develop a preference for alcohol throughout life.

Simon and Julia Brown described how parenting a young child with FASDs can be enjoyable as well as challenging, although parents can feel isolated and frustrated by the lack of professional knowledge about the condition.

They emphasize that parents need knowledgeable professionals who are able to provide access to practical support (e.g. short-break facilities), financial support, emotional support and signposting to other agencies (e.g. the Parent Partnership Service). Parents also need to accept that their child will do most things differently from many other children, and that the support of professionals who understand their problems will help.

Sarah Muir-Timmins and John Timmins reflected that family life with two adopted children who have FASDs requires parents to adopt a particular lens through which to organize and rationalize their expectations. Brief glimpses of 'normal family life' are overshadowed by the need for rigid routine, structure and clarity in order support the needs of two children with disrupted early experiences and FASDs.

They advise that changing their perspective and expectations of family life has enabled their family to enjoy their children, celebrate their achievements and appreciate the positive changes they have brought to their lives.

Kevin Williams reported some startling statistics, trends and outcomes in relation to children in the care system. He advocated that going into care should be a positive experience for the child, whose childhood to date may have been chaotic and traumatic. Through a series of case studies, he illuminated the potential of the fostering and adoption system to not only support, but transform the lives of children and young people with FASDs.

Children with FASDs often begin life with early trauma. They may need to be removed from their biological family due to neglect or abuse. Against this backdrop of family dysfunction, a well-resourced fostering and adoption system can ensure that children with FASDs receive the quality of childhood that every child deserves and that their life chances of a successful adulthood are significantly improved.

Kate Frances reported that in Western Australia, FASDs are not currently recognized as disabilities, and therefore that few professionals working in health and education have the training and skills to support children affected by FASDs. Her research demonstrated, in common with other studies, that professionals working in early childhood settings do not feel equipped to make appropriate referrals for children with FASDs or have the resources to support these children's needs within their settings. Children cannot be provided with the best start when those supporting their earliest education are not suitably trained or skilled to provide early identification, assessment and interventions for their particular needs.

Governments should ensure that their early years workforce is aware of the full range of effects of prenatal alcohol exposure and that professionals working in early years have the necessary training and skills to support both the child and family in a sensitive manner. This will ensure that any necessary referrals can be timely and effective and that the needs of children and families with FASDs will be properly understood.

Carolyn Blackburn reminded readers that the first environment actively shaping the human brain and physical development is the womb, and that a mother's experiences in pregnancy exert a profound influence on child development from conception onwards. Early childhood intervention has the potential to alter the developmental trajectory and support familial relationships for vulnerable children, enhancing both their own potential and the quality of the communities which they inhabit. This can be achieved through preventative, educational and therapeutic measures. Without such intervention children are vulnerable to social and educational exclusion as well as the development of secondary disabilities, including criminal and violent behaviour.

There needs to be a perceptual shift towards viewing child development as commencing at conception and a duty of care placed on professionals in health, education, social care, mental health and social justice, and most importantly policymakers, to familiarize themselves with the harmful effects of prenatal exposure to alcohol and the impact of FASDs on children, family, communities and society so that effective early childhood intervention services can be planned for children with FASDs.

Barry Carpenter discussed how a responsive pedagogy for children and young people may look. As more children receive diagnoses of FASDs, as more teachers seek to engage children with FASDs as active participants in their classrooms, so the void between aspiration and reality will become more apparent. Now is the time to develop a clear rationale and approach teaching children with FASDs to ensure that they are engaged as effective learners.

Quality education, delivered through high calibre teaching and personalized learning, has the capacity to transform the lives of children and young people with FASDs. Many school systems do not have a transparent, tangible pedagogy for these students – now is the time for action.

Jo Egerton reviewed the impact of FASDs as adolescents move on from school and begin to experience adulthood. Based on commentaries and writings by young people with FASDs, their families and the professionals who work with them, the chapter explored outcomes for young people with FASDs, and possible strategies and success stories.

Services, schools and families need to develop a future-orientated perspective from early childhood. Young people with FASDs have a right to a curriculum that is planned to fit them for adulthood – one that is strengths-based, flexible and adaptable, providing concrete experiences, extended practice and opportunities that gradually build and embed essential life skills. The childhood difficulties and vulnerabilities of young people with FASDs are enduring and lifelong; they will need appropriate advocates, support and protection throughout their lives.

Raja A.S. Mukherjee discussed the debates and approaches to the diagnosis of FASDs, offering a detailed analysis of the key features and efficacy of the various tools and tests. What is clear is that there are many challenges to making a diagnosis and, as yet, there is still some way to go. The lack of information around maternal consumption of alcohol during a pregnancy also impacts on the capacity of the physician to make a confirmed diagnosis.

That prenatal alcohol exposure causes damage to brain and body of the unborn fetus is unequivocal. What remains under debate is the extent to which this causes damage and, depending on the manifestations in the child, how this is determined. A range of approaches, ether phenomenological or etiological, are currently used to recognize and manage the effect of prenatal exposure, but there remains scope for further developments in this crucial area.

Christine Rogan and Andi Crawford described how the FASD community and professional stakeholders in Aotearoa New Zealand, together with government-contracted charity, Alcohol Healthwatch, have created a dynamic, economically viable, multidisciplinary capacity for FASD diagnosis and intervention resulting in a more supportive environment for

FASD affected children and families. It has provided efficient, personalized service pathways for at-risk children and outreach into the community.

Evident in this chapter is society's systemic need for FASD diagnostic services, and the moral imperative to fulfil it. Acknowledging and acting on this leads to better informed clinicians and policymakers, and effective screening and diagnosis. Such an approach prevents uneconomic, serial 'revolving door' assessments which are time consuming, often duplicated and costly. This is a model which other countries could explore.

Susan Fleisher focused on a major UK, FASD prevention programme. In pregnancy, women are more likely to turn to midwives for support than to any other health practitioner. Midwives are therefore ideally placed to counsel pregnant women about the impact of prenatal alcohol exposure for their baby. The Baby Bundle Training for Midwives was developed to ensure midwives are adequately prepared to advise women about FASDs.

Midwives are key to FASD prevention. Aside from the massive, lifelong impact of FASDs on the individual, it has been estimated by the USA's Substance Abuse and Mental Health Services Administration that each person with an FASD costs the public purse $2 million across their lifespan to support education, health, social care (including unemployment) and justice. Training and mobilizing midwives and other front-line health workers is the most cost-effective response to reducing the public and personal costs of this entirely preventable condition.

Julian Killingley highlighted that not enough is known within the British legal profession about FASDs, the way it impacts on an individual's intellectual functioning and the resulting potential for mitigating circumstances in criminal defence cases involving individuals with FASDs. This leaves those affected by maternal alcohol consumption vulnerable in court proceedings, particularly where FASDs have not been diagnosed, which is common.

The English legal profession deserves a greater awareness of FASDs, and to realize the potential for mitigating culpability of individuals with FASDs in appropriate cases, especially those carrying indeterminate sentences. Awareness is best raised through conferences, training, continuing professional education programmes and publication.

Alison McCormick considered the effectiveness of the UK Social Care system in meeting the needs of children who have been prenatally exposed to alcohol and their families. Despite their legal obligations, often the UK's Social Services fail to address FASD-related issues such as sharing information about the young person's condition with families, and providing assessment, family support and appropriate services. Consequently, many children with FASDs, brought up in families who lack adequate knowledge of FASDs, go on to develop avoidable secondary disabilities in adolescence and adulthood resulting in family breakdown, imprisonment or hospitalization.

Social services need to fulfil their obligations to the families of children with FASDs by investigating cases where there is suspected maternal alcohol abuse during pregnancy, carrying out assessments, allocating funding, and by working together with families and health and education professionals to ensure effective and appropriate support. Social workers need training so they understand the complexities, impact and management of FASDs and act accordingly.

Tanya T. Nguyen and Edward P. Riley described a wide range of long-lasting impairments associated with FASDs in a variety of neuropsychological domains, including diminished general intelligence, poor learning and memory, impaired executive and visual–spatial function, hyperactivity and attention deficits, and delayed motor and language development.

An understanding of these brain–behaviour relationships in prenatal alcohol exposure is essential in developing a reliable neurobehavioral profile of children with FASDs. Such a profile will aid in the diagnosis of individuals developmentally exposed to alcohol but who may not present with physical characteristics of FAS. A profile will also inform the development of targeted intervention programmes. Developing safe and effective prevention and intervention techniques are among the most important challenges.

Kieran O'Malley addressed the developmental psychiatric disorders associated with FASDs and their proto-conditions, describing their impact, treatment and sequelae. Through a detailed, clinical debate, supported by vignettes illustrating real-life examples, he demonstrated how alcohol abuse and FASDs are the core of a transgenerational problem, and urged interdisciplinary collaboration across the traditional age/service boundaries.

In a radical but penetrating scientific rationale for the transgenerational, we need to acknowledge across gender, age groups and social structure that the prevalence and extent of alcohol abuse is a major public health problem, which requires systemic recalibration to reach resolution.

Therese M. Grant and Stirling K. Clarren discussed perspectives and developments in North America where there is a long-established history of public health campaigns, diagnostic activity and interventions from a range of disciplines in relation to children, young people and adults with FASDs. Prevention approaches to FASDs in public health are now common in the USA and Canada. This has led to frequent endorsement from the US Surgeon General, various political reviews, and initiatives from a range of professions, including the legal profession. Screening and preventions are major features of the dialogue and debate in North America.

The lessons learnt from the public health actions and messages in the USA and Canada could well inform the developments in other countries contemplating how they can reduce alcohol and expand programmes in the face of a rapidly growing binge-drinking culture. Prevention will be far more cost-effective than the unpredictable, but inherent, costs of supporting individuals with FASDs across the lifespan.

Diane Black considered FAS and FASDs in Europe from the first identification by France's Paul Lemoine in 1968 to present European Union (EU) and World Health Organization (WHO) initiatives and strategies in prevention and support. Among stakeholders and policymakers, there is a will for pan-European action, and a European FASD Alliance was founded in 2011 to promote communication and sharing of ideas. The chapter also reviewed research, action and organizations in individual European countries.

The movement to reduce the harm from prenatal alcohol exposure in Europe has been slow compared with action taken on tobacco. More Europe-wide collaboration is needed to build public awareness, prevent FASDs and reduce economic and societal impact. Excellent initiatives on FASDs in individual countries need to be disseminated across Europe and beyond.

Denis Viljoen presented a contemporary perspective on prenatal alcohol exposure in South Africa, within the context of the country's historical relationship with alcohol and the 'epidemic' of FASDs resulting from generalized alcohol abuse. He reviewed activities of the Foundation for Alcohol Related Research (FARR), which have resulted in over 50 reports on FAS/FASD issues (e.g. prevalence, epidemiology, genetics, neurodevelopment and prevention), and current Ministry of Health and research initiatives.

There are lessons for other governments to take forward from South Africa's systemic approach in accepting responsibility for and addressing the challenge of FASDs in national and regional communities.

Elizabeth J. Elliott charts the Australian perspective on FASDs. This has been one of rapid progress in the last ten years, through a range of political, legal and social developments. This has led to initiatives in health, education and social welfare, with a significant leadership role being undertaken by the National Organization for FAS and Related Disorders (NOFASARD).

This chapter powerfully illustrates how many voices, from a range of professional disciplines and life perspectives, can generate enough volume to be heard. The political leadership shown by the Federal House of Representatives, in collaboration with the various leaders in the field of FASDs, will create a future social and political landscape in which provision for this population of children and adults can grow.

Epilogue
FINDING INSPIRATION

'I Will', a poem written by Jennifer Woodward who is diagnosed with a fetal alcohol spectrum disorder

I won't do it right, because I can't.
I will find success, watch me.
I will not feel a thing when it hurts, because I can't.
I will see tomorrow as a new, bright day.
I won't see what I did as wrong, because I can't.
I will stand up and make you see me as a confident person.
I won't ask again, because I can't.
I will not be ashamed to try over and over again.
I won't say yes when what I mean is no, because I can't.
I will shout from the rooftops, 'I'm normal!'
I won't feel bad about myself, but I do.
I will look in that mirror and smile.
I won't try to feel that I need to be perfect, but I do.
I will only do what I can.
I won't say that I'm broken, but I am.
I will find the pieces and put them back together.
Today is your day, my day, their day.
Today we will change the world, shape it and recreate it
To make it fit in our lives.
We are different, but we will stand and together we will
Feel free to be you, them, and me.

INDEX

Abel, E.L. 29–30, 96, 105, 224
Abidin, R. 163, 164
Abkarian, G.G. 228
abstinence 43, 266
Abudabo, S. 249
Acamprosate 256
Accessible Research Cycle (ARC) 132
accommodation 152–3
achievement 5
activity levels 230
Adamson, J. 207, 210, 216
adaptive ability 142, 145, 224
addiction 6
ADH *see* alcohol dehydrogenase
ADHD *see* attention deficit hyperactivity disorder
Adnams, C.M. 91, 129, 229, 289
adolescence 5, 44–5, 143
adoption 7, 71–2, 83, 209, 213–15
adulthood 141–55
advertising 23, 31, 269, 281
affective instability 247
after-school programmes 180
Ainsworth, M.D.S. 169
Akay, M. 59
Alaniz, M.L. 31
Albert, E. 268
alcohol awareness education 7

alcohol consumption 185; Australia 296; documenting 18–19, 190; Europe 279; feminism 15–16; North America 265, 269; patterns 45, 190; social issues 7; United Kingdom 41, 216; *see also* binge drinking
alcohol dehydrogenase (ADH) 292
alcohol dependency 18, 256
alcohol policy 19, 22, 34, 35
alcohol screening 267, 271, 279
alcohol toxicity 16–17
alcohol-related birth defects (ARBD) 4, 40
alcohol-related harm 279
alcohol-related health damage 43–4, 105
alcohol-related neurodevelopmental disorder (ARND) 4, 161, 241
alcohol-related psychiatric problems 44
alcoholic embryopathy 15
Alert Programme 129
alexithymia 246, 247
Allen, G. 104, 107, 108, 113, 114, 117
Althoff, R.R. 247
Altink, M.E. 254
Alton, H. 216
amniotic fluid 60
Anderson, P. 34, 178, 278
Anthony, B. 166
Antrobus, T. 141, 142, 143, 146, 152
anxiety disorders 44, 242, 255

appropriate adults 200
Aragon, A.S. 224, 226, 227, 228, 230
ARBD *see* alcohol-related birth defects
ARC *see* Accessible Research Cycle
Archibald, S.L. 220, 223, 242, 246
Armistead, G. 211, 212, 213, 214
Armstrong, R.W. 266
ARND *see* alcohol-related neurodevelopmental disorder
Aronson, M. 228
ASD *see* autistic spectrum disorders
aspirations 142–3
assessment 117–18, 211–12
assimilation policy 34
assistance 144
Astley, S.J. 97, 162, 169, 220, 221, 223, 230, 270
atomoxetine 254, 255
attachment disorders 6, 8, 72, 106, 129, 169, 242, 249
attention deficit hyperactivity disorder (ADHD) 126, 168, 230, 241, 245; children in care 84; diagnosis 251; family support 67; medication 253–4; pedagogy 123
attention levels 74, 126, 230
attention process training 129
auditory stimuli 56
Australia 91–100, 294–301; alcohol use during pregnancy 16; early childhood intervention 111; education 8; indigenous population 33–5; prevalence 6, 19–20; public policy 22; standard drink 19
autistic spectrum disorders (ASD) 123, 168, 169, 245, 255
Autti-Ramo, I. 111, 164, 221, 223
availability 31
Avaria Mde, L. 229
awareness 3, 109, 175, 209
Azziz-Baumgartner, E. 35

Baby Bundle Training 183–98
Bachman, J.G. 44
Bacon, F. 3
Badry, D. 143

Baer, J.S. 6, 250, 256
BAL *see* Blood Alcohol Level
Baldwin, J. 201
Barr, H.M. 250
Barrow, M. 165
basal ganglia 223
Baumann, P. 282
Baumberg, B. 278
Baxter, S.L. 155
Bearer, C.F. 292
Becker, M. 228
Behavior Rating Inventory of Executive Function (BRIEF) 224
behaviour: difficulties 126; prenatal alcohol exposure 219–32
behaviour management 75
behavioural phenotype 5, 168
Benz, J. 6
Bergmann, K.E. 282
Berman, R.F. 127
Berry, J.G. 35
Bertrand, J. 4
Biederman, J. 254
binge drinking 166; risk 3, 18; social issue 7; South Africa 32, 292; United Kingdom 39, 42, 216, 256; United States 16, 269
Bingham, S. 103, 107, 118
biomarkers 292
birth complications 105
birth weight 17
Bisanz, J. 226
Black, D. 7, 153, 277–84
Blackburn, C. 6, 7, 9, 21, 67, 91, 92, 102–19, 124, 127, 128, 129, 142, 145
Blakemore, C. 53, 61
Blood Alcohol Level (BAL) 43
Bohjanen, S. 91
Bolling, K. 185, 186
Bomber, L. 7
Bookstein, F.L. 221, 245
Boulding, D.M. 154
Bower, C. 9, 18, 91, 296
Bowlby, J. 169
Boyle, C. 102

Bradley, D.M. 229
Brady, M. 34
brain: damage 14, 124, 219; development 104; function 56; prenatal alcohol exposure 16, 219–32; structural abnormalities 4, 17, 220–3, 242
Brazelton, T.B. 115
BRIEF *see* Behavior Rating Inventory of Executive Function
Brien, J.F. 60
Broad, B. 81, 86
Brocklesby, E. 208, 209, 210, 211, 212, 213, 214, 215
Bronfenbrenner, U. 104
Bronstein, L.R. 9
Brown, J. 6, 65–70
Brown, N.N. 201
Brown, R.T. 230
Brown, S. 6, 65–70
Brown, S.E. 6
Brown, T.E. 247, 253
Bruder, M.B. 107, 113, 116
Bucens, I. 33
Bucens, I.K. 297
Bullock, S.L. 40
Burd, L. 162, 230
Burden, M.J. 227, 230, 231
burnout 213
Burns, L. 296, 301
Buspirone 255
Byrne, C. 254

Caetano, R. 30
CAFS *see* child, adolescent and family services
Calhoun, F. 162
CAMHS *see* Child and Adolescent Mental Health Services
Campbell, D. 185, 186
Canada: alcohol screening 271; education 92; prevalence 19, 268–9; public policy 22, 267, 272
carbamazepine 254, 255
care settings 105
care system 21, 81, 169; *see also* adoption; children in care

caregivers 21–2, 213
carers allowance 20
Carlson, G.A. 247, 254
Carney, L.J. 228
Carpenter, B. 3–10, 20, 92, 104, 106, 108, 112, 123–37, 145
Carson, G. 271
Castillo, R.A. 60
caudate nucleus 17, 223
causation 29
CCT *see* Cognitive Control Therapy
central nervous system (CNS) dysfunction 4, 16–17, 54, 219
cerebellum 223
cerebral cortex 220
cerebral palsy 17, 298
charities 112
Chartier, K. 30
Chasnoff, I.J. 224, 271
Chassevent-Pajot, A. 280
Chassin, L. 256
chemosensory stimuli 61
Chermak, G.D. 228
Chersich, M.F. 291
Chess, S. 242
child, adolescent and family services (CAFS) 180
Child and Adolescent Mental Health Services (CAMHS) 72, 252
child development 102–3, 104–6
child protection 212, 214, 252
children of alcoholics (COA) 249
children in care 80–7
Children's Friendship Training 129
Chiodo, L.M. 228, 229
Chionnaith, M.N. 91
chronic anxiety 255
chronic health problems 44
Chudley, A. 176
Chudley, A.E. 4, 5, 165, 267
Chudley, E. 96
citalopram 254
Clark, E. 142
Clarren, S. 143, 185
Clarren, S.G.B. 97, 103

Clarren, S.K. 8, 97, 123, 127, 161, 219, 220, 265–73
classroom strategies 92, 131
Cleaver, H. 3, 208, 211
clinical case management 247–56
clonidine 255
CNS *see* central nervous system
COA *see* children of alcoholics
Coggins, T.E. 229
Cognitive Control Therapy (CCT) 129
cognitive impairment 4, 5, 126, 129, 212, 219
Cohen, D. 249
Coles, C.D. 6, 123, 129, 220, 223, 226, 227, 230
Collins, E. 297
Collins, R.L. 30
colonialism 34, 35
Colvin, L. 15, 295
Common Assessment Framework 211
communication 66, 74, 83, 128
community youth workers 180
comprehension difficulties 212
concentration 74
concept formation 225–6
conduct disorders 123, 254–5
Connor, P.D. 5, 225, 229, 230
Conry, J. 142, 153, 154, 228, 229
constructional apraxia 228
Cooper, G.F. 53, 61
Cooper, M.L. 40
coordination 4
corpus callosum 221
correction services 180
Cosmi, E.V. 59
Coulombre, A.J. 61
Coulter, C.L. 219
Cousins, W. 208
Crawford, A. 7, 174–81
Crawford, K. 91, 92
Crichton, S. 91
criminal intent 199
criminal justice system 8, 21, 108, 153–4, 267
criminal responsibility 199–205

Crocker, N. 227
Croxford, J.A. 289
Cudd, T.A. 166
Cummings, J.L. 224
Cuthbert, C. 104, 111, 112, 113, 118

D2R *see* Dopamine 2 Receptors
Dalen, K. 224
Dalli, J. 279
danger awareness 67, 72, 73
D'Antoine, H. 18, 296
DAP *see* Developmental Assessment Programme
databases 212
dating 147
David, P. 229
DCLD *see* Diagnostic Criteria for Learning Disability
De Beer, M.M. 111, 116
de Chazeron, I. 280
de Crespigny, C. 186, 191
De Nigris, C. 282
De Santis, M. 283
de Vries, J.P.P. 54, 55, 57
DeCasper, A.J. 61
Dehaene, P. 280
Dehaene, S. 232
Denny, C.H. 16
Densmore, R. 241
depression 44, 141, 241
developmental age 125
Developmental Assessment Programme (DAP) 177
Developmental Behaviour Checklist 86
developmental delay 4, 5, 16, 103, 212
developmental profile 125
developmental psychiatric disorders 241–57
Dex, S. 40
dextroamphetamine 253
diagnosis 161–71, 192–3; Australia 298; children in care 85–6; classification systems 243–5; early 20; early childhood intervention 103, 107, 109–10; fetal alcohol syndrome 4; North America 267–8; prenatal behaviour 54; psychiatric

245–7; stigma 6–7, 20, 102, 123, 188; support needs 82; United Kingdom 211–12
Diagnostic Criteria for Learning Disability (DCLD) 168
Diagnostic and Statistical Manual of Mental Disorders (DSM) 243
diagnostic training 21
diffusion tensor imaging (DTI) 219
diminished responsibility 199, 203
Direx, C.E.H. 61
Disability Living Allowance (DLA) 68, 213
dispossession 34, 35
disruptive behaviour disorder 247
Dittrich, W.H. 102
DLA *see* Disability Living Allowance
Doctor, S. 144, 153
Doherty, N.N. 56, 58
Domellof, E. 229
Donaldson, L. 43
dop system 32, 288, 289
Dopamine 2 Receptors (D2R) 242
Dorris, M. 103, 119
Dossetor, D. 123
Down syndrome 58
Drabble, L.A. 271
Drachman, D.B. 61
drinking patterns 40
drug education 210
drug misuse 17, 207
dry communities 23
DSM *see* Diagnostic and Statistical Manual of Mental Disorders
DTI *see* diffusion tensor imaging
du Toit, A. 32–3
Dubovsky, D. 6, 123
Dumaret, A.-C. 249
Dumas, A. 280
Dumont, L. 208, 211, 212
Duncan Smith, I. 107
Dunn, J. 216
Dunst, C.J. 103
Duquette, C. 91
dysexecutive syndrome 126

early childhood education 93, 105, 108
early childhood intervention (ECI) 6–7, 102–19
early intervention (EI) 103
early onset bipolar disorder (EOBD) 247, 254
eating disorders 45
Eaton, L.A. 35
ECI *see* early childhood intervention
Eckardt, M.J. 266
Edmonds, K. 91
education 20–1, 251–2; awareness 3, 109, 175, 209, 266; communication needs 128; community 18; early childhood 110–11; guidance 124; healthcare workers 110; information programmes 117; inquiry approach 132–3; learning needs 5, 8, 124, 130–1; outcomes 81; professional knowledge 115–16; support 69; teacher training 92; *see also* pedagogy; special educational needs
education support strategies 127–8
Egerton, J. 5, 8, 103, 104, 112, 141–55
EI *see* early intervention
elicited startle 57, 58
Elliott, E.J. 4, 6, 7, 9, 14–23, 33, 91, 294–301
Ellis, F.W. 266
emotional dysregulation 5, 127
emotional incontinence 254
emotional maturity 125
employment 142, 146–9; *see also* unemployment
Engagement Profile and Scale 133
environmental supports 249
EOBD *see* early onset bipolar disorder
epidemiological studies 291–2
epilepsy 58
Ernst, C.C. 272
Ervalahti, N. 224
ethyl oleate 292
etiology 3
EU *see* European Union
Eurocare 279
European Union (EU), policy 278–9
Evensen, D. 127

Evenson, D. 216
Every Child Matters 210, 212, 215
evidence-based health care 20–1
Ewing, J.A. 271
exclusions 82
executive function 126, 178, 224, 246
exposure risk history 167
external brain 143
external orientation 201
external stimuli 56

FA *see* fractional anisotropy
Faas, A.E. 61
facial dysmorphology 4, 17, 54, 124–5, 162, 193, 219, 220, 298
FAE *see* fetal alcohol effect
FAEE *see* Free Fatty Ethyl Ester
family income 296
family planning 270
family support 6, 65, 84, 213, 249, 301
Fang, S. 284
FAS *see* fetal alcohol syndrome
FASDs *see* fetal alcohol spectrum disorders
Fast, D.K. 142, 153, 154, 176, 241, 250
fathers 3, 194–5
FECI *see* fetal and early childhood intervention
feminism 15–16, 42
Ferguson, D. 91, 92
Ferguson, D.L. 124
Fergusson, A. 9
fetal alcohol effect (FAE) 161, 175
fetal alcohol spectrum disorders (FASDs): historical context 15; preventable 14, 184; scepticism 17–18
fetal alcohol syndrome (FAS) 4, 54, 161, 183, 219, 241, 297; historical context 15; population perspective 28; social inequality 35–6
fetal behaviour 53–61
fetal brain function 56
fetal breathing movements 59
fetal development 166
fetal and early childhood intervention (FECI) 104, 118
fetal liver function 60

Field, A. 163, 164
Field, F. 107, 114
Fifer, W.P. 61
finance 147, 153
financial support 68
fine motor skills 66
Finland 45
first drink 44–5
Fitzpatrick, J. 295, 298
Fitzpatrick, J.P. 16, 20
Fleisher, S. 4, 7, 110, 183–98
Floyd, R.L. 267, 269, 270
fluency 226
fluoxetine 254, 255
foolish action 200
forensic diagnosis 201–2
Forrester, D. 207, 208, 210, 216
foster care *see* care system
Foudin, L.L. 161
Fox, H.E. 59
fractional anisotropy (FA) 221
fragile X syndrome 168
France 280–1
France, K. 300
Frances, K. 6, 91–100, 115, 116, 117, 118, 308
Free Fatty Ethyl Ester (FAEE) 167
Fried, P.A. 229
friendship 5, 147, 152
front loading 40
frontal lobes 220
Fryer, S.L. 17, 222, 230, 231
Fuchs, D. 142, 152
functional ability 251
functional brain abnormalities 230

GABA *see* gamma-aminobutyric acid
gabapentin 254
Galvani, S. 210
gamma-aminobutyric acid (GABA) 242
Geller, B. 254
gender empowerment 42
gender rights 15
genetic disorders 56
genetic polymorphisms 29
genetics 3, 16

Gere, C. 144, 149
Germany 282
Gibbard, W.B. 125, 126, 127
Gilinsky, A. 189
Gilmour, I. 44
global developmental delay 66, 82
Gmel, G. 44
Goddard, E. 41
Goedhart, G. 284
Gohlke, J.M. 166
Golden, J.L. 6
Goodlett, C.R. 242, 265
Gossage, J.P. 105, 175
Goswami, U. 103
Grant, T.M. 8, 123, 249, 251, 265–73
Gray, D. 34, 35
Gray, R. 3, 4, 5, 27–36, 288
Green, C.R. 224, 227, 229
Green, M. 241
Green, R.F. 29
Greenfield, T.K. 269
Greenough, W.T. 53
Greenspan, S. 200, 201
grey matter 220
Griggs, I. 186
Grittner, U. 42
group homes 153
growth retardation 4, 17, 54, 66, 219, 298
guanfacine 254, 255
Guralnick, M. 6, 103, 104, 113, 133
Gusella, J.L. 229

habituation 57, 58, 242
Hackbarth, D.P. 31
Hagberg, B. 228
Hagerman, R.J. 241, 242, 254
Halliday, J. 296, 298
Halverson, P.T. 227
Hamilton, D.A. 227
Handley, E. 256
Hankin, J.R. 269
Hannigan, J.H. 96, 105, 127, 161, 162, 166, 253
Hanson, K. 40
Hargreaves, D. 133

Harlap, S. 266
harmful drinking 39
Harris, K. 33
Harris, K.R. 297
Harwin, J. 208, 210, 216
Hay, G.C. 31
head circumference 183
health care professionals 18, 108–10, 175, 298–300
health visitors 210
hearing loss 72
Heaton, M.B. 229
Henriksen, T.B. 43
Henshaw, C. 251
Hepper, P. 192
Hepper, P.G. 5, 53–61, 116
Hibell, B. 44
high-risk women 272–3
Hinde, J. 117, 118
hippocampus 223
Ho, R. 15, 175
Hockey, A. 297
hockey-stick hand creases 164
Holmqvist, M. 281
home environment 248
home-based visiting education programmes 108
Hooker, D. 56
Hope, A. 102
Horimoto, N. 54
Hotham, E. 296
Howlin, P. 243
Hoyme, H.E. 4, 162, 164, 241, 267
5HT see 5-hydroxytryptamine
Hudson Breen, R. 142
Huggins, J. 5
Hughes, N. 210
Humphrey, T. 56
Hunter, E. 34
Hutchinson, D. 298
Hutson, J. 167
5-hydroxytryptamine (5HT) 242
hyperactivity disorders 4, 5, 67, 73, 84, 230
hyperkinetic disorders 230, 245

ICD *see* International Classification of Diseases
Ikonomidou, C. 282
Iley, E.P. 165
impulse control 200, 246, 247
inclusion 103
independence 5, 6
information processing 5, 126
information programmes 117
intellectual function 170, 224
intermittent explosive disorder 247
International Classification of Diseases (ICD) 4, 243
intervention 272–3; *see also* early childhood intervention
intimate partner violence 35
IQ 16, 124, 163, 224, 251
isotropic diffusion 221
Italy 6, 19, 282–3

Jacobson, J.L. 162
Jacobson, S.W. 162, 230, 289
Jacquemard, R. 15, 175
James, D. 55, 59
Janzen, L.A. 228, 230
Japan 19
Jirikowic, T. 127, 228, 229
Job, J. 92
Johnson, V.P. 220
joint movement 61
Jones, K.L. 4, 15, 28, 54, 161, 219, 220, 229, 265, 277, 297
Jones, M. 154
Jones, P. 132
Jones, S.C. 186, 191
Jonsson, E. 3, 186, 191
Joshi, H. 40
justice system *see* criminal justice system
juvenile offenders 200

Kable, J.A. 129
Kaemingk, K.L. 227
Kanter, J. 103, 241
Karr-Morse, R. 103, 104, 106, 108
Karshin, C.M. 40
Kellerman, T. 141, 143, 155

Kelly, K. 6, 176
Kelly, S.J. 54
Kelly, Y. 270
Khaole, N.C.O. 292
Killingley, J. 7, 21, 154, 199–205
Kleinfeld, J. 103, 117, 118, 119, 131, 141, 144, 145, 152, 155
Knuiman, S. 283
Kodituwakku, E.L. 252, 253
Kodituwakku, P. 126, 127, 224, 226, 228
Kodituwakku, P.W. 252, 253, 289
Kooistra, L. 230
Kopera-Frye, K. 125
Korkman, M. 228
Kraemer, G.W. 242
Krieger, N. 35–6
Kuendig, H. 43
Kuntsche, S. 42
Kvigne, V.L. 164
Kwate, N.O. 31

LaDue, R.A. 228, 230
Laming, Lord 210
Landegard, M. 164
Landgren, M. 281
language deficits 5, 154, 212, 228–9, 246, 298
language and literacy intervention 129
Larroque, B. 280
Latimer, J. 298
Latino-Martel, P. 280
Laughlan, F. 102
LaVeist, T.A. 31
law 199–200
law-breaking behaviour 17, 141, 200
Layard, R. 216
Leader, L.R. 56, 58
learning disabilities 4, 5, 200–1, 227
learning needs 5, 8, 124, 130–1
Lebel, C. 220, 222
Lecanuet, J.-P. 54
Lee, T.H. 31
Leigh, B.C. 40
leisure time 149–52
Lemoine, P. 4, 15, 54, 161, 241, 277, 280
Lemoine, P.H. 241, 280

Lenz, W. 53
Leslie, M. 91
Leversha, A.M. 175
Lewis, S.J. 3
Li, L. 222
Li, T.K. 29
life goals 145
life skills 142
lip philtrum 162
Lipson, T. 297
Little, J.F. 57
Little, R.E. 266, 269
liver function 16, 43–4, 60
London, L. 32
Looked After Children 82, 207
Loomes, C. 129
Lopez-Claros, A. 42
lorazepam 255
low birth weight 105
Lownsbrough, H. 210
Ludwig, A.K. 282
Lutke, J. 127, 141, 142, 143, 146, 152
Lynch, C. 58
Lynch, R. 108

Ma, X. 222
McCarthy, T. 210
McConville, M. 201
McCormick, A. 6, 207–17
McGee, C.L. 54, 224, 226, 228
MacKinnon, D.P. 269
McLeod, W. 59
MacMahon, B. 29
McNair, L.D. 30
McNicholas, 254
Maggs, J.L. 44
magnetic resonance imaging (MRI) 219
Magnusson, A. 281
Maillard, T. 280
Main, M. 169
Majewski, F. 44, 282
Malbin, D. 118
Malet, L. 280
Malisza, K.L. 230
management plan 20
Manning, M. 164

manual dexterity 131
Marchetta, C.M. 15, 16
Marcus, J.C. 229
Marks, R.E. 175
Marmot, M. 28
Martin, E.A. 166
Martin, J.K. 30
maternal age 3, 16, 105
maternal alcohol consumption 56–7
maternal health 16, 103, 105
maternal illness 56, 58
maternal records 167
maternal risk 105
maternal smoking 58
mathematics processing 125, 232
Mattson, S.N. 3, 4, 5, 6, 54, 162, 220, 221, 223, 224, 225, 226, 227, 228, 230, 245, 252
May, P. 105, 208
May, P.A. 3, 6, 16, 19, 31, 32, 175, 282, 288
medication 253
medication therapy 252
Meewise, M.L. 249
Meier, P. 41
Meintjes, E.M. 232
memory 142, 212
memory deficits 126, 223, 227, 246
Mengel, M.B. 271
Mennella, J.A. 61
mental health problems 6, 7, 17, 141, 155, 193, 241
mentoring 144–5
methylphenidate 245, 251, 253
Mick, E. 254
microcephaly 4, 16, 167, 220, 298
midwives 3–4, 7, 108–9, 183–98, 210
Milberger, S. 254
Miller, P. 40
minimum pricing 23
minimum terms 203
miscarriage 17
misdiagnoses 6, 123
Mitchell, W. 211, 212
mitigation 201
Moessinger, A.C. 53

Mohllajee, A.P. 270
mood disorders 247, 254
mood-swings 127, 247
Moore, T.E. 241
Moore, T.G. 113, 116
Moos, M.K. 270
Morini, L. 283
Morleo, M. 3, 167
Morley, J. 141
Morris, D.S. 30
motor coordination 66, 223
motor function 229
Moussas, G. 29
MRI *see* magnetic resonance imaging
Muggli, E. 18, 296
Muir-Timmins, S. 6, 71–9
Mukherjee, R.A.S. 3, 4, 5, 6, 110, 161–71, 242, 247
Mulder, E.J.H. 59
Mulia, N. 30
multi-system involvement 250–2
multidisciplinary care 174–81
multisensory learning 130
Munro, E. 107, 113, 114, 207, 210, 211, 216
Murphy, J.M. 208
Murphy, P.A. 104, 117
Murray, L. 242
muscle tone 4
Myers, J. 266

N-methyl-D-aspartic acid (NMDA) 242
Nadel, L. 228
Naimi, T. 295
Naltrexone 256
Nanson, J. 247, 253
Nardelli, A. 220, 223
Nash, K. 230
Nathanielsz, P.W. 53
Nava-Ocampo, A.A. 60
Neil, J. 222
Neldam, S. 54
neonatal withdrawal syndrome 5
Nestler, V. 282
Netherlands 283–4

neurobehavioural development 53, 60–1, 105, 219, 224–32
neuroimaging 16
neuroscience 103
New Zealand 6, 174–81
Nguyen, T.T. 5, 219–32
Nijhuis, J.G. 54, 55, 56, 59, 60
Nilsen, P. 281
NMDA *see* N-methyl-D-aspartic acid
Noonan's syndrome 4
Nowick Brown, N. 241, 242, 249, 253
Ntsabula, A. 111
nucleus accumbens 223
nursery places 67

Oberlander, T.F. 254
obesity 44
O'Callaghan, F.V. 295
occupational therapy 67, 252
O'Connor, M.J. 3, 6, 123, 127, 129, 131, 247
Oesterle, S. 44
O'Hare, E.D. 220, 223, 227, 231
Olanzapine 255
O'Leary, C. 91, 229, 298, 301
O'Leary, D. 210
Olegård, R.R. 281
Oliver, C. 168
Oliver, M.L. 31
Olson, H.C. 162, 226, 227, 230
O'Malley, K. 4, 15, 106, 123
O'Malley, K.D. 6, 7, 8, 241–57
O'Malley, S.S. 256
oppositional defiant disorder (ODD) 6, 123
Orakwue, N. 241, 256
organogenesis 270
ownership 146

Padgett, L.S. 129
Page, K. 241, 248, 249
Paley, B. 123, 127, 129, 131
Palmer, C. 31
Palmer, M. 44
palpebral fissure 4, 162
panic disorder 241

Parent Child Assistance Program (PCAP) 251, 272
parental support 21–2
parenting 65–70
parenting capacity 105
Parents' Evaluation of Developmental Status (PEDS) 85
Parents Under Pressure (PUP) 112
parietal lobe 220
partial fetal alcohol syndrome (pFAS) 4
Pascoe, E.A. 31
paternalism 32
Payne, J. 18, 20, 21, 91, 296, 300
PCAP see Parent Child Assistance Program
PDD see pervasive developmental disorder
Peadon, E. 15, 16, 17, 18, 20, 22, 91, 295, 296, 298, 299, 300
pedagogy 9, 123–37
PEDS see Parents' Evaluation of Developmental Status
peer groupings 131
Pei, J.R. 227
perinatal discharge summaries 167
perinatal psychiatry 251
perseverative behaviour 126
personal care routines 146
personal space 127, 146
pervasive developmental disorder (PDD) 247
pFAS see partial fetal alcohol syndrome
pharmacotherapy 253
Phillips, D.E. 229
Pick, J.R. 266
Pienaar, A. 111
Pikkarainen, P.H 60
Pinazo-Duran, M.D. 229
Pine, D. 243
Pitkänen, T. 45
planning skills 224
Plant, M. 7, 39–46, 111
Plant, M.A. 39, 44
Plant, M.L. 39, 45
Plato 3
police interviews 201
policy trends 113–14
Polishuk, W.Z. 56

population health indicators 177
post-adoption support 214
post-partum depression 45, 242, 249
post-traumatic stress disorder (PTSD) 249
poverty 29
pre-drinking 40
Prechtl, H.F.R. 56
preconceptional health care 270
pregnancy: alcohol policy 22; documenting alcohol use 18–19
premature birth 17, 105, 298
Premji, K. 91
prenatal alcohol exposure 4–5, 54
prenatal chemosensory learning 61
prenatal mortality 105
prenatal nicotine 254
prenatal period 53
prenatal stress 249
prevalence 5–6, 19–20, 123, 175, 208, 268–9, 290–1, 297
prevention 22–3, 107, 197, 269–72
problem-solving 224, 230
professional knowledge 115–16
progablin 254
psychiatric disorders 241, 246
psychiatric management 245–7
psychometric screening tests 212
psychotic symptoms 255
PTSD see post-traumatic stress disorder
public health campaigns 7, 266, 269–70, 279
public health nurses 180
public health policies 296, 301
public misconceptions 3
public transport 147
Pulsifer, M.B. 224
PUP see Parents Under Pressure
Purshouse, R. 41

racism 30, 31
Raiha, N.C. 60
railroad ears 164
Raine, A. 245
randomized controlled trials (RCTs) 20, 299

Rasmussen, C. 224, 226, 227
Raul, F. 280
RCTs *see* randomized controlled trials
reflux 73
regulatory disorders 5, 245, 247, 254
rehabilitation 208
rehearsal strategies 129
Reinold, E. 54
resilience 106
resource teachers of learning and behaviour (RTLBs) 180
respite care 213, 214
response inhibition 225, 231
Reyes, E. 250, 256
Rich, S. 251
Richardson, G.A. 227
Riikonen, R. 220, 223
Riley, E. 5, 6
Riley, E.P. 3, 4, 54, 162, 189, 191, 219–32, 242, 245
risk factors 16, 18, 272
Ritalin 251
Roberts, G. 91
Roberts, S.C. 35
Robertshaw, K. 178
Robinson, G.C. 266, 268
Roebuck, T.M. 227, 228, 229
Roebuck-Spencer, T.M. 227, 229
Rogan, C. 7, 174–81
role play 149
Romley, J.A. 31
Rose, G. 28
Rosenthal, J. 28
rote learning 142, 145
Roussotte, F.F. 220, 223
routines 69, 75, 77, 83
RTLBs *see* resource teachers of learning and behaviour
Ruggles Gere, A. 144, 149, 155
Russell, E. 301
Russell, M. 271
Russell, P. xxiii–xxvi
Rutgers, A.H. 169
Ruth Griffiths Scale of Mental Development 85
Ryan, S. 91, 92, 124

Sadler, T.W. 166
safety issues 73
safety skills 129
Saggers, S. 34, 35
Salee, F.R. 254
Salmon, A. 269
Sampson, P.D. 208, 268, 280
Sandys, M. 202
Santhanam, P. 232
Saunders, J.B. 271
Savage, D.D. 253
scaffolding containment system 248–9
scepticism 17–18
Schaal, B. 61
Schofield, G. 81
Schonfeld, A.M. 224, 226
school-based assessment 251
Schulenberg, J. 44
Scianaro, L. 282
screening 269–72
Screiber, M.L. 242
scripting 145
SCRs *see* serious case reviews
SEBD *see* social emotional behavioural disorder
secondary school 8
seizures 4, 242
self-care skills 67, 83, 146, 178
self-identity 152
self-soothing 127, 255
SEN *see* special educational needs
SENCOs *see* special needs coordinators
sensitivity 164
sensory experiences 61
sensory impairments 4, 126
sentencing guidelines 203–4
serious case reviews (SCRs) 207
serotonin-specific reuptake inhibitors (SSRIs) 254
sertraline 254
SES *see* socio-economic status
set-shifting 225–6
sexual behaviour 5, 6
Shahidullah, S. 56, 57
Shapiro, T.M. 31
Shepard, B. 142

Sher, K.J. 44
Shin, S.H. 45
Shiono, P.H. 266
sick populations 28
Sifneos, P. 246
signposting 69
Simitzis, P.E. 61
Simmons, R.W. 229
Sinha, R. 256
Sival, D.A. 56
skills programmes 129
Slack, J. 40
Slinn, J. 145, 146
Sloper, P. 211, 212
Smart Richman, L. 31
Smith, D.W. 4, 15, 54, 161, 219, 220, 229, 241, 265, 277, 297
Smith, N. 136
smoking 58, 187, 278, 296
Smotherman, W.P. 61
social ability 67, 178, 212
social care 207–17
social communication disorder 247
social communication intervention 129
Social Communication Questionnaire 85
social context 40–1
social cues 75
social deprivation 31, 40, 203
social determinants 28
social disadvantage 29
social emotional behavioural disorder (SEBD) 123
social inequality 35–6, 42
social opportunities 149–52
Social Responsiveness Scale 86
social skills 125, 146, 201
social workers 209, 210–11
societal issues 7
socio-economic status (SES) 105
sociocognitive mathematics programme 129
Sokol, R.J. 224, 267, 271
Solomon, J. 169
Sontag, L.W. 54
South Africa 6, 16, 19, 31–3, 111, 288–92
Sowell, E. 242, 245

Sowell, E.R. 220, 221, 222, 223, 231
Spadoni, A.D. 230
Sparrow, J. 115
special educational needs (SEN) 69, 74, 82, 92
special needs 65
special needs coordinators (SENCOs) 180
special schools 133
specificity 164
speech and language therapy 66, 67, 73, 252
spina bifida 283
Spohr, H.L. 142, 164, 167, 168
spontaneous startle 57, 58
SSRIs *see* serotonin-specific reuptake inhibitors
Staggers, S. 116, 117, 118
standard drink 19, 39, 295
startle response 57, 58, 192
Stead, M. 216
Steinhaussen, H.C. 142, 164, 230
stigma 6–7, 20, 102, 123, 188
stillbirth rates 298
Stoler, J.M. 29
Storoz, L. 253
Story Stems Assessment profile 85
Stratton, K. 242, 266, 267, 269
Streissguth, A. 103, 175, 214
Streissguth, A.P. 4, 6, 15, 54, 123, 125, 141, 142, 154, 224, 229, 230, 241, 249, 250, 251, 253, 270
stress 18, 213
stress process model 30
Stromland, K. 229
Strömland, K. 281
Stroop Test 225
subcortical structure 223
Subramaniam, K. 229
substance misuse 141, 210
suicide 6, 17
Sulik, K.K. 166, 266
Sullivan, A. 246, 247
Sullivan, W. 3
supervision 67, 72
support needs 67–9, 208–9, 211

support network 144, 194
Swayze, V.W. 220, 221
Sweden 281

TACT *see* The Adolescent and Children's Trust
taxation 23
teachers 130, 210
teenage pregnancy 40
Templeton, L. 207, 210, 216
temporal lobe 220
Ten Eyck, M. 144
Tenkku, L.E. 30
teratogenicity 16, 162, 166, 196, 219, 242, 265
thalidomide 53
The Adolescent and Children's Trust (TACT) 81, 208
therapy 115, 118–19, 252–3
Thomas, A. 242
Thorne, J.C. 229
Timler, G.R. 129, 229
Timmins, J. 6, 71–9
Tough, S. 40, 45
Toutain, S. 280
training 176, 178, 210–11, 298–9
transgenerational alcohol abuse 250
transition to adulthood 141–55
tricyclic antidepressants 254
Trivette, C.M. 103
Tucker, J.S. 44
Tucker, M. 145
Turk, J. 168, 247
Turner, G. 297
Turney, D. 209, 211, 212
Tutt, R. 102

Uecker, A. 227
ultrasound 54
Umlah, C. 272
unemployment 142
United Kingdom: alcohol culture 216; Baby Bundle Training 183–98; early childhood intervention 111–13; education 91–2, 110, 124; justice system 202–4; perinatal psychiatry 251; social care 207–17; standard drink 19, 39; women's alcohol consumption 39–46
United States: African-American populations 29–31; alcohol use during pregnancy 15–16; binge drinking 16; justice system 202; prevalence 6, 19, 268–9; public policy 22, 266–7
unplanned pregnancies 7, 40, 45, 270, 295

VABS *see* Vineland Adaptive Behaviour Scales
Vagnarelli, F. 283
valproic acid 254, 255
van Balkom, I.D. 283
Vaurio, L. 226
velocardiofacial (22q11) syndrome 168
verbal communication 125, 142
verbal learning 223, 231
vermillion border 4
Vernescu, R. 129
Viljoen, D. 6, 31, 288–92
Viljoen, M.D. 111, 116
Vineland Adaptive Behaviour Scales (VABS) 85, 251
violence 35
Visser, G.H.A. 56
visual processing 131
visual-spatial ability 227, 228
volumetric taxation 23
voluntary confessions 201
Vos, T. 33
vulnerable adults 201

Wade, J. 211
Waldman, B. 61
Wallace, J.M. Jr. 31
Wallace, R.F. 54
Walpole, I.R. 297
warning labels 15, 266, 280
Warren, K.R. 3, 29, 105, 161, 162
Wartnik, A.P. 176
Wass, T.S. 229
water diffusion 221
Watkinson, B. 229
Wechsler Intelligence Scales 85, 247
weight gain 66

Wells, D.L. 61
Wells, K. 208
Werner, E.E. 251
Westcott, S. 103, 118, 131
white matter 220, 221–2
Whitebread, D. 103, 107, 118
Whitehurst, T. 102, 110
WHO *see* World Health Organization
Wight Felske, A. 143
Wild, R. 34
Wilens, T.E. 253
Wiley, M.S. 103, 104, 106, 108
Willford, J.A. 227
Williams, K. 7, 80–7, 208
Williams, M.S. 129
Williams, P. 107, 109, 115, 119
Williams, R.J. 268
Williams, S. 44
Williams syndrome 4
Williamson, J. 39
Willoughby, K.A. 223, 227
Wilsnack, R.W. 39, 44
Wilsnack, S. 44
Wilson, D. 203
Wilson, J.G. 270
Wilson, M. 34
Winstone, A. 9, 110
Winstone, A.M. 189
Wisconsin Card Sorting Task 226
Wise, S. 108
Wisniewski, K. 220
Woods, A. 296
Woodward, J. 313-4
working memory 129, 227, 230–1
World Health Organization (WHO) 279
Wouldes, T. 175
Wozniak, J. 254
Wozniak, J.R. 222

Yang, Y. 17, 220
York, J.L. 44

Zahidi, S. 42
Zammit, S. 296